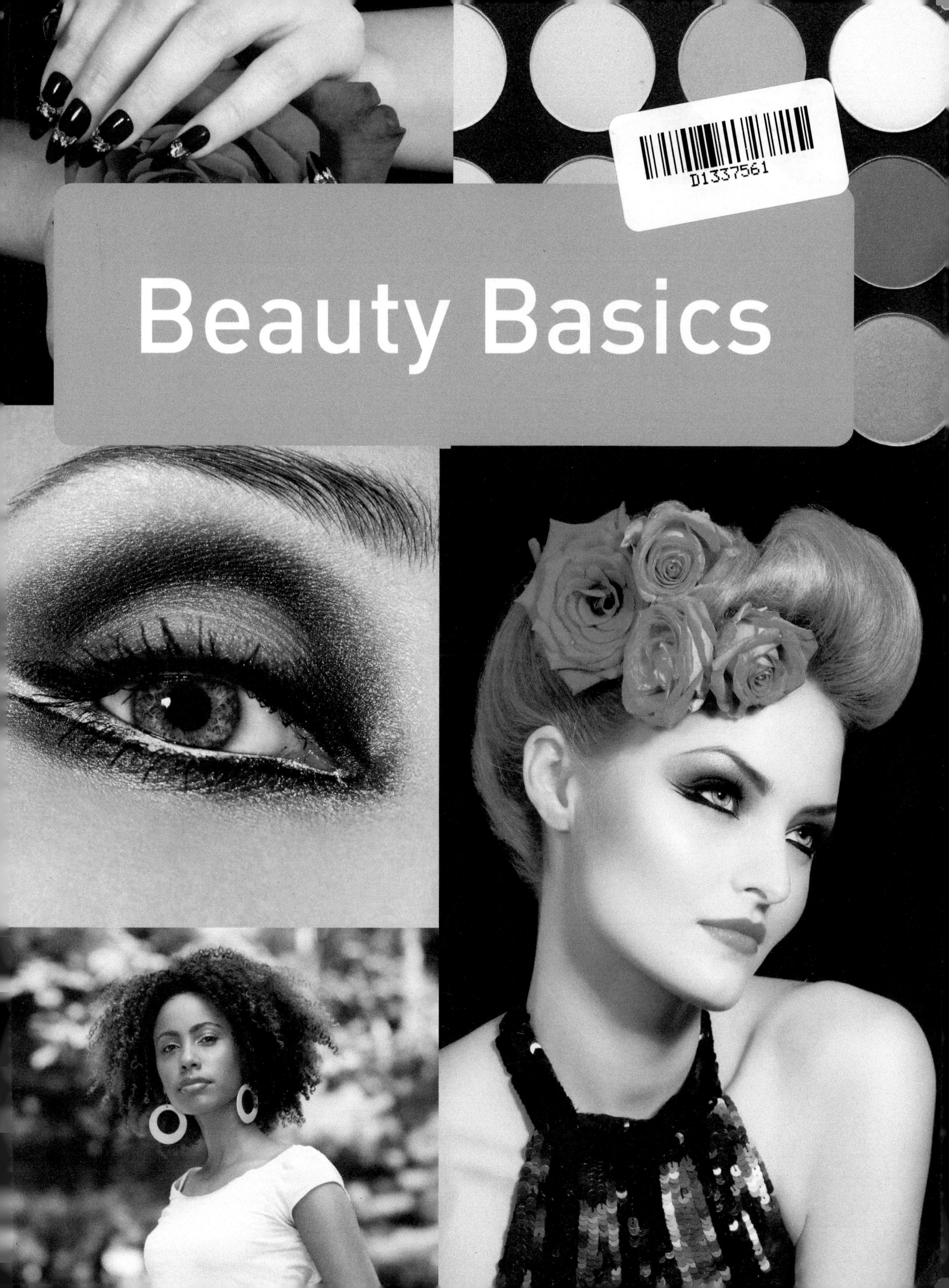
Beauty Basics
D1337561

HAIRDRESSING AND BEAUTY THERAPY TITLES

Hairdressing

Student textbooks

Begin Hairdressing: The Official Guide to Level 1 3e *Martin Green*

Hairdressing – The Foundations: The Official Guide to Level 2 6e *Leo Palladino and Martin Green*

Professional Hairdressing: The Official Guide to Level 3 7e *Martin Green and Leo Palladino*

The Official Guide to the City & Guilds Certificate in Salon Service 1e *John Armstrong with Anita Crosland, Martin Green and Lorraine Nordmann*

The Colour Book: The Official Guide to Colour for NVQ Levels 2 and 3 1e *Tracey Lloyd with Christine McMillan-Bodell*

eXtensions: The Official Guide to Hair Extensions 1e *Theresa Bullock*

Salon Management *Martin Green*

Men's Hairdressing: Traditional and Modern Barbering 3e *Maurice Lister*

African–Caribbean Hairdressing 3e *Sandra Gittens*

The World of Hair Colour 1e *John Gray*

The Cutting Book: The Official Guide to Cutting at S/NVQ Levels 2 and 3 *Jane Goldsbro and Elaine White*

Professional Hairdressing titles

Trevor Sorbie: The Bridal Hair Book 1e *Trevor Sorbie and Jacki Wadeson*

The Art of Dressing Long Hair 1e *Guy Kremer and Jacki Wadeson*

Patrick Cameron: Dressing Long Hair 1e *Patrick Cameron and Jacki Wadeson*

Patrick Cameron: Dressing Long Hair 2 1e *Patrick Cameron and Jacki Wadeson*

Bridal Hair 1e *Pat Dixon and Jacki Wadeson*

Professional Men's Hairdressing: The Art of Cutting and Styling 1e *Guy Kremer and Jacki Wadeson*

Essensuals, The Next Generation Toni and Guy: Step by Step 1e *Sacha Mascolo, Christian Mascolo and Stuart Wesson*

Mahogany Hairdressing: Steps to Cutting, Colouring and Finishing Hair 1e *Martin Gannon and Richard Thompson*

Mahogany Hairdressing: Advanced Looks 1e *Martin Gannon and Richard Thompson*

The Total Look: The Style Guide for Hair and Make-up Professionals 1e *Ian Mistlin*

Trevor Sorbie: Visions in Hair 1e *Trevor Sorbie, Kris Sorbie and Jacki Wadeson*

The Art of Hair Colouring 1e *David Adams and Jacki Wadeson*

Beauty therapy

Beauty Basics: The Official Guide to Level 1 REVISED 3e *Lorraine Nordmann*

Beauty Therapy – The Foundations: The Official Guide to Level 2 5e *Lorraine Nordmann*

Professional Beauty Therapy – The Official Guide to Level 3 REVISED 4e *Lorraine Nordmann*

The Official Guide to the City & Guilds Certificate in Salon Services 1e *John Armstrong with Anita Crosland, Martin Green and Lorraine Nordmann*

The Complete Guide to Make-up 1e *Suzanne Le Quesne*

The Encyclopedia of Nails 1e *Jacqui Jefford and Anne Swain*

The Art of Nails: A Comprehensive Style Guide to Nail Treatments and Nail Art 1e *Jacqui Jefford*

Nail Artistry 1e *Jacqui Jefford*

The Complete Nail Technician 2e *Marian Newman*

Manicure, Pedicure and Advanced Nail Techniques 1e *Elaine Almond*

The Official Guide to Body Massage 2e *Adele O'Keefe*

An Holistic Guide to Massage 1e *Tina Parsons*

Indian Head Massage 2e *Muriel Burnham-Airey and Adele O'Keefe*

Aromatherapy for the Beauty Therapist 1e Valerie Worwood

An Holistic Guide to Reflexology 1e *Tina Parsons*

An Holistic Guide to Anatomy and Physiology 1e *Tina Parsons*

The Essential Guide to Holistic and Complementary Therapy 1e *Helen Beckmann and Suzanne Le Quesne*

The Spa Book 1e *Jane Crebbin-Bailey, Dr John Harcup, and John Harrington*

SPA: The Official Guide to Spa Therapy at Levels 2 and 3, *Joan Scott and Andrea Harrison*

Nutrition: A Practical Approach 1e *Suzanne Le Quesne*

Hands on Sports Therapty 1e *Keith Ward*

Encyclopedia of Hair Removal: A Complete Reference to Methods, Techniques and Career Opportunities, *Gill Morris and Janice Brown*

The Anatomy and Physiology Workbook: For Beauty and Holistic Therapies Levels 1–3. *Tina Parsons*

The Anatomy and Physiology CD-Rom

Beautiful Selling: The Complete Guide to Sales Success in the Salon *Ruth Langley*

The Official Guide to the Diploma in Hair and Beauty Studies at Foundation Level 1e *Jane Goldsbro and Elaine White*

The Official Guide to the Diploma in Hair and Beauty Studies at Higher Level 1e *Jane Goldsbro and Elaine White*

Beauty Basics

The official guide to beauty therapy at level 1

REVISED THIRD EDITION

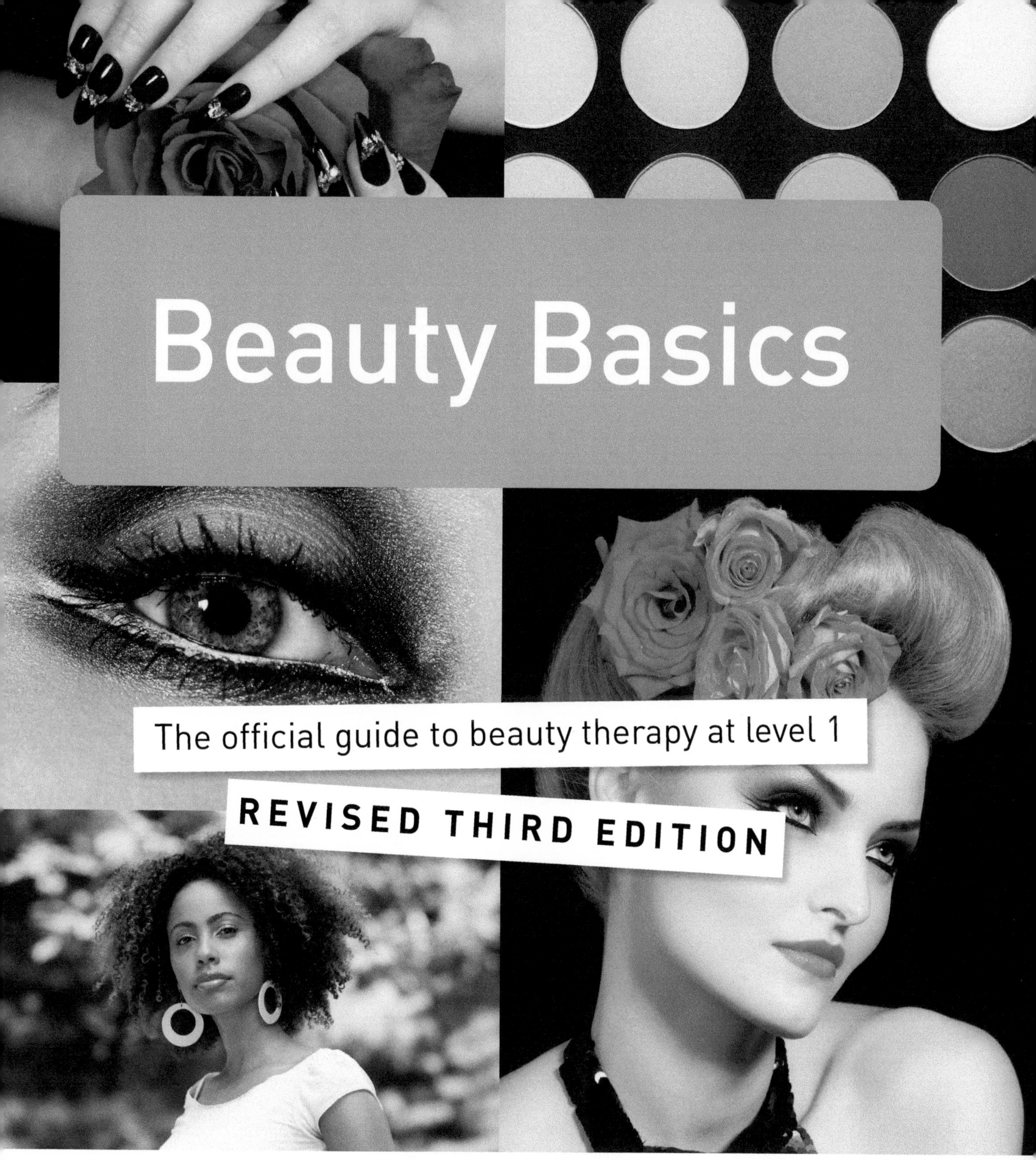

LORRAINE NORDMANN

CENGAGE Learning

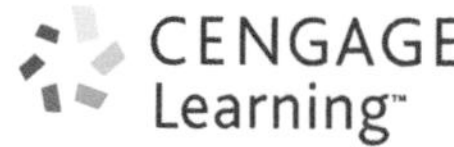

Australia • Brazil • Japan • Korea • Mexico • Singapore • Spain • United Kingdom • United States

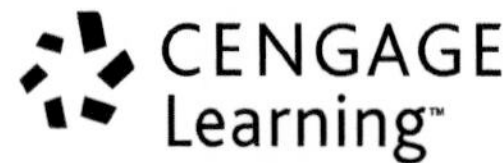

Beauty Basics
Revised Third Edition
Lorraine Nordmann

Publisher: Melody Dawes
Development Editor: Lauren Darby
Publishing Assistant: Claire Whittaker
Content Project Editor: Sue Povey
Production Controller: Eyvett Davis
Typesetter: MPS Limited
Cover design: HCT Creative

British Library Cataloguing-in-Publication Data
A catalogue record for this book is available from the British Library.

ISBN: 978-1-4737-1060-3

Cengage Learning EMEA
Cheriton House, North Way, Andover, Hampshire SP10 5BE
United Kingdom

Cengage Learning products are represented in Canada by Nelson Education Ltd.

For your lifelong learning solutions, visit **www.cengage.co.uk**

Purchase your next print book or e-book at **www.cengagebrain.com**

Printed in the United Kingdom by CPI Antony Rowe
Print Number: 08 Print Year: 2021

Contents

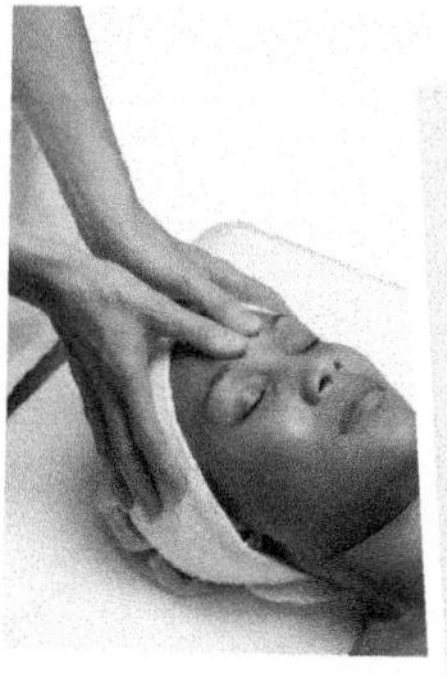
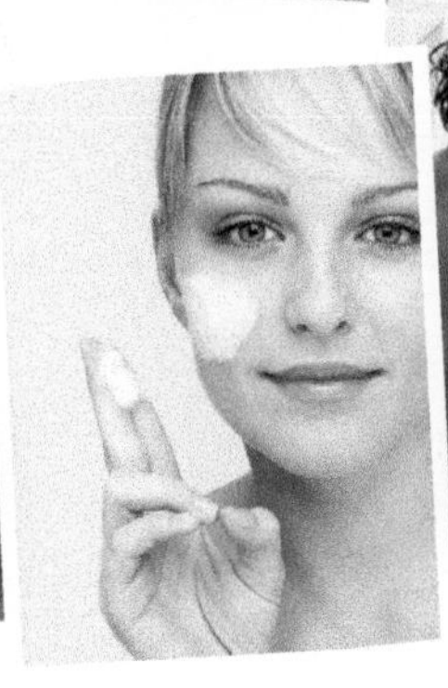
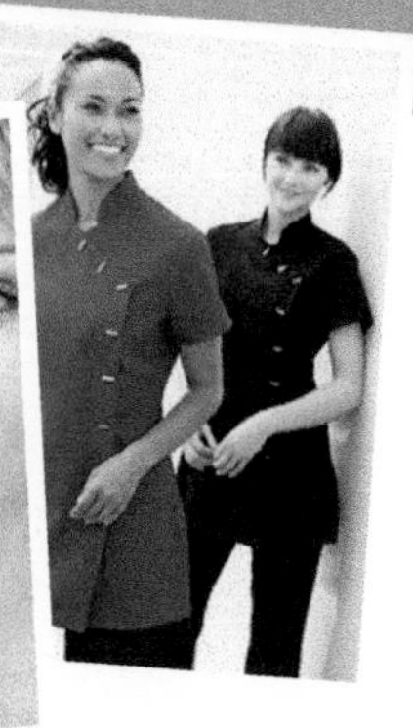

4 Preparing and maintaining the salon treatment work area 58

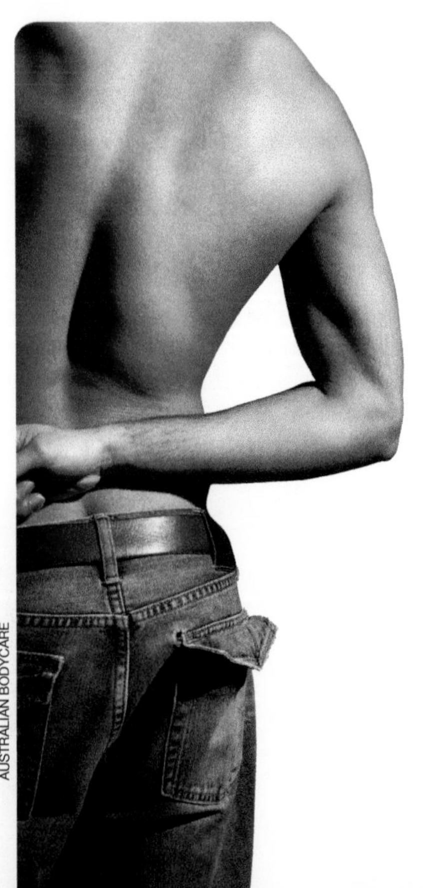
AUSTRALIAN BODYCARE

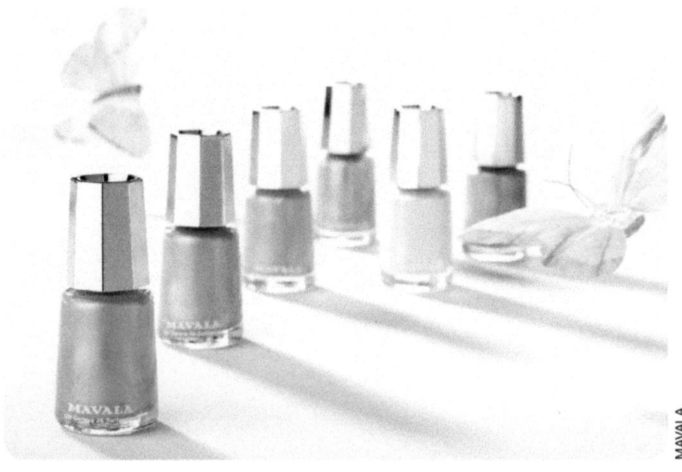

MAVALA

5 Salon reception duties 107

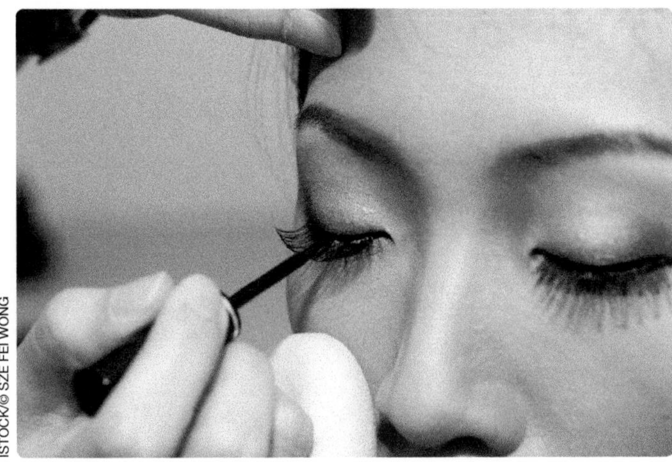
ISTOCK/© SZE FEI WONG

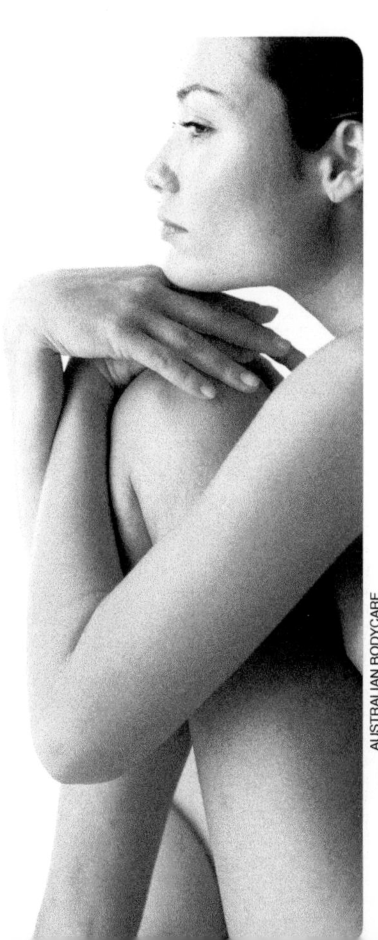
AUSTRALIAN BODYCARE

8 Nail services 193

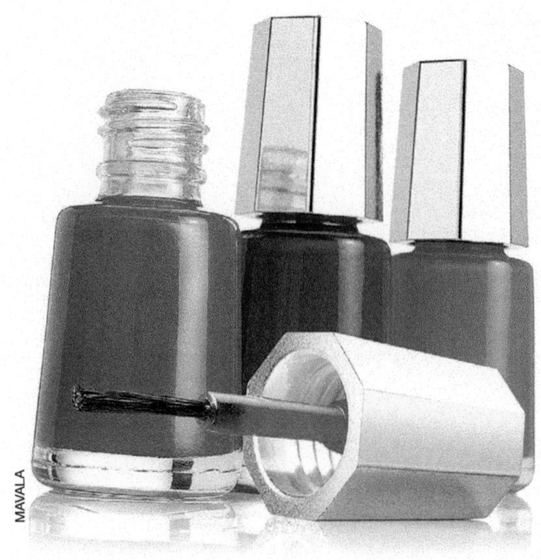
MAVALA

About VTCT

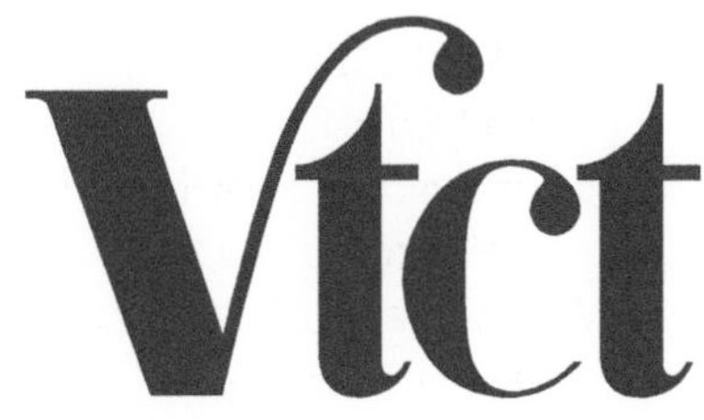

VTCT is a government approved specialist awarding organisation responsible for qualifications in the beauty therapy, complementary therapy, hairdressing, sports, fitness, hospitality and catering sectors.

VTCT has been in existence for over 50 years, and in fact it was VTCT who originally coined the phrase *Beauty Therapy*. VTCT has remained at the forefront of developing the vocational system of qualifications in the UK and internationally.

VTCT invests in many charitable projects which support education and training in the beauty therapy industry. VTCT is the main sponsor and organiser of Worldskills UK (Beauty Therapy competitions) and VTCT also fund the development of the European and British Standard for Beauty Salon Services. In addition, VTCT donates charitable funds to disfigurement charities, prison education and other worthwhile causes linked to the beauty therapy sector.

VTCT has the widest and most diverse range of qualifications in the beauty industry and are leading on many new initiatives in education, including online assessment and registration, e-portfolio and e-resources.

VTCT develops innovative, fit for purpose qualifications via beauty therapy technical expert panels made up of employers, industry experts and educationalists from all over the UK.

About this book

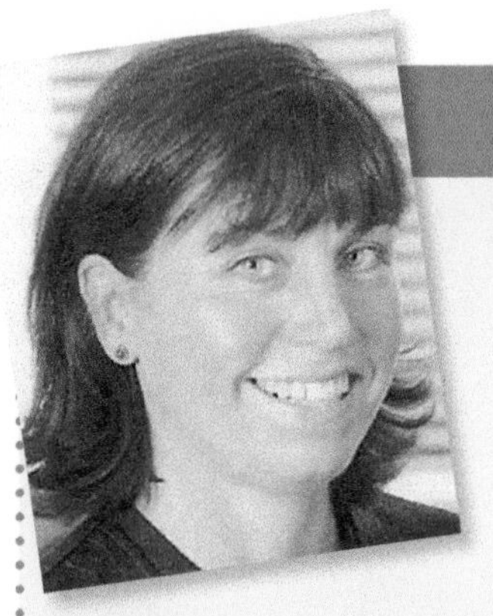

Janice Brown

Director of HOF Beauty (House of Famuir Ltd)

My career journey has taken me from working in and later managing a group of salons, through, sales, teaching, training, research and development and I am currently director of HOF Beauty Ltd. Along the way I have specialized in electrolysis and other hair removal methods. I am the co-author of *The Encyclopedia of Hair Removal* along with Gill Morris. I am proud to say that I have been able to make a real difference to people's lives by helping to correct skin, body and hair growth issues. I hope I have also been able to inspire and encourage fellow beauty therapists through the training I have provided. In the course of my career I have been fortunate enough to travel the world and work with wonderful people. Beauty therapy for me is not only a career but is a true passion.

Industry Role Models feature throughout the book and are your insight into the exciting beauty industry. Their profile is included at the start of the chapter and they provide subject specific tips that are both practical and inspiring.

ACTIVITY

List some examples of what being courteous means to you, when dealing with a client. Consider the scenarios below and state how you would deal with each in a courteous manner:

- A client arriving at reception when you are already busy with another client
- A client arriving late for a service
- A client receiving a service for the first time

Activity boxes feature within all chapters and provide additional tasks for you to further your understanding.

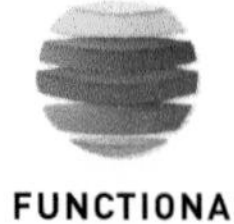

FUNCTIONAL SKILLS

Functional skills icons show where your information communication technologies (ICT), maths, and English skills can be developed by using the suggestions or activities suggested.

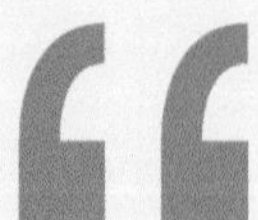

By creating the right atmosphere on arrival at the salon, giving excellent service and paying attention to the client's needs you will encourage the client to return to you for their beauty therapy services.

Janice Brown

Role Model quotes are included throughout a number of core chapters. Each quote provides valuable insight into the world of work, providing helpful and practical advice about working in such a varied and innovative industry.

BEST PRACTICE

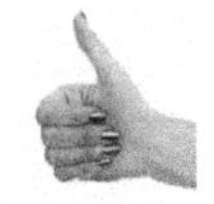

All staff should be aware of any promotions that their business is offering so that they can build on a client's initial interest in a product or service and turn it into a sale.

Best Practice boxes suggest good working practice and help you develop your skills and awareness during your training.

ALWAYS REMEMBER

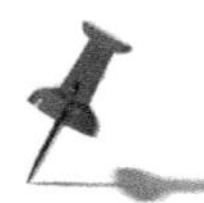

Psoriasis

With the skin disorder psoriasis, cell division occurs much more quickly, resulting in clusters of dead skin cells appearing on the skin's surface.

Always Remember boxes draw your attention to key information or helpful hints that will help you prepare for assessment.

TOP TIP

Whilst training at your work placements it is vital to improve your confidence and practical skills 'on the job'. This will increase your CV and as a make-up artists help you to build an impressive portfolio.

Top Tips share the author's experience and provide positive suggestions to improve knowledge and skills for each unit.

EQUIPMENT AND MATERIAL LIST

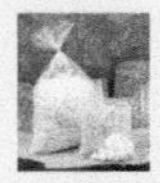

Clean, dampened and clean, dry cotton wool
With sit-up and lie-down positions and an easy-to-clean surface

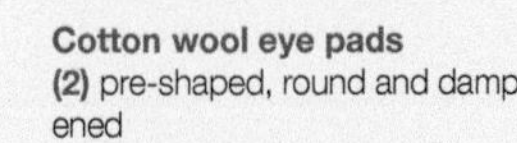

Cotton wool eye pads
(2) pre-shaped, round and dampened

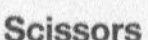

Scissors
To cut cotton wool eye pads (if cotton wool discs are not used)

YOU WILL ALSO NEED:

Disposable tissue roll Such as bedroll

Towels (2) Freshly laundered for each client

Flat mask brushes (3) Disinfected

Trolley To display all facial treatment products to be used in the facial service

Client's record card To record all the details relevant to the client's service

Facial toning lotions (a selection) To suit various types of skin

Equipment Lists help you prepare for each practical treatment and show you the tools, materials and products required.

HEALTH & SAFETY

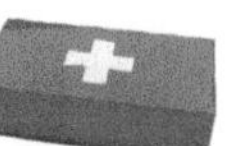

Skin protection

Although the skin is structured to avoid penetration of harmful substances by absorption, certain chemicals can be absorbed through the skin. Always protect the skin when using potentially harmful substances, and wear gloves when using harsh chemical cleaning agents.

Health & Safety boxes draw your attention to related health and safety information essential for each technical skill.

Sample client record card

<table>
<tr><td>Date</td><td colspan="2">Beauty therapist name</td></tr>
<tr><td colspan="2">Client name</td><td>Date of birth (Identifying client age group)</td></tr>
<tr><td colspan="2">Home address</td><td>Postcode</td></tr>
<tr><td>Landline phone number</td><td>Mobile phone number</td><td>Email address</td></tr>
<tr><td>Name of doctor</td><td colspan="2">Doctor's address and phone number</td></tr>
<tr><td colspan="3">Related medical history (Conditions that may restrict or prohibit service application.)</td></tr>
<tr><td colspan="3">Are you taking any medication? (This may affect the condition of the skin or skin sensitivity.)</td></tr>
</table>

Client record cards illustrate what you need to assess and gain from the client at consultation and also provide guidance on information following a treatment.

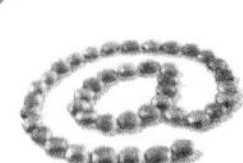

COURSEMATE

CourseMate video boxes highlight certain techniques which are available to view online.

Step-by-step: Deep cleansing

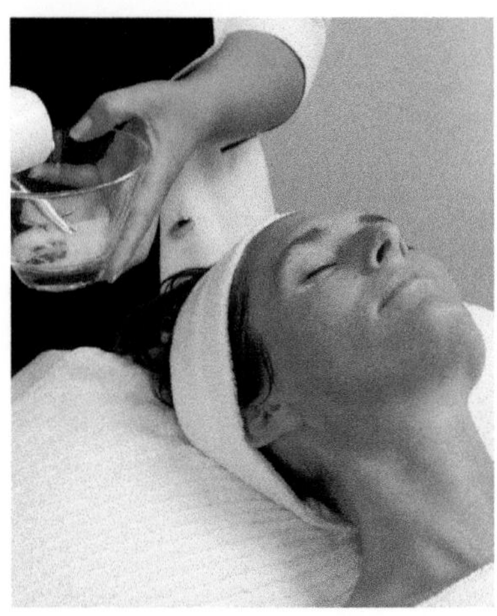

1 Select a cleansing medium to suit your client's skin type. The procedure for application is the same as that for the superficial cleanse.

Step-by-step sequences demonstrate the featured practical skills using colour photographs to enhance your understanding.

ASSESSMENT OF KNOWLEDGE AND UNDERSTANDING

Having covered the learning objectives for **making sure your own actions reduce risks to health and safety**, test what you need to know and understand by answering the following short questions below.

Actions to avoid health and safety risks

1 What are your main legal responsibilities under the Health and Safety at Work Act (1974)?

2 Name four different pieces of legislation relating to health and safety in the workplace.

3 What is the purpose of a salon health and safety policy? What sort of information does it include?

4 What is the importance of personal presentation in respect of your salon workplace policy?

5 Why is your personal conduct important to maintain the health and safety of yourself, colleagues and clients?

6 Why must regular health and safety checks be carried out in the workplace?

Assessment of knowledge and understanding questions are provided at the end of all core chapters. You can use the questions to prepare for oral and written assessments and help test your own knowledge throughout. Seek guidance from your supervisor/assessor if there are areas you are unsure of.

About the author

Lorraine Nordmann has worked in the beauty therapy industry for the past 30 years and has witnessed significant technological advances to both the client and industry. Her commitment to the industry and passion for learning is evident in every page of her publications. As well as this revised Level 1 book, Lorraine is also the author of *Beauty Therapy: The Foundations* and *Professional Beauty Therapy*, covering the latest industry standards at Levels 2 and 3.

Lorraine Nordmann

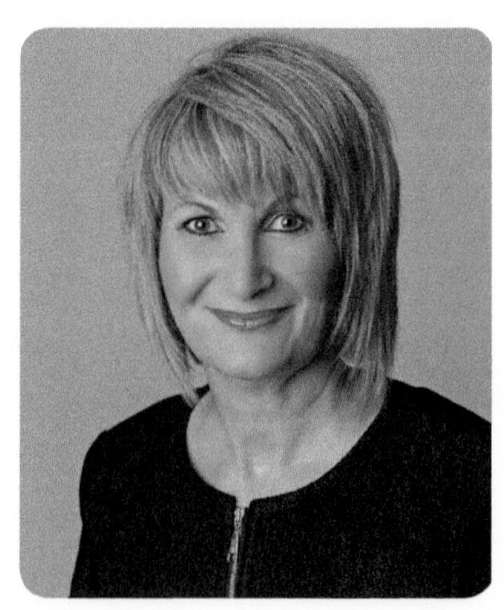

About the website

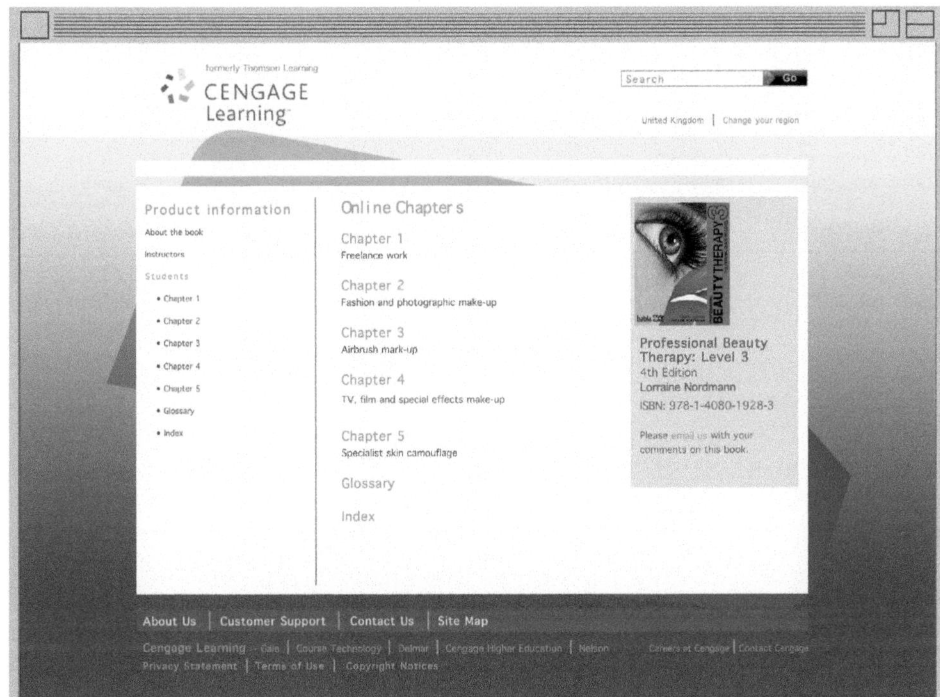

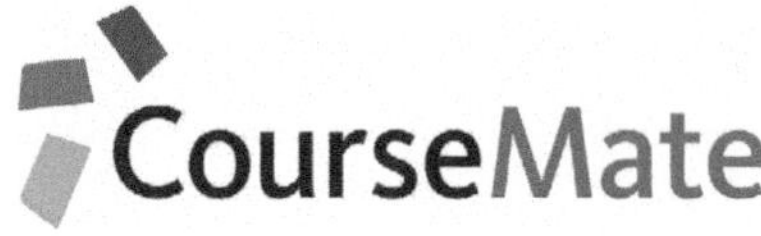

Use the *Beauty Basics Level 1* CourseMate alongside the *Beauty Basics: The Official Guide to Level 1, Revised Third Edition* textbook for a complete blended learning solution!

This highly interactive resource brings course concepts to life and is designed to support lecturers and students through the range of online resources which can be perfectly integrated into the classroom to cover the guided learning hours for each unit.

For Students:

- Searchable eBook
- Step-by-step videos
- Interactive multiple choice quizzes
- Interactive activities and games

For Lecturers:

- Lessons plans
- PowerPoint slides
- Activity handouts
- 'Engagement Tracker' tools so students' progression and comprehension can be fully monitored

For more information please email emea.fesales@cengage.com

Acknowledgements

The author and publishers would like to thank the following:

For providing the cover image:

Shutterstock

For providing pictures for the book:

Absolute Aesthetics
www.absoluteaesthetics.co.uk
Alamy
Australian Bodycare
Babor
BABTAC
Beauty Express Ltd
City & Guilds
Dermalogica, The International Dermal Institute www.dermalinstitute.co.uk
Dr A L Wright
Dr John Gray, *The World of Skincare*
Dr M H Beck
Ellisons
Habia
Health and Safety Executive
House of Famuir, www.hofbeauty.co.uk
HMSO
HSE
Istock photo
Julia Francis and photgrapher Thomas Sergeant www.juliafrancis.co.uk
Korres Natural Products, www.korres.com
Mavala
Mediscan
Wellcome Photo Library
Salon system (Beauty Express Ltd)
Salon Iris, www.saloniris.co.uk Silhouette-Dermalift
Simon Jersey Ltd, www.simonjersey.com
Sister PR Sorisa
Studex UK Ltd, www.studex.com
The Colour Wheel Company www.colourwheelco.com
The Sanctuary at Covent Garden Ltd, www.thesanctuary.co.uk
Unilever
www.shavata.co.uk Wellcome Photo Library
World of Beauty by Katy, Park Road, London

For their help with the photoshoot:

Mike Turner, www.miketurner-photography.co.uk

For their contribution as industry role models:

Wendy Turner
Sally Penford
Sally Biles
Joanne Mackinnon
Vicky Kennedy
Janice Brown
Sally-Anne Braithwaite
Julia Francis
Jacqui Jefford

1 Introduction

This book is aimed to support those entering the Beauty Therapy industry. The content covers current practical skills and knowledge that are required when working as a beauty therapist qualified at NVQ Level 1, a work-related qualification. If you are in Scotland you may be studying the SVQ Level 4. The book is also useful as a reference text for non-NVQ qualifications such as VRQs and for all those aiming to work in the beauty industry in the future.

What is an NVQ?

NVQ stands for National Vocational Qualification – Vocational means work related and is competency based. NVQs are available in different levels, allowing progression. Achieving this qualification means that you are work ready, having been trained and continually assessed whilst employed in the workplace. NVQs are referred to as *'job ready'* qualifications.

In Scotland an NVQ is known as an SVQ (Scottish Vocational Qualification).

What is a VRQ?

You may be studying towards an Award, Certificate or Diploma Vocational Related Qualification – a VRQ. These are *'preparation for work'* qualifications. Preparation for work qualifications provides knowledge, understanding and capability to do the job without the ability to be immediately ready for work.

Qualifications in beauty therapy may be gained through different government-approved awarding organisations. These are listed below with their website addresses and include:

- VTCT – www.vtct.org.uk
- CGLI – www.cityandguilds.com
- Edexcel – www.edexcel.com
- ITEC – www.itecworld.co.uk

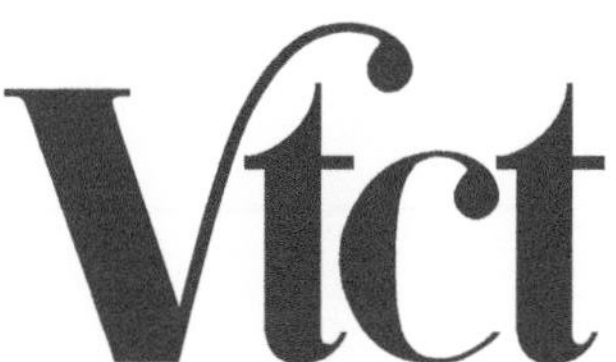

You can also complete CIBTAC and CIDESCO qualifications, which are internationally recognized.

Whoever you study with, each awarding organisation for *'job ready'* qualifications is required to cover the same standards of skills and knowledge, referred to as National Occupational Standards (NOS) describing what an individual needs to do, know and understand.

The Standards are provided by the government approved standards setting body for hairdressing, beauty therapy, nails and spa therapy, Habia (Hairdressing and Beauty Therapy Industry Authority). This ensures an employer can be confident of the skills an employee will be able to perform competently at the NVQ/SVQ level they have achieved, whichever awarding organisation has accredited it.

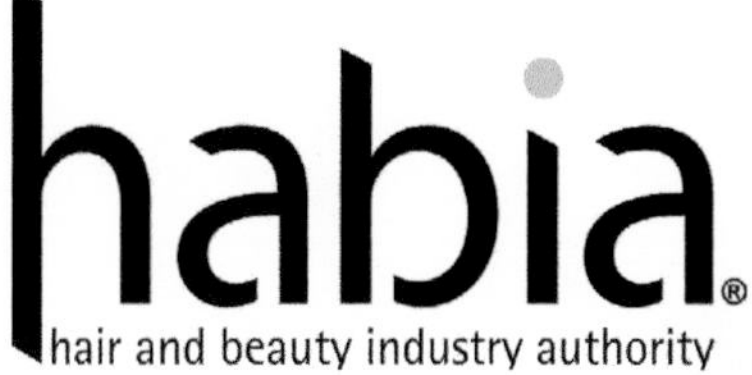

TOP TIP

Beauty therapy standards for NVQ/SVQ Level 1/4
The National Occupational Standards for Beauty Therapy are usually found in your awarding body's candidate logbook. They can also be obtained from the Habia website.

Your choice of how to study towards your qualification may be either in a college or employed in a beauty therapy business while training.

When training, you will assist with beauty salon services including: reception, facials, make-up, nails services and preparing and maintaining the beauty therapy work areas. You must carry out all related health and safety responsibilities at all times. Good working relationships are essential and you will demonstrate your effectiveness in this area while participating in everyday workplace situations.

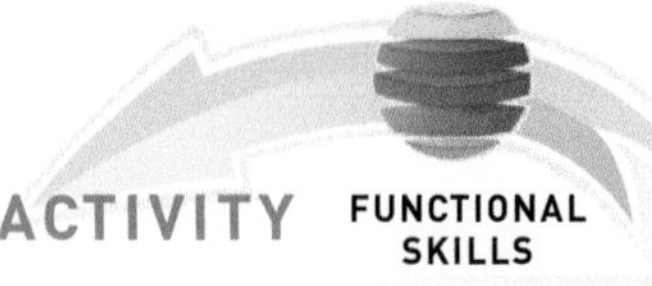

ACTIVITY FUNCTIONAL SKILLS

1 What is the title of the qualification you are studying towards? i.e. NVQ /SVQ Level 1/4 in Beauty Therapy.
2 Who is the awarding organisation for this qualification? i.e. VTCT; CGLI; Edexcel.
3 What will you be qualified to do when you have achieved the qualification?
4 What progression choices are there for you to consider when you have qualified?

Assessment

For NVQ/SVQ qualifications you will be assessed against targets that have been set individually for you. Your assessment will be by an assessor and will be ongoing throughout your training programme. Your assessor will be very experienced in beauty therapy and as well as assessing they will support you as you work towards achieving your NVQ/SVQ. You will be assessed when you reach a level of competence, this is when you feel confident that you can perform the practical skills '*what you need to do*' to the necessary standard and have the necessary level of knowledge for 'what you need to know'. Remember the standards are listed in your candidate logbook and on the Habia website.

Your assessor will provide feedback following every assessment and will provide guidance on where you need to develop your skills/knowledge further if you are not competent.

NVQ/SVQ qualification structure

The structure of an NVQ/SVQ is a similar format for all occupational sectors, e.g. hairdressing. It is made up of a number of units and outcomes.

A unit covers different areas of your work.

A unit is made up of **outcomes** '*what you must do*' and there are a different number of outcomes for each unit.

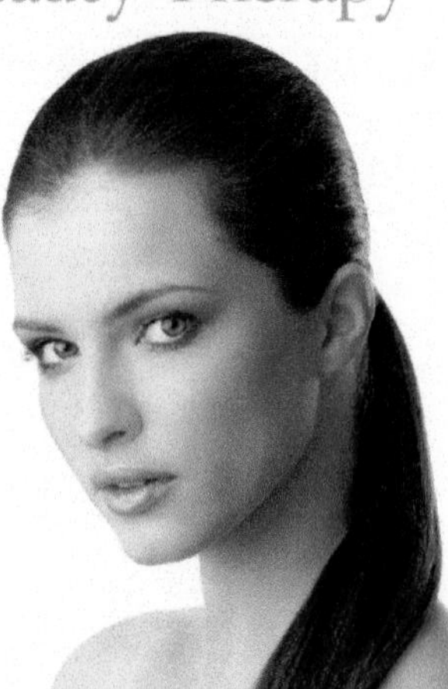

CITY & GUILDS

Level 1 candidate logbook

ALWAYS REMEMBER

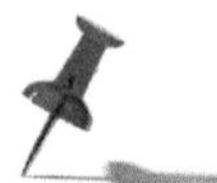

Qualification level

The level given to a qualification is decided by its difficulty, the knowledge and skills required and the level of independence required of the candidate when carrying out the unit outcomes.

Unit credit value

As well as level, which shows how difficult it is, each qualification unit has a 'credit value'. So as you achieve each unit you are awarded a number of credits based upon how long it takes to complete. One credit currently equals 10 hours of learning. Each qualification will have a different credit length related to how long it will take to complete and makes up the type of qualification.

Award 1–12 credits

Certificate 13–36 credits

Diploma 37+ credits

The credit value you earn when learning may be transferred between qualifications as you progress in your training.

It is necessary for you to be able to meet the expected standard of competence for all outcomes to be assessed as competent. Your assessor will observe you while working when you are being assessed – this is called an *observation*.

The outcomes for each NVQ/SVQ Level 1/4 unit are listed in each chapter of Beauty Basics.

Each unit also has range requirements – '*what you must cover*' –these are different assessment requirements to be covered when completing each skill.

It is necessary for you to be able to cover the range requirements meeting the expected standard of competence for each outcome to be assessed as competent.

The range for each NVQ/SVQ Level 1/4 unit is listed in each chapter of Beauty Basics.

From the **range** statement, you must show that you:

- have participated in all the listed **opportunities** to learn
- have agreed and reviewed your progress towards both productivity and personal development **targets**
- have offered **assistance** to both an individual colleague and in a group of your colleagues.

You will need to collect evidence to show how you have met the standard for developing and maintaining your effectiveness at work.

Finally, as well as being competent at practically carrying out the task, you must understand why you are doing it so each unit has knowledge requirements – '*what you must know*'. This is assessed through short written tests, assignments and oral questions.

Written tests

Written tests require you to answer questions that show you understand the subject. These may be completed on a computer, online.

Oral questions

Oral questions are where your assessor asks you questions to test what you know.

Some units are mandatory and some are optional.

Mandatory Mandatory units are those *you must do*

Optional Optional units are those *you can choose to do*.

For NVQ/SVQ Level 1/4 Beauty Therapy there are **three** mandatory and **four** optional units:

Mandatory units
Make sure your own actions reduce risks to health and safety
Contribute to the development of effective working relationships
Prepare and maintain salon treatment work areas

ALWAYS REMEMBER

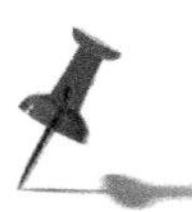

If you were ever unhappy with the outcome of an assessment decision, you can appeal. Your centre will explain this procedure to you.

ALWAYS REMEMBER

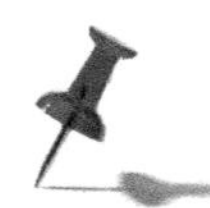

Your portfolio is your responsibility so it is important to keep everything in it up-to-date.

ACTIVITY

1 What do you understand by the term 'professional'?
2 In the workplace, is there a role model you aspire to? What skills make them special?

Working relationships

First impressions really count so try to be open, friendly and relaxed so that you put your clients at ease. Photo shoots start early in the morning and I am usually the first person they meet on set so it is important we get off on the right foot, no matter how tired we all are!

Wendy Turner

Optional units
Assist with salon reception duties
Assist with facial skincare treatments
Assist with day make-up
Assist with nail services

To achieve your NVQ/SVQ Level 1/4 qualification you must achieve **five** units, **three** mandatory units and **two** optional units.

Beauty Basics follows the NVQ/SVQ Beauty Therapy skill and knowledge requirements for all the mandatory and optional units.

Previous experience

Your assessor may need to be informed if you already have beauty therapy skills that you have gained previously. This may affect what you need to study, practice and when you are ready to be assessed. Evidence will need to be presented to prove your competence as requested by your assessor.

Regularly another person appointed as *internal verifier* will check the quality of the assessment process. They may look at you while you are being assessed practically or sample other forms of assessment evidence. An *external verifier* may also check the standard of your work. This is a person appointed by the awarding body who visits the centre again checking the quality of the assessment process and that it meets the requirements for offering the qualification.

Certification

All your evidence gained as you study towards your NVQ/SVQ Level 1/4 qualification is placed in a portfolio (a folder in which you present your evidence of competence for each unit). This may be either paper-based or electronic. When this is complete it will be checked by the internal verifier and possibly the external verifier and if all evidence is in place you will be issued with your certificate.

As well as targets related to your qualification you will have targets related to employability skills. Some of these skills will be assessed. Meeting these will help you to achieve your potential, benefiting you – to be the best you can be in the workplace and benefiting the business through the employment of good staff.

Employability skills

These include:

- acting professionally and having a professional appearance at all times
- being polite and helpful with all the people that you come into contact with every day
- being able to keep things confidential when required
- having a 'positive' attitude, wanting to do well and succeed – personal problems should not affect your work role

- learning and taking advice from experienced staff
- being reliable – not letting others down
- having very good communication skills.

Communication

Being able to 'connect' with your client is invaluable as a therapist. Try to see the world through the other person's eyes, think about how they might feel and adapt your communication as necessary. For instance, if it is their first ever skin treatment, are they shy or embarrassed? How can you help them to feel more at ease?

Sally Penford

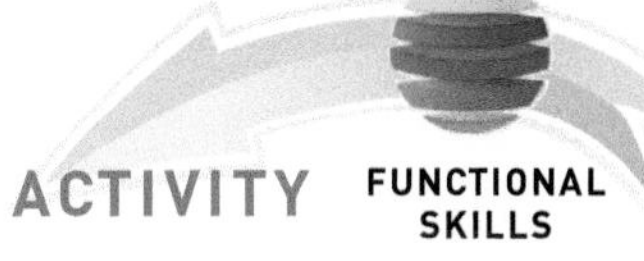

ACTIVITY FUNCTIONAL SKILLS

Employability skills

Habia have produced a table which highlights the essential employability skills and qualities required to make a successful employee. Below is a list of the headings for the skills they discuss.

Research each skill/quality heading and in your own words explain what you understand each to mean. Discuss your ideas with your assessor to check your understanding.

Willingness to learn	
Teamwork	
Flexible working	
Customer care	
Positive attitude	
Personal and professional ethics	
Self-management	
Creativity	
Communication skills	
Leadership	

TOP TIP

Employability skills

Employability skills will be assessed as part of every assessment you undertake as you are being prepared for employment in beauty therapy.

ACTIVITY

Demonstrate what value you add to the business – every day

Use your initiative – don't wait to be asked. This helps things run smoothly and you will become an asset to the business.

Give examples of you using your initiative that makes that difference!

Know you targets

In order to develop personally and to improve your skills professionally, it is important to have personal targets against which you can measure your achievement.

When you have successfully completed your NVQ/SVQ in Beauty Therapy at Level 1/4 you may gain employment or progress your training, gaining a further or higher-skilled qualification.

Employment opportunities

- assistant beauty therapist in the beauty therapy workplace supporting others delivering services
- assistant receptionist, supporting senior reception staff not necessarily in the beauty therapy industry.

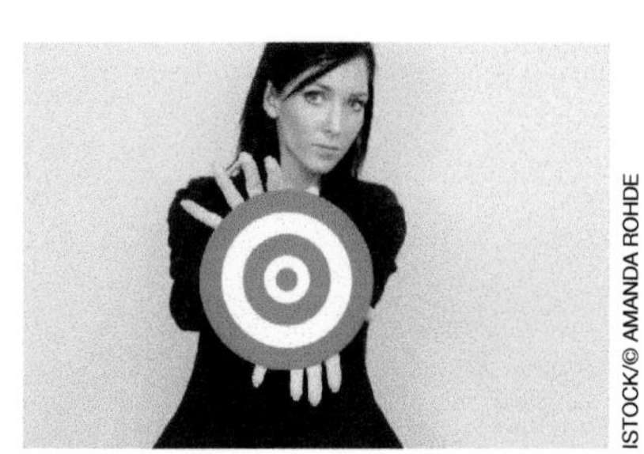

Target

Progression opportunities

- NVQ/SVQ Level 2/5 beauty therapy route studying practical skills including facials, waxing, manicure, pedicure and eye services
- NVQ/SVQ Level 2/5 make-up route studying practical skills including facials, make-up and eye services
- NVQ/SVQ Level 2/5 nail services route studying practical skills including manicure, pedicures, nail art and nail enhancements.

While training it is important to keep yourself up-to-date, keep aware of any industry trends and develop your knowledge to help you make the correct choice at the next stage in your career path.

> "Your initial NVQ course is just the start of your learning. You should continue improving your skills by attending other training, trade exhibitions, and by giving and receiving services. Your learning never stops!
>
> **Sally Biles**

TOP TIP

Keep up-to-date – the industry is dynamic and constantly changing

- **Visiting trade shows provides an excellent opportunity to keep up-to-date with new products, equipment and services as well as subscribing to professional trade magazines.**
- **This is known as Continuing Professional Development (CPD).**
- **Keep your clients motivated when discussing new industry developments.**

On achievement of your NVQ/SVQ Level 2/5 qualification you may find employment related to your chosen training route.

Employment opportunities

- business owner
- freelance working for yourself
- specialist in an area of beauty therapy, e.g. eye services
- junior beauty therapist/make-up artist/nail technician in a salon
- modelling agency make-up artist
- make-up/nail technician promotional work
- retail in cosmetics and skincare referred to as a make-up consultant.

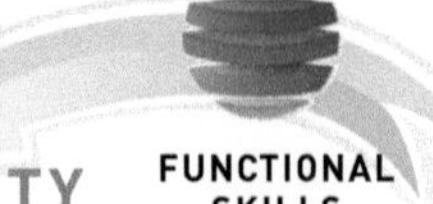

ACTIVITY FUNCTIONAL SKILLS

Where do you see yourself?

While studying NVQ/SVQ Level 1/4 start to research what part of the industry in the future you would like to work in.

Prepare some questions that will help you make the correct choice.

Ask the questions to senior staff working in the different employment routes, i.e. beauty therapy, make-up and nail services to help you in your decision-making.

What do you enjoy doing, are you passionate about any aspect of the industry? have you excelled in any area, receiving good feedback? answers to these questions may help you decide.

Industry role models

In the beauty therapy, make-up and nail industry there are many role models who have a great amount of experience which has helped raise the status of the beauty industry. They are inspirational to meet and work with and all share a common passion for their work.

Industry role models have contributed 'tips of the trade' in Beauty Basics sharing their expertise and valuable knowledge. They include:

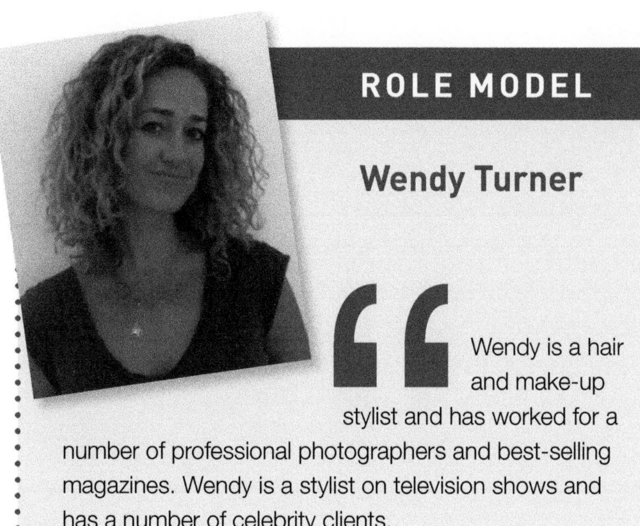

ROLE MODEL

Wendy Turner

Wendy is a hair and make-up stylist and has worked for a number of professional photographers and best-selling magazines. Wendy is a stylist on television shows and has a number of celebrity clients.

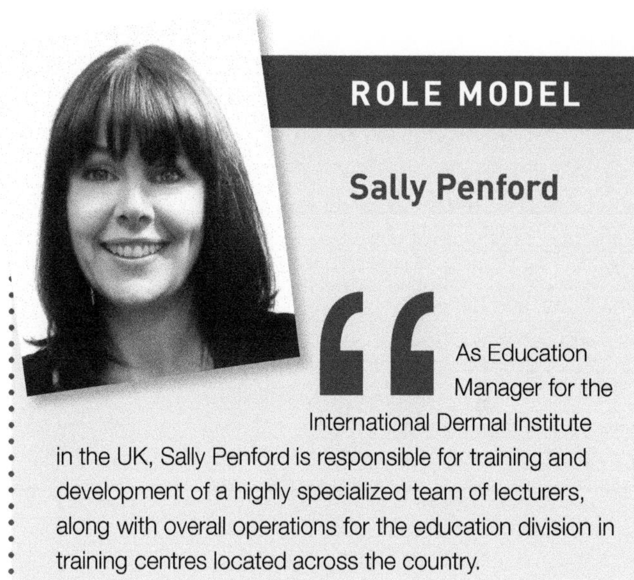

ROLE MODEL

Sally Penford

As Education Manager for the International Dermal Institute in the UK, Sally Penford is responsible for training and development of a highly specialized team of lecturers, along with overall operations for the education division in training centres located across the country.

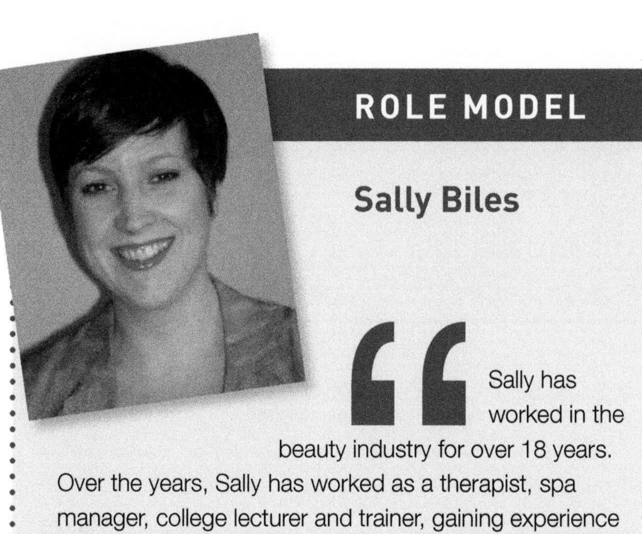

ROLE MODEL

Sally Biles

Sally has worked in the beauty industry for over 18 years. Over the years, Sally has worked as a therapist, spa manager, college lecturer and trainer, gaining experience and knowledge. Sally is currently working at the Sanctuary in Covent Garden and is responsible for training and service development.

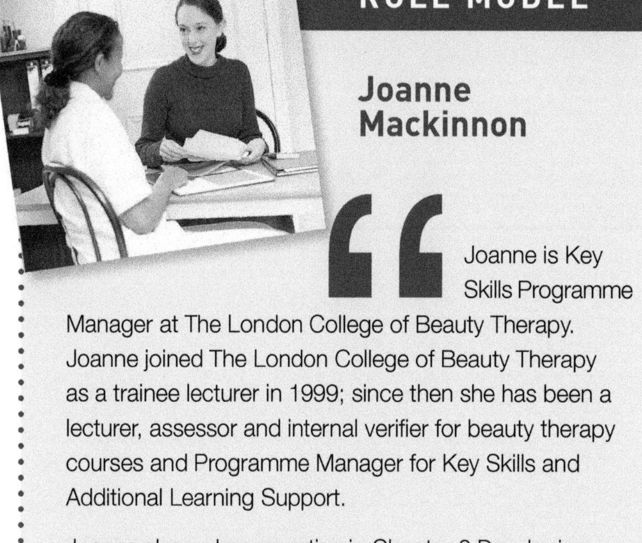

ROLE MODEL

Joanne Mackinnon

Joanne is Key Skills Programme Manager at The London College of Beauty Therapy. Joanne joined The London College of Beauty Therapy as a trainee lecturer in 1999; since then she has been a lecturer, assessor and internal verifier for beauty therapy courses and Programme Manager for Key Skills and Additional Learning Support.

Joanne shares her expertise in Chapter 3 Developing positive working relationships.

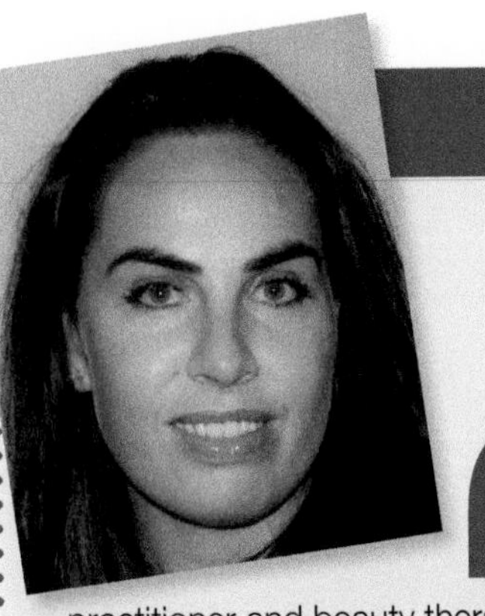

ROLE MODEL

Vicky Ann Kennedy

Vicky is a paramedical skin practitioner and beauty therapist and has been the principle owner of a very successful beauty clinic since 1991. She trained at Bolton College under Lorraine Nordmann, and became Student of the Year in her final year.

Vicky shares her expertise in Chapter 4 Preparing and maintaining the salon treatment work area.

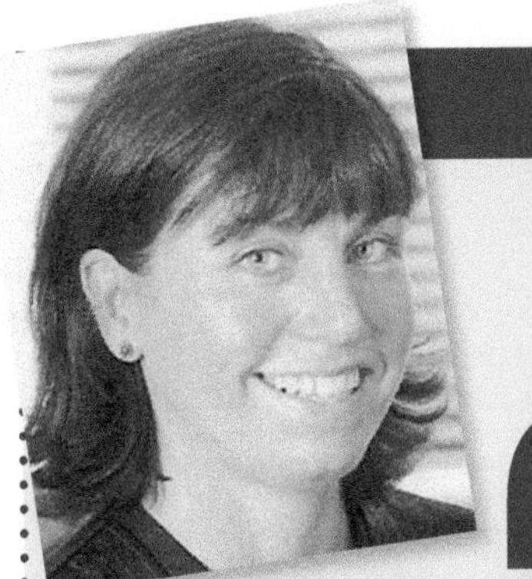

ROLE MODEL

Janice Brown

Janice is Director of Beauty (House of Famuir Ltd). Her career journey has taken her from working in and later managing a group of salons, through sales, teaching, training, research and development. Janice is the co-author of the *Encyclopaedia of hair removal* along with Gill Morris.

Janice shares her expertise in Chapter 5 Salon reception duties.

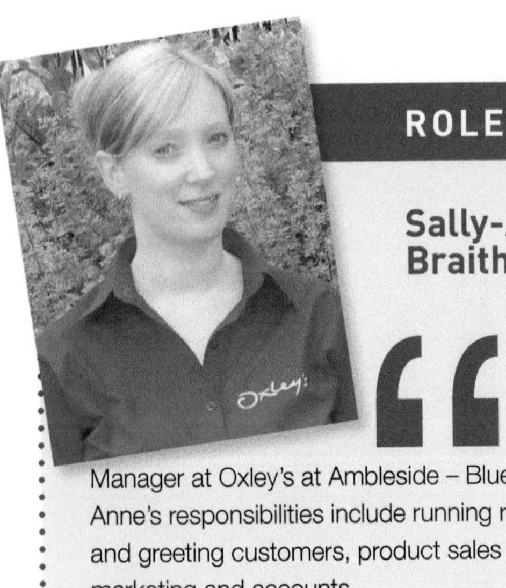

ROLE MODEL

Sally-Anne Braithwaite

Sally-Anne is Front of House Manager at Oxley's at Ambleside – Blue Fish Spa. Sally-Anne's responsibilities include running reception, meeting and greeting customers, product sales and helping with marketing and accounts.

Sally shares her expertise in Chapter 6 Facial skincare.

ROLE MODEL

Julia Francis

Julia is a professional make-up artist and body painter. Julia is also an experienced teacher and make-up consultant and has been conducting workshops for many years.

Julia shares her expertise in Chapter 7 Assist with day make-up.

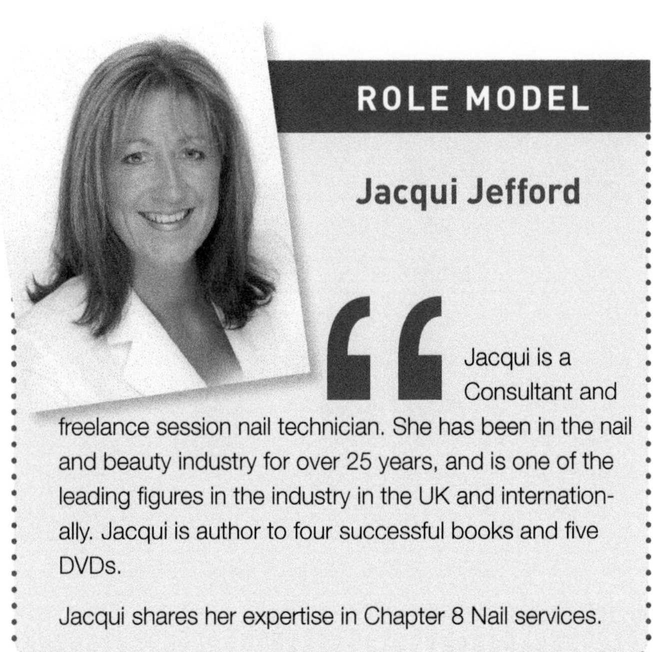

ROLE MODEL

Jacqui Jefford

" Jacqui is a Consultant and freelance session nail technician. She has been in the nail and beauty industry for over 25 years, and is one of the leading figures in the industry in the UK and internationally. Jacqui is author to four successful books and five DVDs.

Jacqui shares her expertise in Chapter 8 Nail services.

As you can see *Beauty Basics Level 1* will support you as you begin a learning journey enabling you to work in a rewarding job, full of variety with career possibilities that are endless!

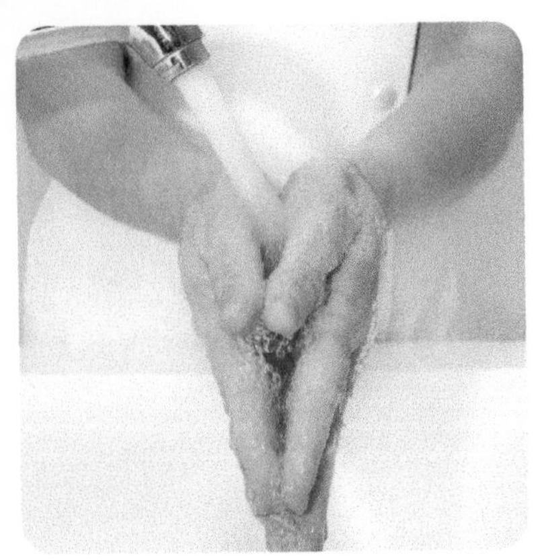

2 Health and Safety

Learning Objectives

This chapter covers the **Make sure your own actions reduce risks to Health and Safety** unit.

This chapter is all about how to make sure that your workplace is a safe working environment at all times and a safe working practice occurs at all times to ensure the safety of yourself, clients, colleagues and any other visitors to the workplace. It also covers the necessary health and safety duties and responsibilities for everyone in the beauty therapy workplace.

You will be assessed while carrying out your health and safety responsibilities.

No range has been identified for this unit.

Health and safety practice should be considered at all times within every service.

There are **two** learning outcomes which you must achieve competently:

1 **Identify the hazards and evaluate the risks in the workplace**

2 **Reduce the risks to health and safety in the workplace**

ALWAYS REMEMBER

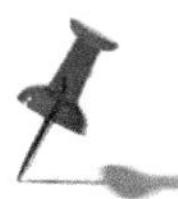

Health and Safety Executive (HSE) guidance

It is very important you understand the following terms:

Hazard – a hazard is something that has potential to cause harm.

Risk – a risk is the likelihood of the hazard's potential being realized.

Control – the means by which risks identified are removed or reduced to acceptable levels.

Remember every day in every workplace situation you must avoid a hazard/risk occurring through safe working practices.

ACTIVITY

List **three** hazards that present a 'high' risk in the beauty therapy workplace.

What action would you take within your area of responsibility, for each to prevent them becoming a risk?

Outcome 1: Identify the hazards and evaluate the risks in your workplace

Learn how to identify hazards and assess the risks in the workplace by:

1. Identifying which workplace instructions are relevant to your job.
2. Identifying those working practices in your job which could harm you or others.

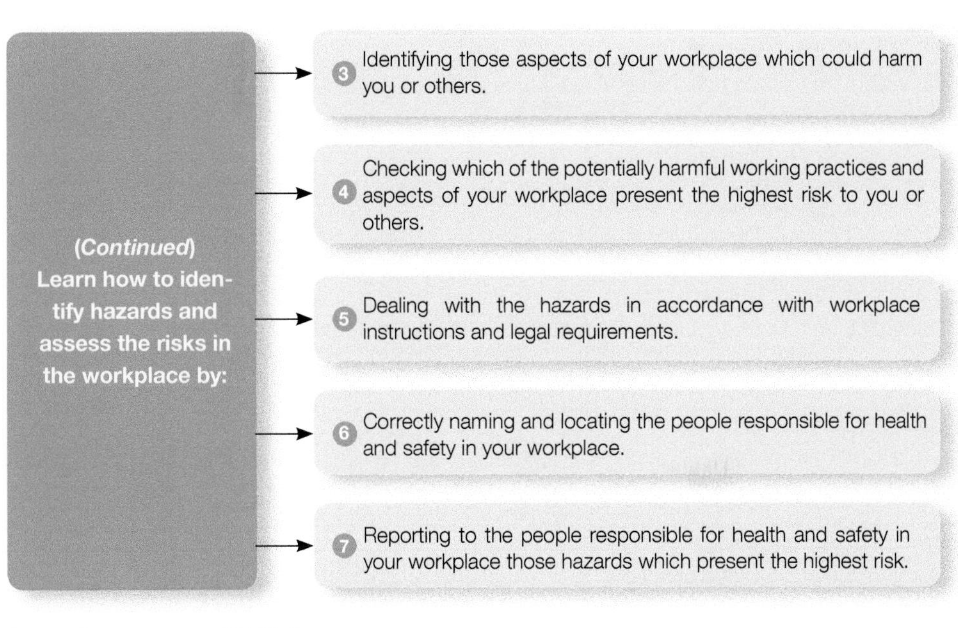

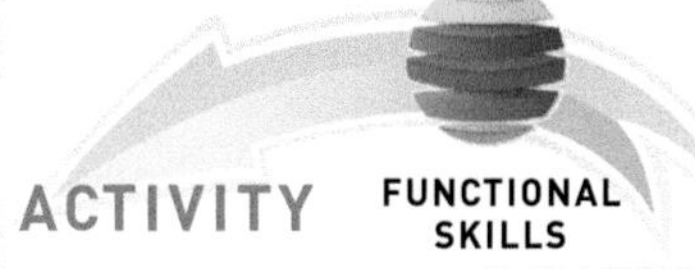

ACTIVITY FUNCTIONAL SKILLS

Keep up-to-date

Health and safety information is always being updated. Keep yourself up-to-date

Visit habia.org to find out more about current beauty therapy health and safety legislation (or laws) and the minimum requirements that you must meet.

Legal responsibilities

If you cause harm to your client, or put a client at risk, you will be held legally responsible and have legal action taken against you called **prosecution**, with the possibility of being fined and at worst imprisoned.

There is a good deal of health and safety legislation, you will need to know relating to beauty therapy. Information is widely available and you must be aware of your responsibilities and also your rights which are there to safeguard you. It is important that you receive guidance, training and read all relevant documents provided relevant to your job role and responsibilities. The HSE provides guidance and information on all aspects of health and safety legislation.

In addition, as the standards-setting body for beauty therapy, the hair and beauty industry authority Habia provide health and safety working guidelines and legislative requirements. **Codes of practice** are available from Habia these share best and mandatory (must do) working practice approved by both industry experts and health and safety advisors. Approved codes of practice are recognized by the HSE.

ALWAYS REMEMBER

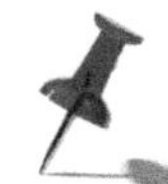

Mandatory means something that you must do – it is not an option. The word mandatory is also referred to in the units that you must study to achieve your Level 1 qualification. These are referred to as mandatory units.

Outcome 2: Reduce the risks to health and safety in the workplace

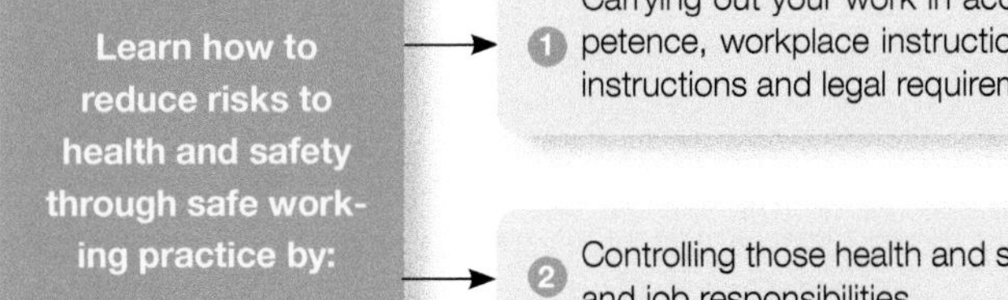

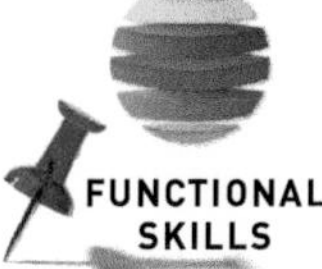

ALWAYS REMEMBER FUNCTIONAL SKILLS

Legislation

Legislation is law that **must** be put into place in the workplace. This is not a choice, you are required by law to meet their requirements. It is important to know how health and safety workplace legislation or law applies to you. For more information you can visit the HSE and Habia websites to:

- find the legislation relevant to the beauty therapy industry
- read the Habia codes of practice, available for different skills
- watch out for any changes in the law
- know where you can go for more advice and guidance.

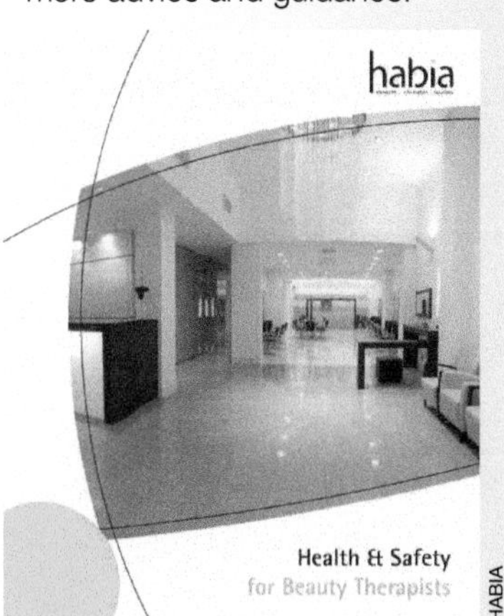

Habia health and safety guidance documentation for beauty therapists

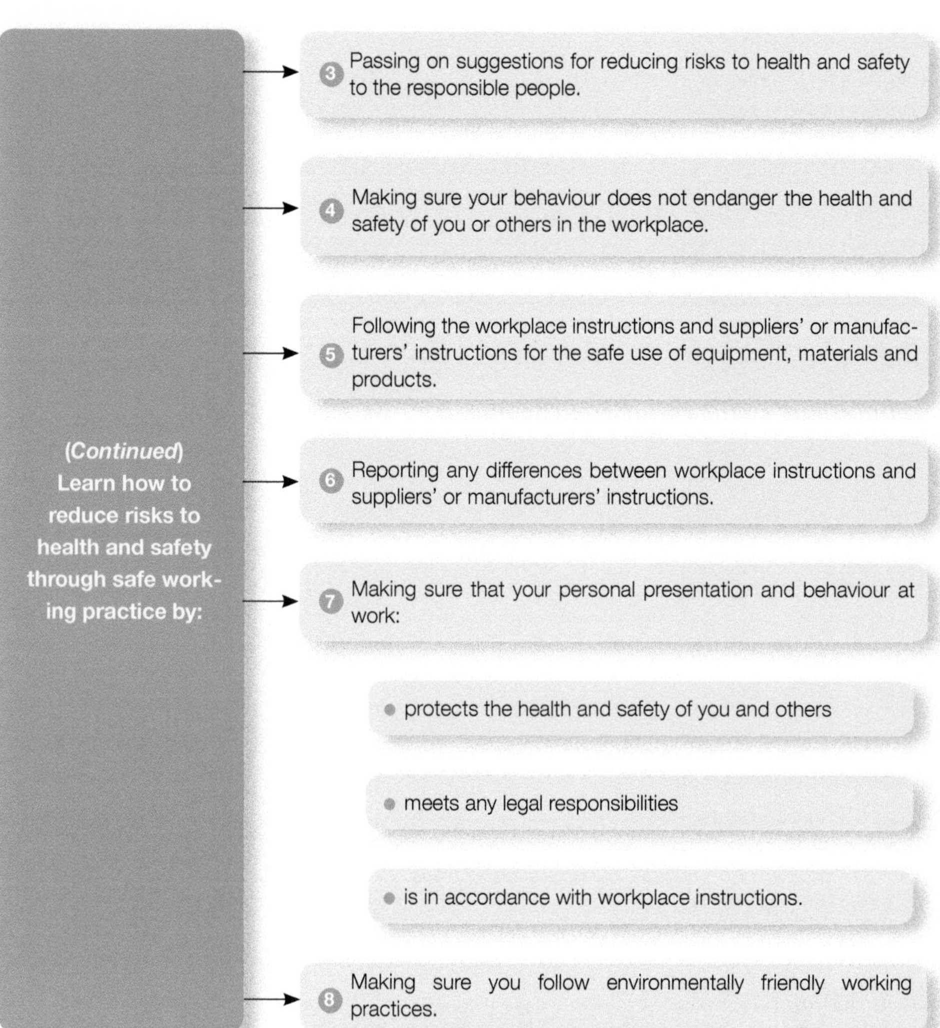

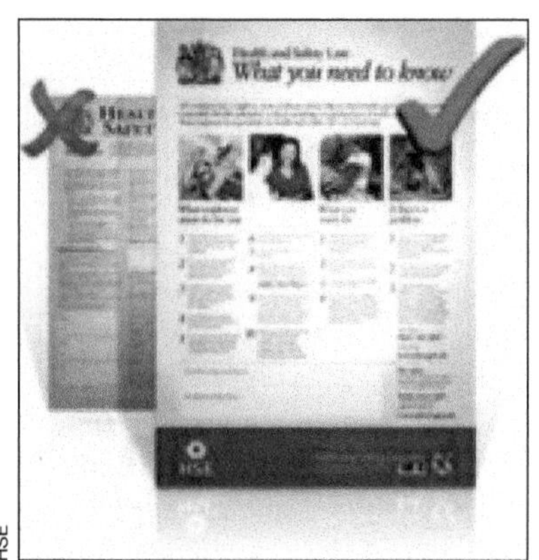

HSE

Health & Safety executive poster

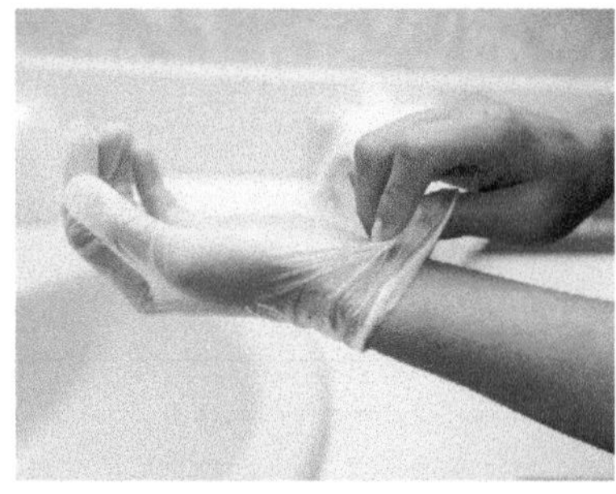

Ensure you follow health and safety guidelines when carrying out services. An example is the wearing of Personal Protective Equipment (PPE) when required.

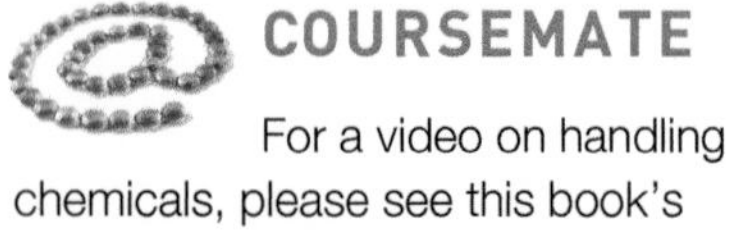

COURSEMATE

For a video on handling chemicals, please see this book's accompanying CourseMate

The Health and Safety at Work Act (1974) (HASAWA) The **Health and Safety at Work Act (1974)** is always being reviewed to make sure it continues to meet the needs of the workplace and is the main piece of legislation affecting all health and safety issues. It lays down the minimum standards of health, safety and well-being required in each area of the workplace. It is the employer's legal responsibility to put into action the Act and make sure, so far as is reasonably possible, the health and safety at work of the people for whom they are responsible and those who may be affected by the work are cared for.

Enforcement of health and safety legislation, (to confirm it is being put into practice) is divided between the local authorities (LAs) and the Health and Safety Executive (HSE). Both bodies provide support and guidance on all aspects of health and safety legislation.

If non-compliance or any area of dangerous work practice is observed, an improvement notice is issued and it is the responsibility of the employer to remove this danger within a stated period of time. Failure to comply with this will lead to prosecution. A business can be forced to stop providing a particular product or service or closed completely until all danger to employees/clients has been removed. Such workplace closure involves the issuing of a prohibition notice.

Each employer of more than five employees is required to put together a written **health and safety policy** for their business. The health and safety policy lists how health and safety is managed for that business, who does what, when and why. It is necessary to identify

responsible persons. The policy must be issued and discussed with each employee, this means you, at induction when you start work and should outline the health and safety responsibilities employees are required to undertake. It should include things such as:

- how chemical substances should be handled, stored and disposed of
- details of what is stored in the stock cupboard or dispensary
- details and records of the checks made by a qualified electrician for electrical equipment
- names and addresses of key holders for the business
- escape routes and emergency evacuation procedures e.g. in the event of an emergency i.e. fire
- whom the responsible person is to report emergencies and major risks to.

The health and safety policy should be looked at regularly to make sure it continues to meet the legislation guidelines, including any updates. Regular health and safety training should be provided and recorded. Also, checks should be made and procedures looked at to make sure that health and safety is being satisfactorily controlled and poor practice, which is a 'risk' is not taking place.

As an employee you must work with your employer to ensure a safe and healthy workplace is provided. As soon as an employee observes a **hazard** (remember anything that has potential to cause harm) this must be reported to the correct person or organization body i.e. HSE so that the problem can be put right. Hazards include:

- obstructions to corridors, stairways and fire exits (an obstruction is anything that blocks the traffic route in the salon work environment)
- trailing wires
- spillages and breakages.

Deal with low risk hazards within your responsibility, following **workplace policy** and legal requirements.

If there are fewer than five employees, relevant health and safety arrangements and procedures should be in place to meet the needs of all health and safety law. In 1992, European Union (EU) instructions updated the legislation on health and safety management. Current legislation (at the time of writing – 2009) is outlined below.

The Health and Safety at Work Act covers many other smaller regulations also which are discussed.

Health and safety rules and regulations and examples of how they are met to be displayed in the workplace include:

- the fire evacuation procedures
- Public Liability insurance certificate. This is an insurance to protect employers and employees against the possibility of death or injury to a third party e.g. client whilst in the workplace
- Health and Safety (Information for Employees) Regulations (1989) poster updated April 2009. The previous poster can continue to be displayed until 2014
- health and safety policy (dependent upon employee numbers)
- risk assessment records and guidance.

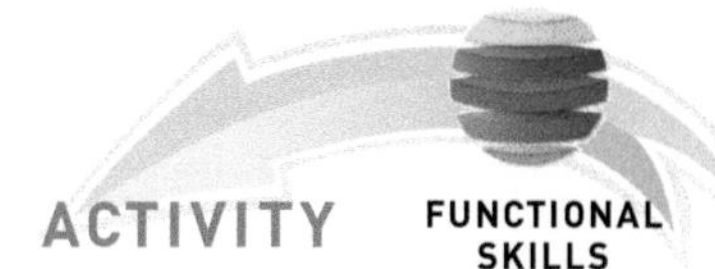

ACTIVITY FUNCTIONAL SKILLS

Health and safety workplace policy rules

Write down rules which you have been instructed apply to you in your workplace's health and safety policy. The health and safety policy identifies how health and safety is managed: who does what, when and why. What do you do?

HEALTH & SAFETY

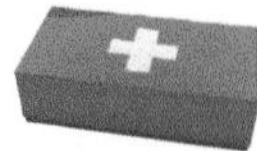

Health and safety law notice

Every employer is required by law to display a health and safety law poster in the workplace. This explains the responsibilities of employers and also employees, what action to take if a health and safety problem arises and employment rights. A leaflet is available called 'Your health and safety – a guide for workers'. Both poster and leaflets are available from the HSE.

ALWAYS REMEMBER

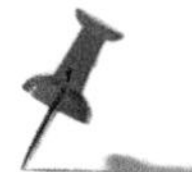

HASAWA remember!

- co-operate with your employer to provide a safe, secure and healthy workplace for all
- deal with or inform the responsible person of any potential hazard or welfare concern immediately that you become aware of it
- only carry out activities that you are qualified and competent to do so

ALWAYS REMEMBER

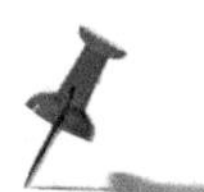

Public liability insurance is an insurance which covers any damage to a client (or other visitor to the workplace) and their property.

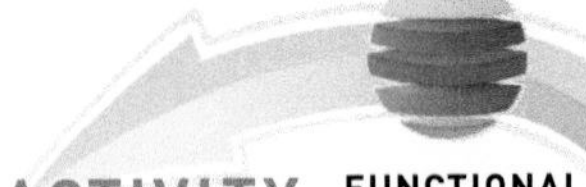

ACTIVITY

Where are the following items of health and safety legislation found in your workplace?

- the fire evacuation procedures
- public liability insurance certificate
- health and safety (Information for Employees) Regulations poster

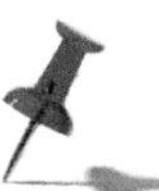

ACTIVITY FUNCTIONAL SKILLS

Risk assessment

We all have a part to play in risk assessment.

Can you think of a particular risk associated with a task you undertake in the workplace?

Answer the following questions when you have identified the risk

- what is the hazard associated with the risk?
- who is at risk from the hazard
- how do you reduce or prevent the risk occurring, what action/s do you take.

ALWAYS REMEMBER

PPE remember!

- if required you have to wear the provided PPE appropriate to the activity
- follow your training on how PPE is to be worn, removed and disposed of
- make employers aware of any shortage in supplies

TOP TIP

Working temperature on arrival at work

The working temperatures is required to be a minimum of 16C within one hour of employees arriving for work. If the temperature is too warm or too cold, temperature stress can occur.

The Management of Health and Safety at Work Regulations (1999) These require employers to make formal arrangements for maintaining and improving safe working conditions and practices in compliance with the Health and Safety at Work Act. This includes training for employees to ensure they are competent and to regularly monitor risk in the workplace (including product use), known as risk assessment. Employers with five or more employees need to record important risk assessment findings. Employers need to:

- identify and record any potential hazards
- assess the possible risks associated with the hazard
- identify who may be at risk from the hazard
- identify how the risk is to be reduced or removed and put emergency procedures in place
- train staff to identify and **control risk**
- regularly look at or review the risk assessment process.

The Personal Protective Equipment (PPE) at Work Regulations (2002) The **Personal Protective Equipment (PPE) at Work Regulations (1992)** require employers to identify – through a **risk assessment** – those activities or processes which require special protective clothing or equipment to be worn. Personal Protective Equipment (PPE) includes aprons, gloves and particle masks. This clothing and equipment must then be made available, and must be suitable for its purpose and in sufficient supplies. Employees must wear the protective clothing and use the protective equipment provided for their own safety and well-being, and make employers aware of any shortage so that supplies can be maintained and be always available.

Training should be provided on the correct use application, removal and disposal of PPE. If not used the reason should be investigated as this can then become a risk.

PPE should be 'CE' marked – that it meets the Personal Protective Equipment at Work Regulations 2002, and satisfies basic safety requirements.

The Workplace (Health, Safety and Welfare) Regulations (1992)
The **Workplace (Health, Safety and Welfare) Regulations** cover a broad range of basic health, safety and welfare (well-being) issues and require all in the workplace to maintain a safe, healthy and secure working environment. These regulations aim to make sure that the **environmental conditions** of the workplace meet the health, safety and welfare needs of all the employees including those with disabilities, and adaptations should be made where practicable. The Equality Act 2010 requires the access and facilities provided at the workplace premises must be equal for all, regardless of age, disability, gender reassignment, marriage and civil partnerships, pregnancy and maternity, race, religion or belief, sex or sexual orientation. The regulations include legal requirements in relation to the following aspects of the working environment:

- maintenance of the workplace and equipment to meet a safe standard
- ventilation systems must ensure the air is changed regularly and hazardous vapours and materials are removed.
- lighting satisfactory to enable people to move safely and perform tasks competently
- cleanliness of equipment, furnishing and fittings and correct handling and disposal of waste materials

- safe workplace premises layout, dimensions safe for people to move about and suitable for services being carried out
- workstations should be suitable for people using them, and the work being carried out. Adequate postural support should be provided
- safety protection: from falls and falling objects, objects should be stored safely
- windows, doors, gates and walls should be safe and fit for purpose
- escalators and moving walkways should operate safely and have appropriate safety mechanisms
- sanitary conveniences, i.e. toilets available for all staff and clients: suitable and sufficient
- washing facilities: hot and cold running water should be available with soap and a hygienic means of drying hands
- drinking water: adequate supply
- facilities for changing and storage of clothing should be adequate and secure
- facilities for staff to rest and eat meals should be suitable
- fire exits are clearly located and accessible. Fire fighting equipment should be available and maintained.

Manual Handling Operations Regulations (1992) The **Manual Handling Operations Regulations (1992)** apply in all occupations where lifting using the body referred to as manual lifting occurs, the aim being to avoid injury to the body, to the skeleton or muscles, and prevent the risk of repetitive strain disorders and injury caused by continuous poor working practice. The employer is required to carry out a risk assessment of all activities undertaken which involve manual lifting. Risk assessment records must be available for audit when required.

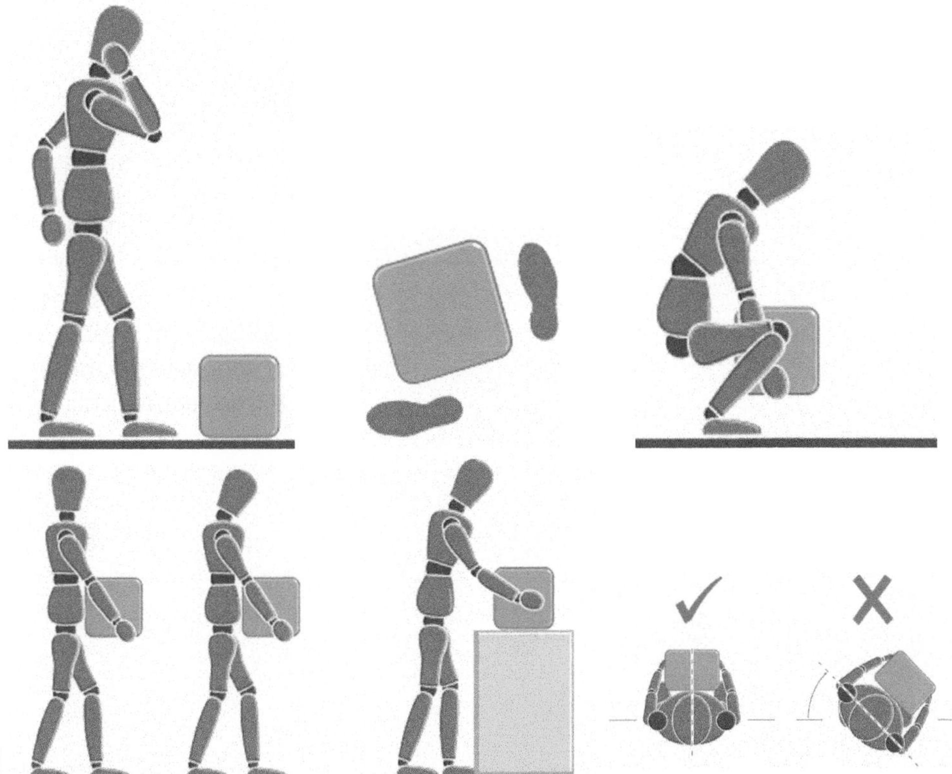

HMSO

Best practice for manual handling

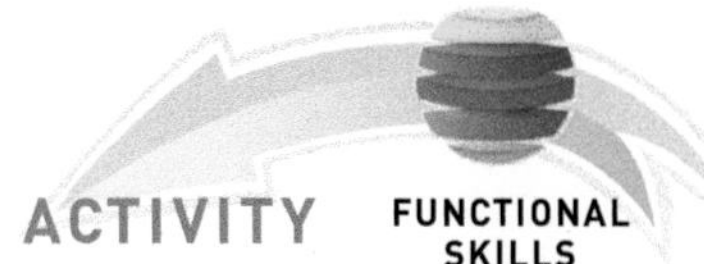

ACTIVITY FUNCTIONAL SKILLS

Workplace regulations

Obtain a copy of the *Workplace (Health & Safety & Welfare) Regulations 1992 HSE Approved Code of Practice*. Look through the code of practice guidelines, and ensure your workplace practice complies with the code.

ACTIVITY

Moving objects in the salon

What equipment or objects may you be required to move in the salon? Name three examples and they should be safely lifted and handled. Which legislation are you complying with when lifting and moving objects in the workplace?

HEALTH & SAFETY

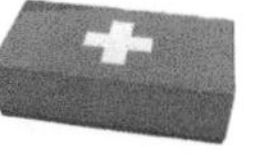

Broken goods

When you unpack a delivery, make sure the product packaging is undamaged, to avoid possible personal injury from broken goods.

ALWAYS REMEMBER

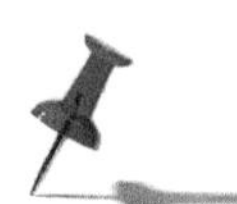

W(HS&W)R remember!

- follow all your responsibilities to maintain a safe, healthy and secure working environment for all in the work place
- inform the responsible person of any concerns you have in relation to meeting health and safety legislation requirements

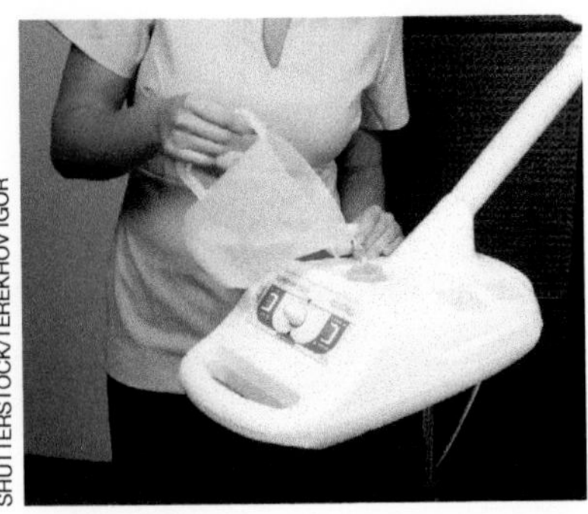
SHUTTERSTOCK/TEREKHOV IGOR

Filling the water reservoir in the steam unit with distilled water

Always take care of yourself when moving goods around the salon. Assess the risk. Do not struggle or be impatient: get someone else to help. When **lifting**, reduce the risk where possible break up larger items into more manageable loads; lift from the knees, not the back. When **carrying**, balance weights evenly in both hands and carry the heaviest part nearest to your body.

ALWAYS REMEMBER 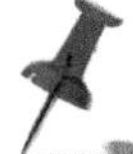

Manual Handling Operating Regulations remember!

- always assess the risk before you proceed
- get assistance if required
- break up the load
- follow the recommended safe lifting procedure

ALWAYS REMEMBER 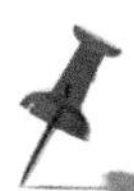

PUWER remember!

- only use equipment that you are trained and qualified to use
- use equipment for its intended purpose
- inform the responsible person if you detect any fault

Provision and Use of Work Equipment Regulations (PUWER) (1998) The **Provision and Use of Work Equipment Regulations (PUWER) (1998)** lay down the important health and safety controls on the provision and use of work equipment for both new and second-hand. They state the duties for employers and for users, including the self-employed and employees. They identify the requirements in selecting equipment and in maintaining it so that it is fit for purpose. They also discuss the information provided by equipment manufacturers, and instruction and training in the safe use of equipment. Specific regulations look at the dangers and possible risks of injury that could occur during use of the equipment and not using it for its intended purpose. Suitable safety measures must be in place, including making protective devices available and use of warning signage as appropriate.

ACTIVITY

Display Screen Equipment

Research the recommended guidelines which you should follow when using DSE to avoid the risk of injury or harm. An example is provided:

- take short regular breaks and change activity to avoid fatigue

Health and Safety (Display Screen Equipment) Regulations (1992) The **Health and Safety (Display Screen Equipment) Regulations (1992)** cover the use of display screen equipment and computer screens. They specify acceptable levels of radiation given off from the screen and recommend correct posture, seating position, suitable working heights and rest periods required when using the computer. Employers have a responsibility to meet the requirements of this regulation to monitor the well-being of their employees in avoiding the possible risks of eyestrain, mental stress and muscle strain.

HEALTH & SAFETY 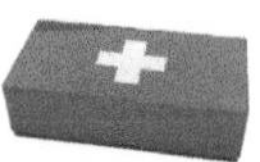

COSHH in practice

Some ingredients you may come into contact with can lead to skin allergies and the inflammatory skin disorder dermatitis; respiratory disorders including asthma; general feelings of ill-health such as headaches and nausea; cross contamination from contact with blood and tissue fluid which can lead to infection. Stay safe – always follow recommended health and safety practice.

Control of Substances Hazardous to Health (COSHH) Regulations (2002) The **Control of Substances Hazardous to Health (COSHH) Regulations (2002)** aim to ensure employers consider the substances used in their workplace and assess their possible risks to health. Many substances that seem quite harmless can prove to be hazardous if used or stored incorrectly.

Employers are responsible for assessing the risks from hazardous substances and controlling contact with them to prevent ill health. Any hazardous substances identified must be formally recorded in writing. Safety precaution procedures should then be put in place and training given to employees ensuring that procedures are understood and will be followed correctly.

Hazardous substances are shown by the use of known symbols, examples of which are shown below. Any substance in the workplace that is hazardous to health must be identified on the packaging and stored and handled correctly.

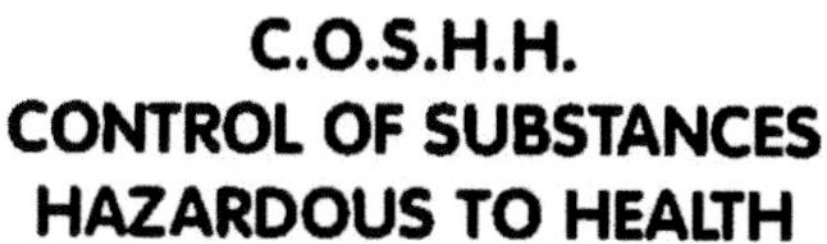

C.O.S.H.H.
CONTROL OF SUBSTANCES HAZARDOUS TO HEALTH

Health and Safety Information for the Beauty Salon and Beauty Therapist.

Compiled by The Sterex Academy

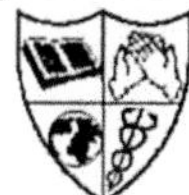

Contents:

50 x Product assessment record forms
1 x 'How to' fill in/use your product assessment record forms
1 x Daily/monthly/quarterly/annual Check List
1 x Ellisons Booklet COSHH and the Beauty Salon.

BEAUTY EXPRESS LTD. COURTESY OF HSE

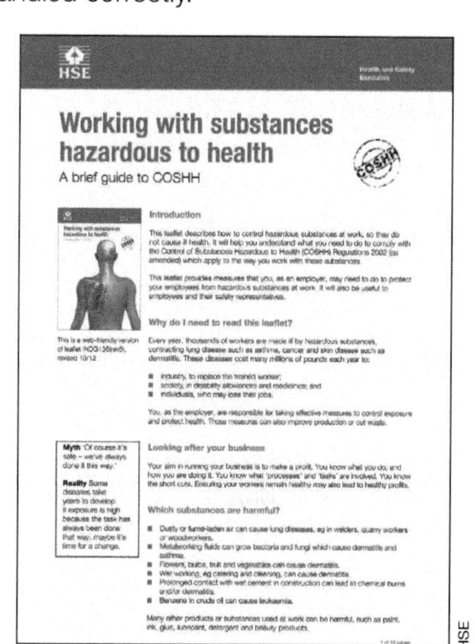

HSE

Working with substances hazardous to health

A brief guide to COSHH

Introduction

Why do I need to read this leaflet?

Looking after your business

Which substances are harmful?

HSE

COSHH regulations

COSHH information packs available from beauty suppliers, providing MSDS information.

Each beauty product supplier is legally required to make guidelines available on how materials should be used and stored. These are called material safety data sheets (MSDSs) and will be supplied on request.

Hazardous substances can enter the body through the:

- eyes
- skin
- nose (called **inhalation**)
- mouth (called **ingestion**).

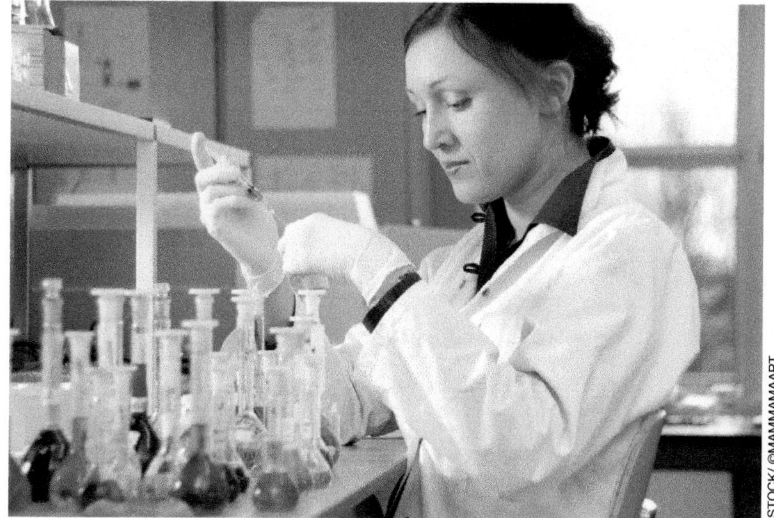

ISTOCK/ ©MAMMAMAART

Cosmetic products must be safe for use in their formulation

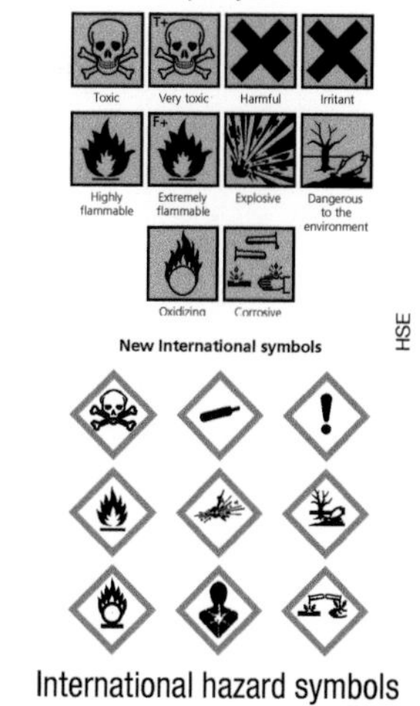

HSE

International hazard symbols

ACTIVITY

Hazard Symbols

What do each of the above International hazard symbols mean?

HEALTH & SAFETY

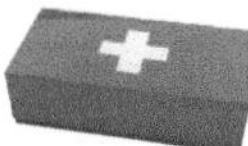

COSHH assessment

All hazardous substances must be identified and recorded when completing the risk assessment.

High-risk products should, where possible, be replaced with lower-risk products.

COSHH assessments should be reviewed on a regular basis and updated to include any new products. Ensure you are aware of any COSHH updates that may affect your daily activities.

ACTIVITY

Hazardous substances

Potentially hazardous substances include:

- aerosols
- disinfectants
- nail polish remover.

Can you add further items to this list?

TOP TIP

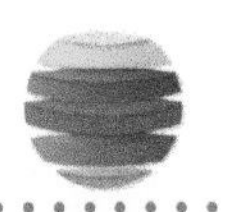

FUNCTIONAL SKILLS

COSHH and beauticians – key messages
Information for people in the beauty industry, including the controls required for specific tasks or services, is available on the HSE website in a section called, COSHH and your industry.
Do you know how COSHH affects you?

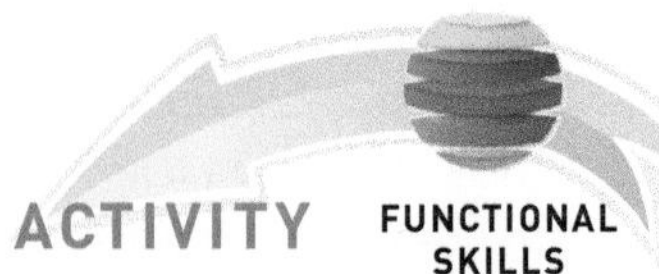

ACTIVITY FUNCTIONAL SKILLS

Identifying hazards
Make a list of potential electrical hazards in the workplace e.g. damaged plugs. Who should these be reported to if you discover them?

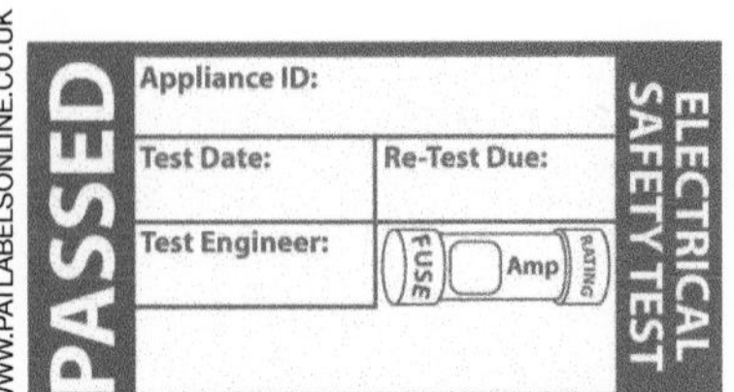

Pat test sticker records the date when equipment is tested. Green indicates it has met the safety requirements. A red sticker indicates it has failed it.

ALWAYS REMEMBER

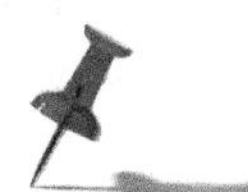

Remember EAWR !

- Never use equipment you are not trained or qualified to use
- Always visually check it appears safe to use, before use
- Report immediately any faulty equipment and remove from use
- Always use equipment for its intended purpose following manufacturers instructions

ALWAYS REMEMBER

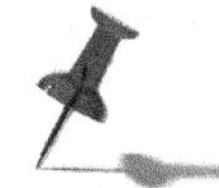

COSHH remember!
Following training guidelines on how you should handle hazardous substances

- What PPE are you required to wear? if advised you must wear it!
- Where should hazardous substances be stored?
- What is the procedure for disposal of hazardous substances?
- Do you need to wear PPE during this activity?
- What do the different hazard symbols inform you of?

Cosmetic Products (Safety) Regulations (2008) The **Cosmetic Products (Safety) Regulations (2008)** combines earlier regulations and includes current European directives. As part of consumer protective legislation protecting those buying the products, it requires that cosmetics and toiletries are safe in their formulation and are safe for use for their intended purpose as a cosmetic before being placed on the market and meet labelling requirements. The product must be accurately described to the consumer.

Electricity at Work Regulations (1989) The **Electricity at Work Regulations (1989)** state that every piece of electrical equipment in the workplace must be tested by a qualified electrician. This is called portable appliance testing or (PAT). A written record of testing must be kept and made available for inspection. A list of all salon electrical equipment should be available with its unique serial number and date of purchase/usage and disposal. Often this testing is an annual occurrence but will depend upon usage.

A trained member of staff should regularly check all electrical equipment for safety. This is recommended every 3 months.

Although it is the employer's responsibility to ensure all equipment is safe to use, it is also the responsibility of the employee to check that equipment is safe before use, and never to use it if it is faulty. This complies with the requirements of public liability insurance. Failure to do so could lead to an accident which would be considered neglectful termed negligent or careless.

If faulty equipment must be labelled to ensure that it is not used by accident.

Accidents

Accidents in the workplace usually occur through carelessness by employees or unsafe working conditions.

Any accidents occurring in the workplace must be recorded on a **report form**, and entered into an **accident book**. Anything recorded in the accident book should be looked at regularly to see where improvements to working practice can be made. The **accident form** requires more details than the accident book. You must note:

- the date and time of the accident
- the date of entry into the accident book
- the name of the person or people involved
- the details of how the accident occurred
- the injuries received and the action taken
- what happened to the person immediately afterwards (e.g. went home or to hospital)
- name and address of the person who provided first aid service
- the signature of the person making the entry in the accident book.

In the instance of an accident, first aid should only be carried out by employees qualified to do so.

Breakages and spillage Accidents can damage stock, resulting in breakage of containers and spillage of contents. Breakage of glass can cause cuts; spillages can cause somebody to slip and fall. Any breakages or spillages should therefore be dealt with immediately and in the correct way. Remember to always deal with a hazard within your responsibility – a hazard is anything that has potential to cause harm.

You must decide whether the spillage could become a hazard to health and what action is necessary. To whom should you report it? What equipment is required to remove the spillage? How should the materials be disposed of? Always consider your COSHH data and check to see how the product should be handled and disposed of if this is relevant to your job role.

Reporting of Injuries, Diseases and Dangerous Occurrences Regulations (RIDDOR) (1995) The **Reporting of Injuries, Diseases and Dangerous Occurrences Regulations (RIDDOR) (1995)** requires the reporting and recording of work-related deaths and serious major injuries, cases of diagnosed industrial disease and certain 'dangerous occurrences' (near miss accidents).

Deaths and serious major injuries occurring in the workplace related to a work activity must be reported. It is a legal requirement to notify the HSE Incident Contact Centre (ICC) and this must be immediately, by telephone, followed by a written report on HSE notification form, within 10 days of the incident. This action is completed by the person in a position of control for the workplace. If a person is absent from work for 7 consecutive days due to injury this must also be reported within 15 days of the accident. In all cases where personal injury occurs, an entry must be made in the workplace accident book. It is a legal requirement to keep an accident book. Occupational diseases such as dermatitis (see page 40) must also be reported. Where visitors to the work premises, such as clients, are injured and taken to hospital, the same reporting systems apply. This information assists the HSE in investigation of serious accidents. The HSE website provides guidance of what constitutes a reportable major injury, occupational disease and dangerous occurrence.

First aid The **Health and Safety (First Aid) Regulations (1981)** state that workplaces must have first aid provision. Employers must have appropriate and adequate first aid arrangements in the event of an accident or illness occurring. It is recommended that at least one person holds an HSE-approved basic first aid qualification.

All employees should be informed of the first aid procedures, including:

- where to find the first aid box
- who is responsible for the upkeep of the first aid box
- which member of staff to tell in the event of an accident or illness occurring
- the staff member to tell in the event of an accident or emergency.

HEALTH & SAFETY

First aid

- This should only be given by a qualified first aider.
- A first aid certificate is only valid for 3 years after qualifying and must then be renewed. This may mean further updating first aid training.
- Know what action you can take within your responsibility in the event of an accident occurring.
- An accident book should be available to record details of any accident that has occurred.

HEALTH & SAFETY

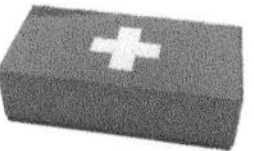

Breakages and spillages

When dealing with hazardous breakages and spillages, the hands should always be protected with gloves. To avoid injury to others, broken glass should be put in a secure container prior to disposing of it in a waste bin, in compliance with waste disposal regulations.

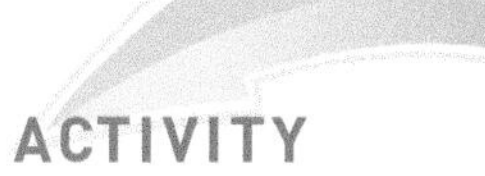

ACTIVITY

Accidents

Discuss possible causes of accidents in the workplace. How could these accidents be prevented? Who would you report an accident or injury to in the workplace and when?

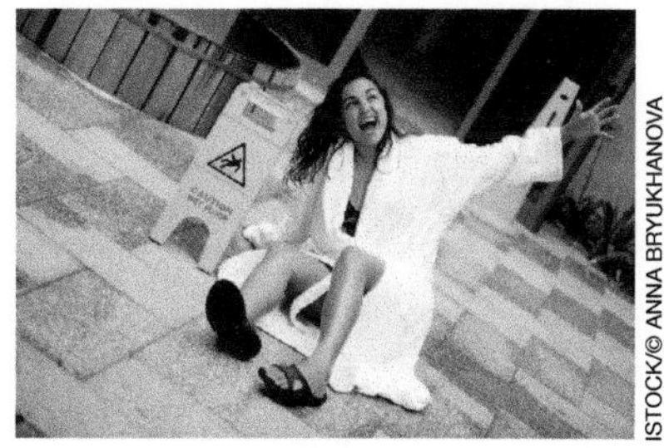

ISTOCK/© ANNA BRYUKHANOVA

HEALTH & SAFETY

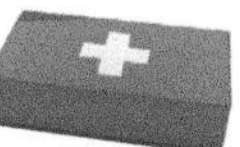

First aid

What is adequate will depend upon each workplace and requires an assessment of first aid needs. **HSE First aid at work The Health and Safety (First-Aid) Regulations 1981. Guidance on Regulation**

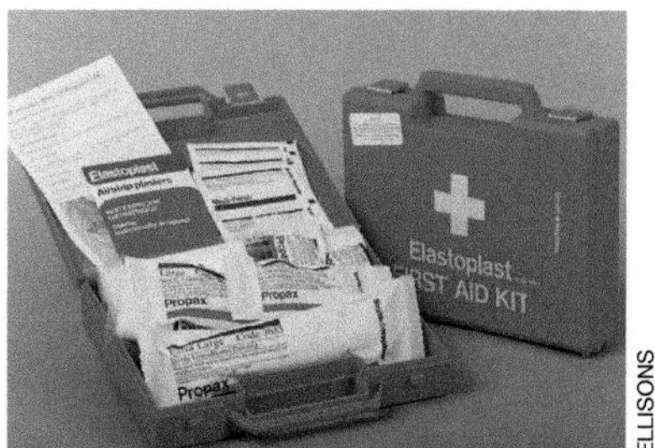

ELLISONS

First aid kits these should only be used by those qualified to carry out first aid

TOP TIP

First aid booklet
HSE guidance publication Basic advice on first aid at work can be stored in the first aid box informing of what actions to take in the event of an emergency but is not a substitute for first aid training.

An adequately stocked first aid box that is suitable for the health and safety first aid for your workplace should be available.

Basic items include:

- basic first aid guidance leaflet (1)
- assorted individually wrapped sterile adhesive dressings (20)
- individually wrapped sterile triangular bandages (6)
- safety pins (6)
- sterile eye pads, with attachments (2)
- medium-sized individually wrapped sterile unmedicated wound dressings, 10 cm x 8 cm (6)
- large individually wrapped sterile unmedicated wound dressings 13 cm x 9 cm (2)
- extra large sterile individually wrapped medicated wound dressings 28 cm x 17.5 cm (3)
- individually wrapped medical wipes.

Where clean tap water is not readily available, sterile water should be stored in sealed containers for bathing eyes.

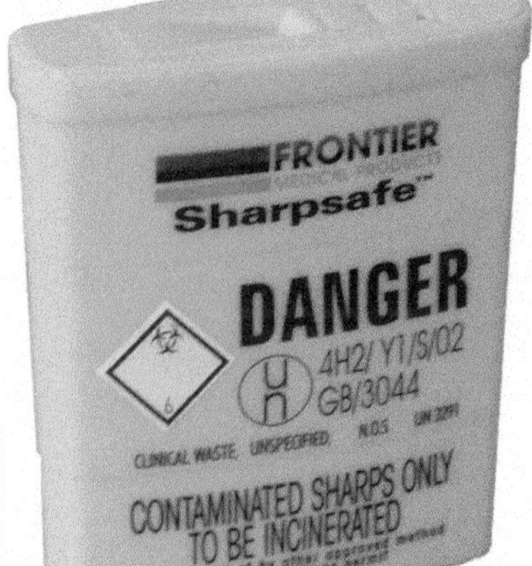

BEAUTY EXPRESS LTD

Used Sharps container

Disposal of waste

Waste Waste should be sorted and disposed of according to its risk and in an environmentally friendly way. Remember, recycle your waste and packaging wherever possible. Waste which is general, not hazardous, should be disposed of in an enclosed waste bin fitted with a polythene bin liner that is durable enough not to tear. The bin should be regularly cleaned and disinfected in a well-ventilated area: wear protective gloves while doing this. When the bin is full, the liner can be sealed using a wire tie and placed ready for refuse collection. If the bin liner punctures, the damaged liner and waste should be placed inside a second bin liner Hazardous waste must be disposed of following the COSHH procedures and training by the employer.

Clinical (contaminated) waste is waste derived from human tissues. This includes blood and tissue fluids. **Clinical waste**, such as wax strips, should be disposed of as recommended by the Environment Agency in accordance with the **Controlled Waste (Amendment) Regulations (1993)**. Items which have been used to pierce the skin, such as electrical epilation needles, should be safely discarded in a disposable **sharps container** as shown.

Certain services carried out in beauty therapy, such as ear piercing, create an additional risk because they might produce blood and body tissue fluid which could lead to contamination and cross-infection. Inspection of the premises is necessary before such services can be offered to the public. An environmental health inspector can visit the workplace to ensure the guidelines listed in the **Local Government (Miscellaneous Provisions) Act (1982)** relating to this service area are being met in terms of levels of hygiene and competence in training. If all requirements are being met, a certificate of registration will be awarded.

Fire

The **Regulatory Reform (Fire Safety) Order (2005)** replaces all previous legislation relating to fire, including fire certificates which are no longer valid. This law applies to England and Wales only. Northern Ireland and Scotland have their own similar legislation.

The Regulatory Reform (Fire Safety) Order (2005) places responsibility for fire safety onto the 'responsible person' which is usually the employer. The 'responsible person' will have a duty to ensure the safety of everyone who uses their premises and those in the immediate vicinity who may be at risk if there is a fire. The 'responsible person' must carry out a fire safety risk assessment.

Fire risk assessments will include:

- identifying and removing any barriers that may hinder fire evacuation
- ensuring that suitable fire detection equipment is in place, such as a **smoke alarm**
- making sure that all escape routes are clear and clearly signposted
- testing fire alarm systems regularly to ensure they work properly.

All staff must be trained in fire and emergency evacuation procedures for their workplace. The **emergency exit route** will be the easiest route by which staff and clients can leave the building safely. Fire action plans should be clearly displayed to show the emergency exit route. Firefighting equipment should be available and maintained, to be used only by those trained to use it.

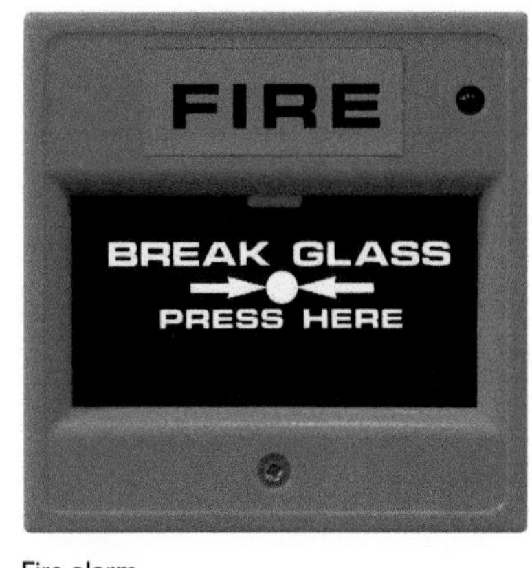

Fire alarm

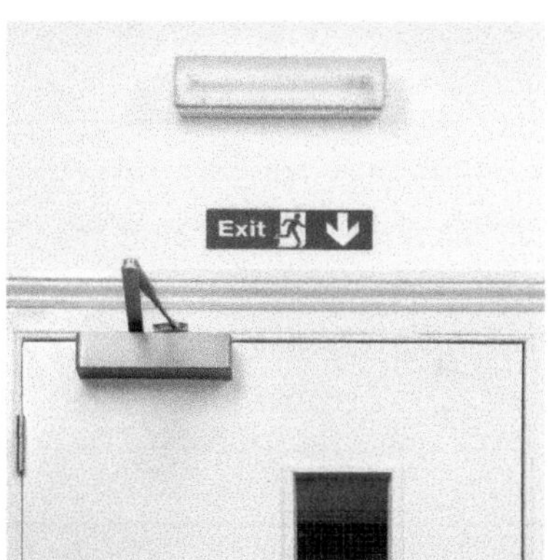

Fire exit door

Firefighting equipment Firefighting equipment must be available, placed in a specified area. The equipment includes fire extinguishers, blankets, sand buckets and water hoses. Firefighting equipment should be used only when the cause of the fire has been identified – using the ***wrong*** fire extinguisher could make the fire worse.

Fire classifications include class A, B and C. Symbols are used to identify these classifications and choice of fire extinguisher as shown below:

Class D Fires involve metals.

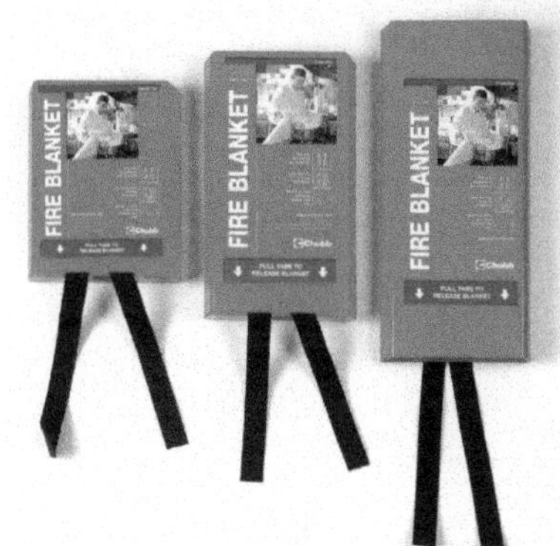
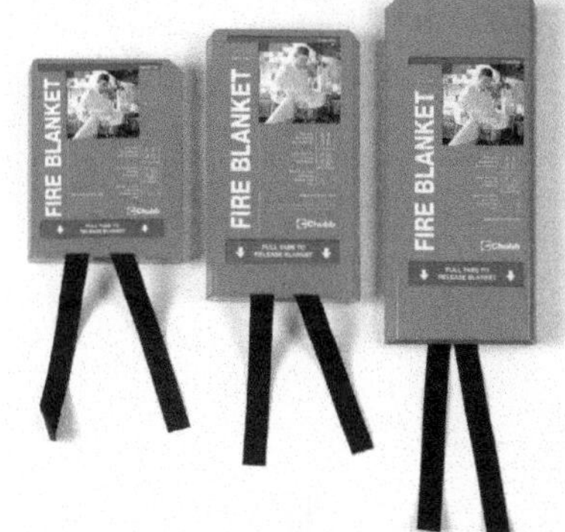

Fire blankets

Class A Fire – Carbonaceous materials such as paper and wood.

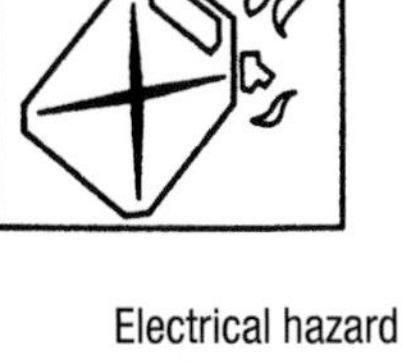

Class B Fire – Flammable liquids such as petrol, oil and paints.

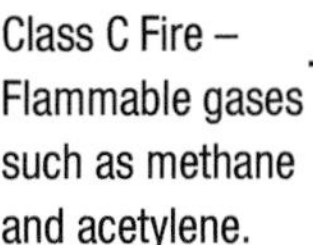

Class C Fire – Flammable gases such as methane and acetylene.

Electrical hazard symbol – For extinguisher products safe on electrical fires.

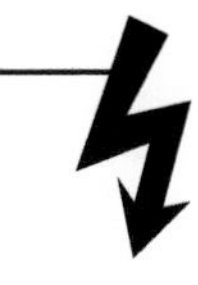

Fire extinguisher symbols

ACTIVITY

Fire drill

Each workplace should have a fire drill regularly. This allows staff to remain confident in the procedure practise so that they know what to do in the event of a real fire. It may make you aware of areas for improvement also. What is the fire drill procedure in your workplace?

HEALTH & SAFETY

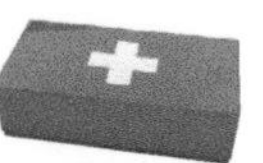

Fire!

If there is a fire, never use a lift. A fire quickly becomes out of control. You do not have very long to act!

Fire drill notices should be visible to show people to the emergency exit route.

HEALTH & SAFETY

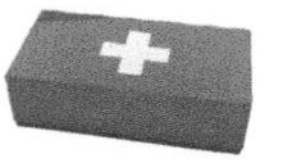

Fire exits

Fire-exit doors must be clearly marked, remain unlocked during working hours and be free from any barriers.

ACTIVITY

Fire extinguisher – when to use?

What is the fire extinguisher colour code shown on the fire extinguisher(s) in your workplace?

What does this mean it can be used upon?

ACTIVITY

Causes of fires

Can you think of several possible causes of fire in the salon? How could each of these be prevented?

HEALTH & SAFETY

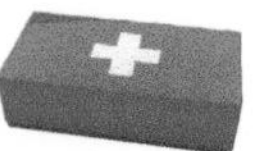

Using fire extinguishers

The vapours released when using vaporizing liquid extinguishers 'starve' a fire of oxygen. They are therefore dangerous when used in confined spaces, as people need oxygen too!

Never use firefighting equipment unless you are trained in its use.

Fire extinguishers Fire extinguishers are available to tackle different types of fire. These should be located in a set place known to all employees. It is important that these are checked and maintained as required.

Fire blankets are used to smother a small, localized fire or if a person's clothing is on fire. **Sand** is used to soak up liquids if these are the source of the fire, and to smother the fire. **Water hoses** are used to extinguish large fires caused by paper materials and the like – buckets of water can be used to extinguish a small fire. *Remember the electricity should always be turned off at the mains first!*

Never put yourself at risk – fires can spread quickly. Leave the building at once if in danger and raise the alarm by telephoning the emergency services on the emergency telephone numbers, **999** or **112**.

ALWAYS REMEMBER

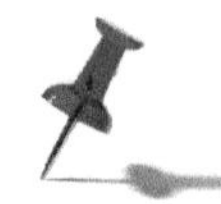

Fire extinguishers

Label colour indicates the use of particular fire extinguishers. Make sure you know the meaning of each of the colours.

KNOW YOUR FIRE EXTINGUISHER COLOUR CODE

Cylinder Colour Coding and Contents

Classification of Fire Risk	WATER	FOAM	CO_2	DRY POWDER	VAPOURISING LIQUIDS	WET CHEMICAL
	Unsafe all voltages Wood, Paper Textiles etc.	Unsafe all voltages Flammable liquids	Safe all voltages Flammable liquids	Safe all voltages Flammable liquids	Safe all voltages Flammable liquids	Unsafe all voltages Wood, Paper Textiles etc.
A Paper, Wood, Textile and Fabric	✓	✓		✓	✓	✓
B Flammable Liquids		✓	✓	✓	✓	
C Flammable Gases			✓	✓	✓	
Electrical Hazards			✓	✓	✓	
Vehicle Protection		✓		✓	✓	

COLOUR CODING IN ACCORDANCE WITH BS EN3: 1996 - PORTABLE FIRE EXTINGUISHERS
FLAMMABLE GAS FIRES MUST BE EXTINGUISHED BY THE EMERGENCY SERVICES ONLY

Fire extinguisher label colour code

Cause of fire and choice of fire extinguisher

Cause	*Extinguisher type*	*Lable colour code*
Electrical fire, flammable gases	Carbon dioxide (CO_2) extinguisher	Black
Solid material fire (paper, wood, etc.)	Water extinguisher	Red
Flammable liquids	Foam extinguisher	Cream
Electrical fire flammable liquids	Dry-powder extinguisher	Blue
Flammable metal fires	Vaporizing liquid	Green
Wood, paper, textiles and cooking related fires	Wet chemical	Yellow

Other emergencies

Other possible emergencies that could occur relate to fumes and flooding. Know where the water and gas stopcocks are located. In the event of a gas leak or a flood, the stopcocks should be switched off and the appropriate emergency service contacted. Never switch on an electric switch as this could cause a spark and ignite the gas!

In the event of a bomb alert, staff must be trained in the appropriate emergency procedures. This will involve recognition of a suspect package, how to deal with a bomb threat, evacuation of staff and clients and contacting the emergency services. Your local Crime Prevention Officer (CPO) will advise on bomb security.

Environmentally friendly working practices Being environmentally friendly, also known as 'eco- friendly' or 'green', means that you consider how you can help to minimize harm to the environment and put this into practice in your everyday working practice. Think about how you work, use and dispose of products within your workplace. Are you always environmentally friendly? Below are some ideas how your workplace can help your workplace to become more environmentally friendly.

- do not allow taps to run unnecessarily
- use biodegradable, recycable, packaging for disposal of non-contaminated waste
- for hospitality drinks rather than use disposable plastic cups change to cups and glasses that can be washed
- dispose of chemicals safely, not down the sinks
- use wooden spatulas from sustainable wood sources that can be maintained at sufficient levels without harm
- use recycled consumable materials where possible, e.g. bed-roll, tissues and cleaning products
- use light bulbs that reduce energy use. Switch off lights in rooms not being used and also equipment when not in use – if safe to do so
- turn down the heating thermostat rather than opening windows, this will save money too
- buy in bulk, reducing trips to the wholesaler, and buy locally
- consider promoting fair trade products where possible, to support ethical trading

ACTIVITY

Health and safety awareness
Where can you find the following in your workplace:

1. fire extinguisher(s)?
2. information sheets stating how products should be stored/used. MSDS (Material Safety Data Sheets)?
3. health and safety workplace information?
4. first aid kit?
5. sterilization/disinfection equipment?
6. PPE?
7. the fire exit(s)?
8. accident book?
9. sharps box and waste bags for contaminated waste?

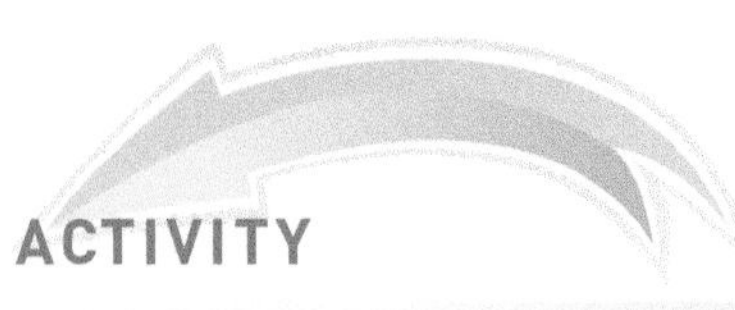

ACTIVITY

Noise levels

Assess the noise level at your workplace. Are there any intrusive noise levels preventing normal communication i.e., do voices need to be raised? This could occur if you had loud background music during promotional events for example.

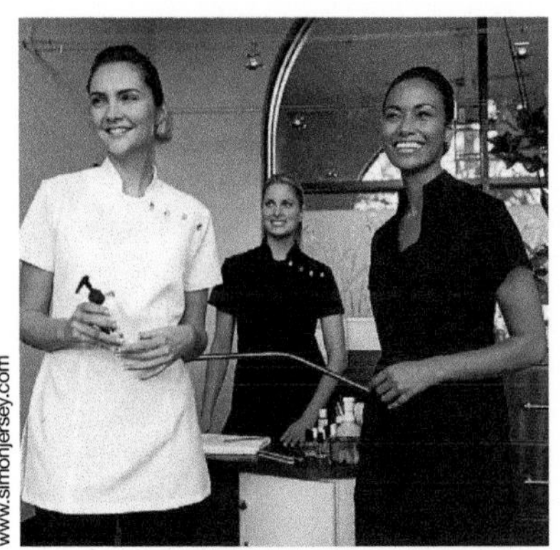

Beauty workwear

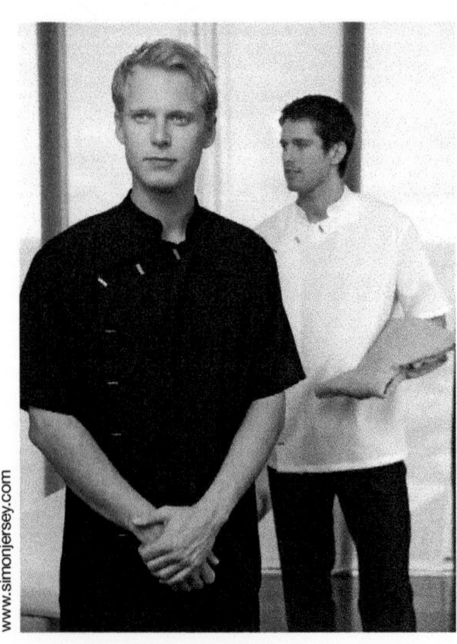

Small steps can make a big difference.

Control of Noise at Work Regulations (2005) Loud noise can damage hearing. Noise is measured in decibels (db). A-weighting is sometimes written as 'dB(A)' which is average noise level. C-weighting is 'dB(C)' – noise which is at its highest point, e.g. explosives.

As an employer a safe working environment should be provided with noise levels kept within safe levels. This does not include low-level noise. As in all **workplace practices**, noise levels can be classified as a risk. If a risk is identified, action should be taken to correct it. This could be a PPE hearing protection. Information, instruction and training must be provided which is monitored.

Insurance

Insurance must cover all activities in the workplace. **Public Liability Insurance** protects employers and employees against the cost of death or injury to a third party while on the premises. This does not relate to claims by employees. Professional indemnity insurance extends public liability insurance to cover named employees against claims.

Product and **Service Liability Insurance** is usually included with your public liability insurance but should be checked with the insurance company. Product Liability Insurance covers you for risks which might occur as a result of the products you are using and/or selling.

It is a legal requirement under the **Employers' Liability (Compulsory Insurance) Act (1969)** that every employer must have **Employers' Liability Insurance**. This provides financial compensation to an employee should they be injured as a result of an accident in the workplace. This certificate must be displayed indicating that a policy of insurance has been obtained.

Personal health, hygiene requirements and presentation

Your appearance enables the client to make a judgement about both you and the workplace, so make sure that you create the correct impression! Employees in the workplace should always reflect the desired image of the profession that they work in.

Personal presentation

Assistant beauty therapist As a beauty therapist qualified to Level 1 you will be required to wear a clean protective overall as you will be preparing the working area for client services and may be involved in preparing clients and performing basic skills in facial, nail and make-up services. What image does your workplace create, relaxing, bright and lively?

Workwear is available in a range of fabrics but a cotton overall is ideal; air can circulate, allowing perspiration to evaporate, discouraging body odour. The use of a light colour such as white immediately shows the client that you are clean. Workwear might comprise a dress, in a length suited to a work role, a jumpsuit or a tunic top, with co-ordinating trousers varied in length. Fresh, clean overall protective workwear should be worn each day.

Make-up artists work with different cosmetic mediums throughout the day and in order to maintain a professional appearance throughout the day, black is a popular colour worn as a tunic or T-shirt top with trousers.

Receptionist If receptionists are employed solely to carry out reception duties, they may wear a different salon dress/uniform, to those worn by the practising beauty therapists. As the receptionist will not be as active, it may be appropriate for them to wear a smart jacket or cardigan. If on the other hand they are also carrying out services, the standard salon overall must be worn.

General rules for employees

Make-up An appropriate make-up should be worn according to your work role, and always use the correct skincare cosmetics to suit your skin type. A healthy facial appearance will be a positive advertisement for your work. First impressions count!

Jewellery Keep jewellery to a minimum, such as a wedding ring, a fob watch and small stud earrings. Facial piercings are increasingly popular, worn as a form of self expression, but the acceptability and wearing of facial piercings will be discussed as part of your workplace policy on appearance and dress code in order to maintain a professional appearance.

Nails Beauty therapist work requires nails to be short, neatly manicured and free of nail polish unless the employee's main duties involve nail services or reception duties. Nail polish contains ingredients which can cause an allergic reaction in some people. Nail length can interfere with the application of the service, such as facial cleansing. Also, nail polish will generally spoil when in contact daily with different cosmetics. Make-up artists, however, often wear nail art as an additional expression of their creativity.

Shoes Ideally you should wear flat, well-fitting, comfortable shoes that enclose the feet fully but allow the toes to spread. Remember that you will be on your feet for most of the day and this action will help prevent future foot and postural disorders caused by ill-fitting shoes!

Ethics

Beauty therapy has a **code of ethics**. This is a code of behaviour and expected standards for the professional beauty therapist to follow, which will help keep the reputation of the beauty therapy industry and ensure best working practice for the safety of the industry and members of the public. Beauty therapy professional bodies produce codes of practice for their members. A business may have its own code of practice. Although

Code of Ethics

1 Towards BABTAC

a) By not bringing the profession as a whole into disrepute.

b) By protecting collective morality. Members should not professionally associate themselves with any person or premises which may be deemed to be unprofessional or disreputable, as such an Association which may put the good name of the therapist and of BABTAC at risk.

2 Towards clients (concerned with the individual therapist/client relationship)

a) Appointments must be kept. If unforeseen circumstances arise every effort must be made to make the client aware of the treatment cancellation.

b) Client confidentiality – personal information should be kept private and only used for the specific purpose for which it is given, namely, to enable the therapist to carry out a safe and effective treatment.

c) Information concerning the client and views formed must be kept confidential. The member should make every effort to ensure that this same level of confidence is upheld by receptionists and assistants where applicable.

d) Client treatment details should remain confidential. Possible exceptions are the following;

i) The client's knowledge and written consent are obtained.

ii) There is a necessity for the information to be given, for example if the client is being referred onto another professional.

The exceptions are:

iii) If the therapist is required by law to disclose the information.

iv) If the therapist considers it their duty for the protection of the public.

If a therapist has information of a criminal nature the member is advised to take legal advice.

An excerpt from *The BABTAC Handbook*, code of ethics, www.babtac.com/www.babtac.com
BABTAC, The British Association of Beauty Therapy and Cosmetology

HEALTH & SAFETY

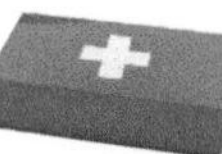

Aprons and the Personal Protective Equipment (PPE) at Work Regulations (1992)
For certain services, such as waxing services, it is necessary to wear a protective apron over the overall. Assistant beauty therapists may also wear an apron while preparing and cleaning the working area, to protect the overall and keep it clean.

HEALTH & SAFETY

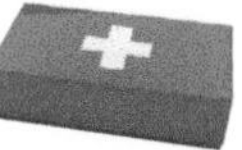

Workplace policy skin adornment
Employers will advise you on personal presentation requirements in relation to facial piercings and skin tattoos.

ACTIVITY

Personal appearance

1 Collect pictures from various suppliers of overalls. Select those that you feel would be most practical for a Level 2 beauty therapist, make-up artist or receptionist. Briefly describe why you feel these are the most suitable.

2 Design various hairstyles, or collect pictures from magazines, to show how the hair could be smartly worn by a beauty therapist with medium-length to long hair.

ACTIVITY

Code of ethics
As a professional beauty therapist it is important that you follow the to a code of ethical practice. This helps to maintain the standards of the industry. You may wish to join a professional organization, which will issue you with a copy of its agreed standards.

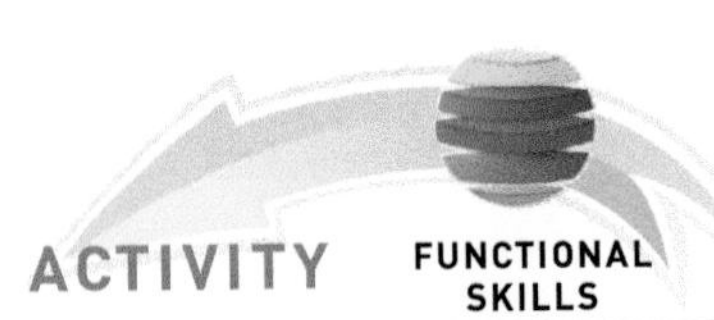

ACTIVITY FUNCTIONAL SKILLS

Staying healthy

Ask your tutor for guidelines before beginning this activity.

1 Write down all the foods and drinks that you most enjoy. Are they healthy? If you are unsure, ask your tutor.
2 How much exercise do you take weekly?
3 How much sleep do you regularly have each night?
4 Do you think you could improve your health and fitness levels?

not a legal requirement, this code may be used in criminal proceedings as evidence of unacceptable practice.

Diet, exercise and sleep

A beauty therapist requires strength and energy. To achieve this you need to eat a healthy, well-balanced diet, take regular exercise and have enough sleep, recommendations are between 7–8 hours a night.

Posture

Posture is the way you hold yourself when standing, sitting and walking. *Correct* posture enables you to work longer without becoming tired, it prevents muscle tiredness, repetitive strain injury (RSI) and stiff joints, and it also improves your general physical appearance.

Good standing posture If you are standing with good posture, these terms will describe you:

- head up, centrally balanced
- shoulders slightly back, and relaxed
- chest up and out
- abdomen flat
- hips level
- fingertips level
- bottom in
- knees level
- feet slightly apart and weight evenly distributed.

Good sitting posture Sit on a suitable chair or stool with a good back support and:

- sit with the lower back pressed against the chair back
- keep the chest up and the shoulders back
- share the body weight evenly along the thighs
- keep the feet together, and flat on the floor
- do not slouch, or sit on the edge of your seat.

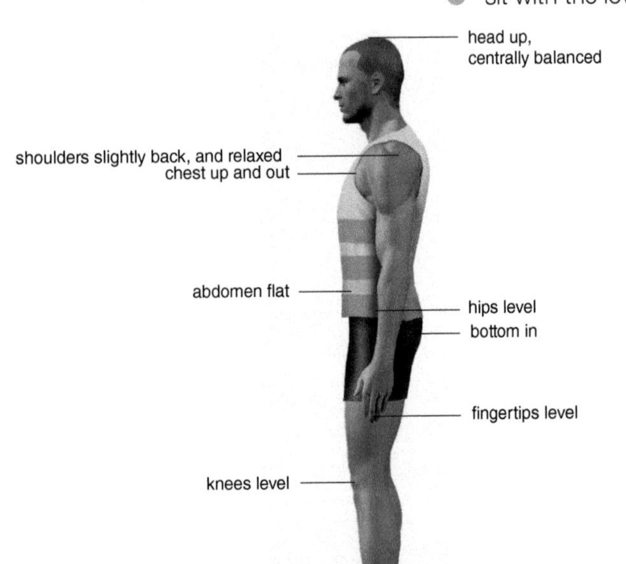

Good standing posture

Personal hygiene

It is vital that you have a high standard of personal **hygiene** as you are going to be working very near to people.

Bodily cleanliness is achieved through daily showering or bathing. This removes the stale sweat, dirt and bacteria which cause body odour. An antiperspirant or deodorant may be applied to the underarm area to reduce sweating called perspiration and the smell of sweat. Clean underwear should be worn each day.

Hands Your hands and everything you touch are covered with germs. Although most are harmless, some can cause ill-health or disease. Wash your hands regularly, especially after you have been

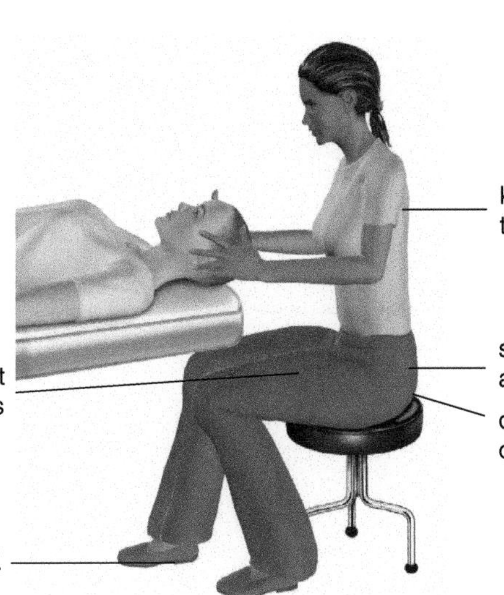

Good sitting posture

to the toilet and before eating food. You must also wash your hands before and after treating each client, and during a service if necessary. Washing the hands before treating a client minimizes the risk of cross-infection and presents to the client a hygienic, professional, caring image. Disinfecting hand gel may also be applied to the clean hands before services are delivered. Even if wearing gloves the hands must be cleaned thoroughly first before their application.

Skin on the hands should be regularly checked for dryness or soreness. If this occurs hand maintenance systems should be reviewed including PPE.

ACTIVITY

The importance of posture

1 Which services will be performed sitting, and which standing?
2 In what way do you feel your services would be affected if you were not sitting or standing correctly?

HEALTH & SAFETY

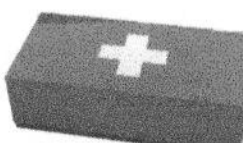

Repetitive strain injury (RSI)

If you do not follow correct postural positional requirements when performing services, muscles may become overstretched and overused resulting in repetitive strain injury (RSI). This may result in you being unable to work in the short term, and possibly long term in the occupation.

Step-by-step: How to wash your hands

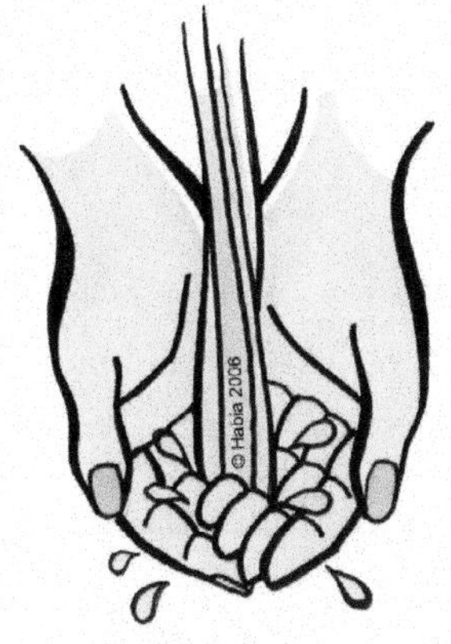

1 Wet your hands, wrists and forearms thoroughly using running water

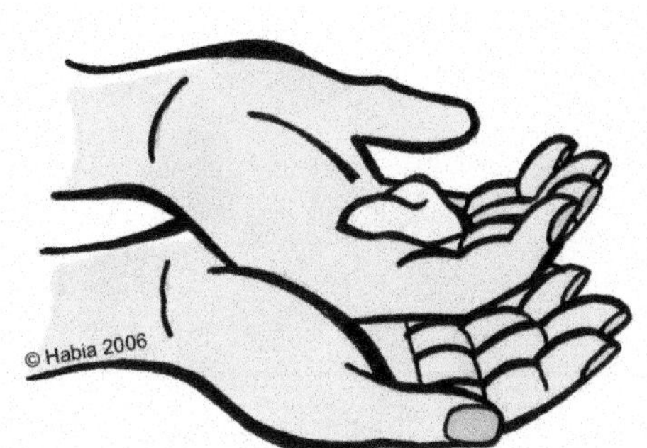

2 Apply around 3ml to 5ml of liquid soap

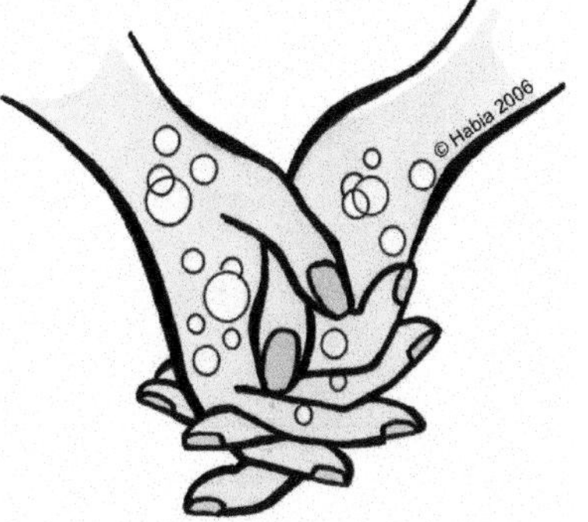

3 Start the lathering process, rubbing palm to palm

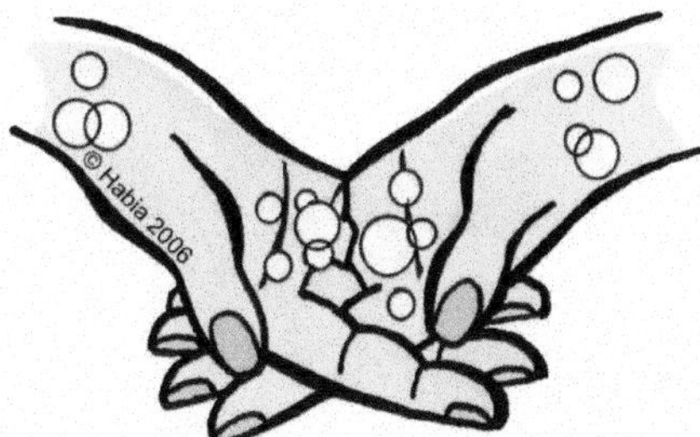

4 Interlock fingers and rub, ensuring a good lather

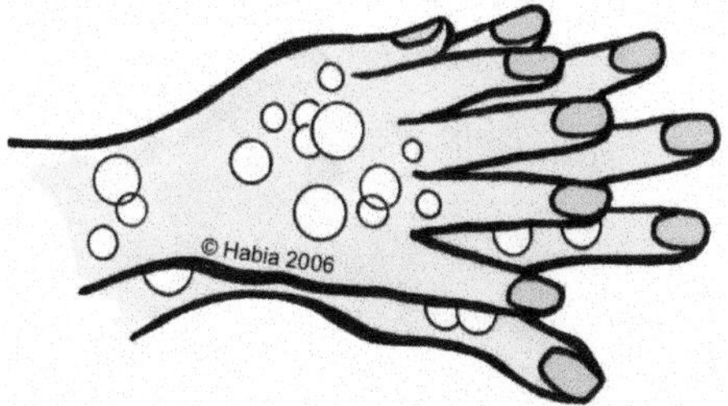

5 Rub right hand over back of left, then left over right hand

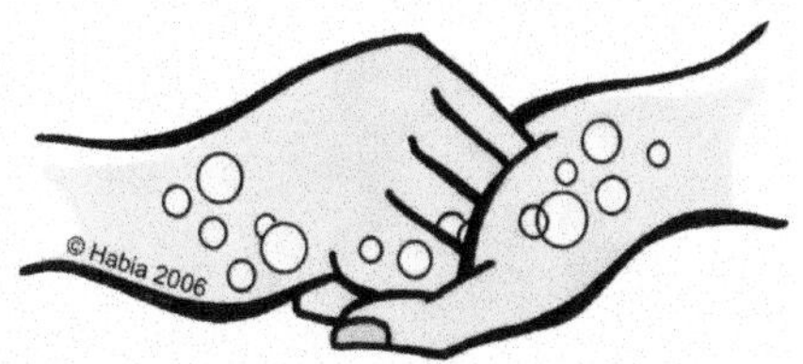

6 Rub with fingers locked in palm of hand ensuring fingertips are cleaned

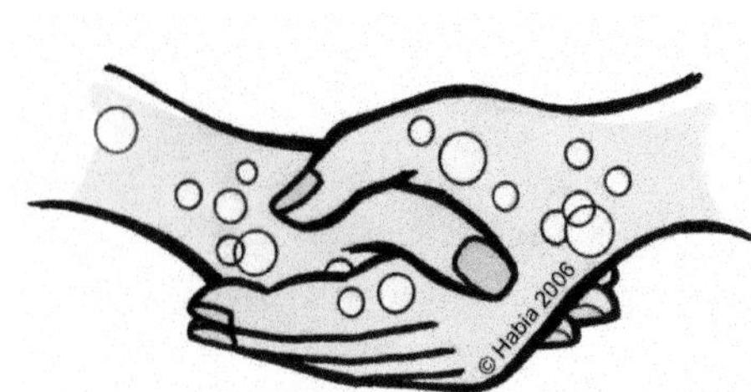

7 Lock thumbs and rotate hands

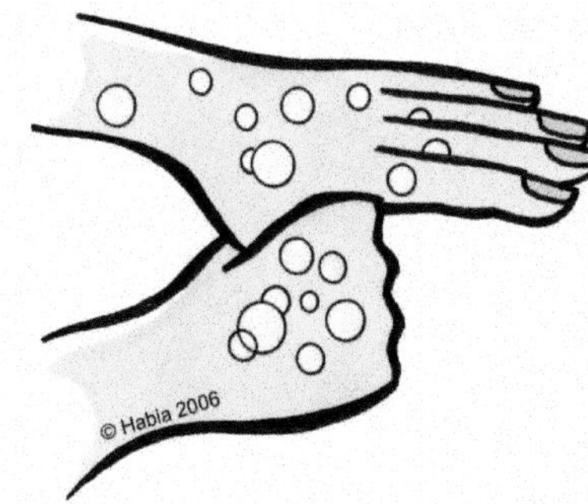

8 Grasp thumb with hand and rotate, repeat with opposite thumb

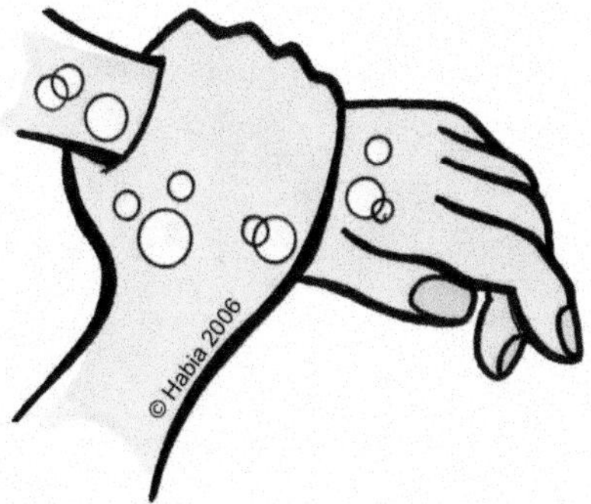

9 Rotate hand around wrist, repeat on opposite wrist

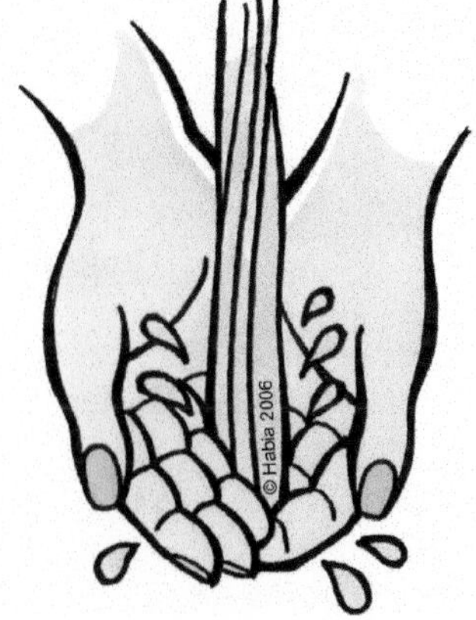

10 Rinse hands and wrists thoroughly using running water

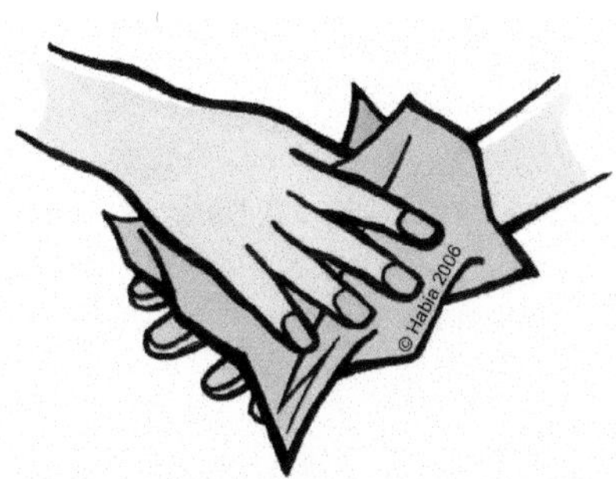

11 Dry the hands and wrists thoroughly

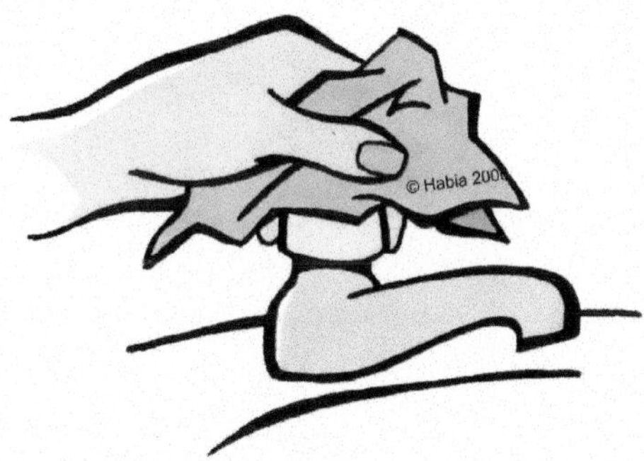

12 Turn off the tap using a paper towel

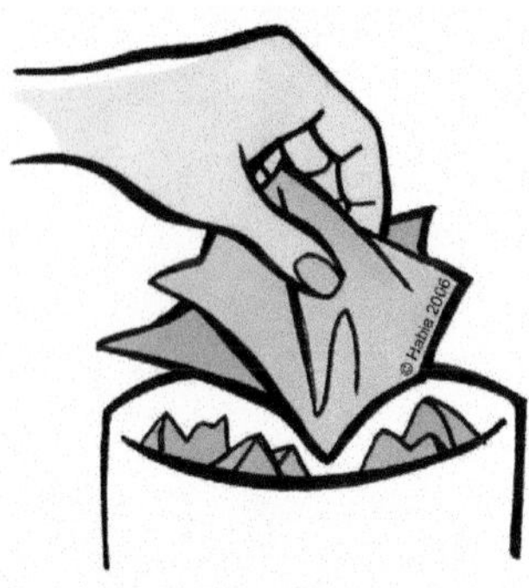

13 Dispose of paper towel without touching any part of the waste bin

ACTIVITY

Hand hygiene

What further occasions can you think of when it will be necessary to wash your hands when treating a client?

HEALTH & SAFETY

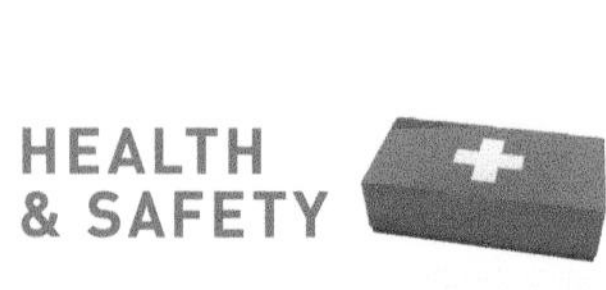

Soap and towels

Wash your hands with liquid soap from a sealed dispenser. This should take 10–20 seconds. Don't refill disposable soap dispensers when empty: if you do they will become a breeding ground for bacteria.

Disposable paper towels or warm-air hand dryers should be used to thoroughly dry the hands.

Protecting yourself

You will be wise to have the relevant inoculations, including those against tetanus and hepatitis, to protect yourself against ill-health and even death.

Protecting the client

If you have any cuts or abrasions on your hands, cover them with a clean dressing to minimize the risk of secondary infection. Disposable gloves may be worn for additional protection.

Certain skin disorders are contagious. Beauty therapists suffering from any such disorder must not work, but must seek medical advice immediately.

Protective face masks may be worn when working closely with the client.

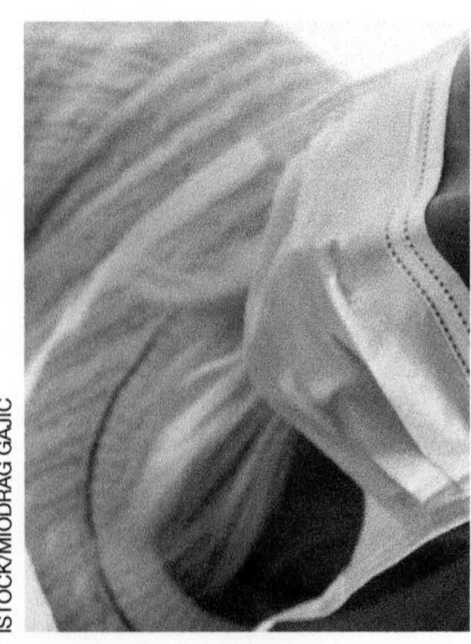

Face masks may be worn when working in close proximity to the client

Feet Keep your feet fresh and healthy by washing them daily and then drying them thoroughly, especially between the toes to avoid foot disorders developing such as athlete's foot. Deodorizing foot powder may then be applied.

Oral hygiene Avoid bad breath by brushing your teeth at least twice daily and flossing the teeth frequently. Use breath fresheners and mouthwashes as required to freshen your breath. Visit the dentist regularly, to maintain healthy teeth and gums. Avoid eating strong-flavoured foods, e.g. onions and garlic, which could cause offence, when in close contact with clients

Hair Your hair should be clean and tidy. Have your hair cut regularly to maintain its appearance, and shampoo and condition your hair as often as needed.

If your hair is long, wear it off the face and have it taken to the crown of the head. Medium-length hair should be clipped back, away from the face, to prevent it falling forwards.

TOP TIP

Fresh breath

When working, avoid eating strong-smelling highly spiced food. This includes the day before with strong smelling foods like garlic.

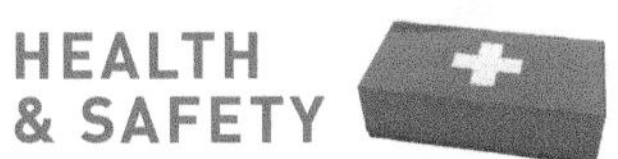

Long hair

If long hair is not taken away from the face, you will be tempted to move the hair away from the face repeatedly with the hands, and this in turn will require that the hands be washed repeatedly. Always secure hair away form the face to avoid contamination of the hands.

ACTIVITY

Avoiding cross-infection

1 List the different ways in which infection can be transferred in the salon.
2 How can you reduce the possibility of cross-infection occurring in the workplace?

Hygiene in the workplace

Infections Effective hygiene is necessary in the salon to prevent *cross-infection* and *secondary infection.* These can occur through poor practice, such as the use of tools and equipment that are not sterile. Infection of the skin can be recognized by redness and inflammation, or the presence of pus.

Cross-infection occurs because some microorganisms (germs i.e. bacteria, viruses and fungi) are contagious – they may be transferred through personal contact or by contact with an infected instrument that has not been disinfected or sterilized.

Secondary infection can occur as a result of injury to the client during the service or, if the client already has an open cut, if bacteria penetrate the skin and cause infection. **Sterilization** and disinfection procedures (below) are used to minimize or destroy the harmful microorganisms which could cause infection – **bacteria**, **viruses** and **fungi**.

Infectious diseases that are contagious contra-indicate beauty service: they require medical attention. People with certain other skin disorders, even though these are not contagious, should likewise not be treated by the beauty therapist, as the service might lead to secondary infection.

HEALTH & SAFETY

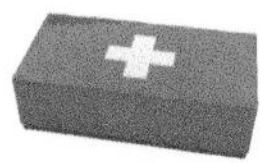

Sterilization record

Ultraviolet (UV) light is dangerous, especially to the eyes. The lamp must be switched off before opening the cabinet. A record must be kept of usage, as the effectiveness of the lamp decreases with use.

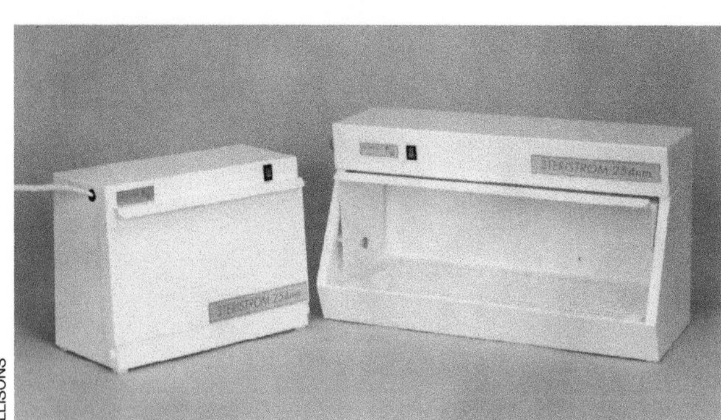

ELLISONS

An ultraviolet light cabinet

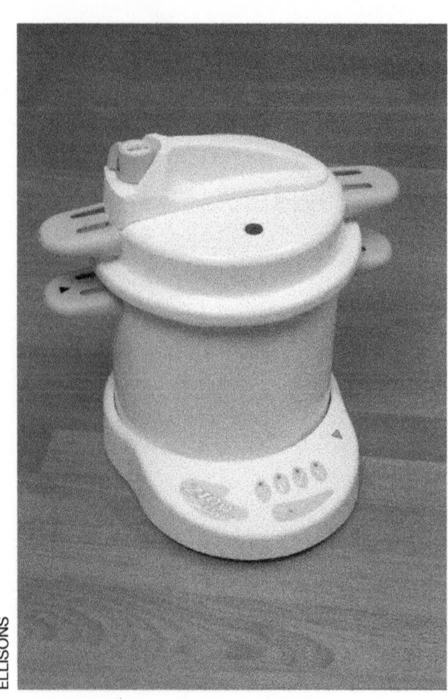

ELLISONS

An automatic medical autoclave

HEALTH & SAFETY

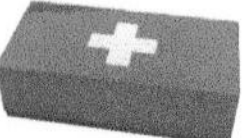

Aseptic conditions

This is the situation you should try to ensure occurs in the workplace by eliminating bacteria. All service procedures must be **aseptic**, e.g. wearing PPE, hand hygiene, correct methods of waste disposal, etc.

Sterilization and disinfection **Sterilization** is the total destruction of all living microorganisms in metal tools and equipment. **Disinfection** is the destruction of most living microorganisms in non-metal tools, equipment and work areas. Sterilization and disinfection techniques practised in the beauty salon involve the use of ***physical*** agents such as radiation and heat and ***chemical*** agents such as antiseptics and disinfectants.

Radiation – a quartz mercury-vapour lamp can be used as the source for ultraviolet (UV) light, which minimizes harmful microorganisms. However, UV light is less effective and cannot be relied upon for complete sterilization. Radiation only destroys microorganisms on the surface that the UV rays strike, requiring the object to be turned. For each surface of the object 20 minutes exposure is required. A UV cabinet is a good place to store previously sterilized objects.

The UV lamp must be contained within a closed cabinet. This cabinet is an ideal place for storing sterilized objects.

Heat – dry and moist heat can both be used in sterilization. One method is to use a dry **hot-air oven**. This is similar to a small oven, and heats to 150–180°C. It is rarely used in the salon.

More practical is a **glass-bead sterilizer**. This is a small, electrically heated unit that contains glass beads: electrically heated in an insulated unit to between 190–300°C. these beads transfer heat to objects placed in contact with them. This method of sterilization is suitable for small tools such as tweezers and scissors. All objects should be cleaned before being placed in the glass-bead sterilizer to remove surface dirt and debris.

Water is boiled in an **autoclave** (similar to a pressure cooker): is a popular moist heat method of sterilization because of the increased pressure, the water reaches a temperature of 121–134°C. Autoclaving is the most effective method for sterilizing objects in the salon.

Disinfectants and antiseptics If an object *cannot* be sterilized, it should be placed in a chemical **disinfectant** solution. A disinfectant destroys most microorganisms, but not all. Hypochlorite is a disinfectant – bleach is an example of a hypochlorite. Hypochlorite is suitable for cleaning work surfaces but is particularly corrosive and unsuitable for use with metals – use as directed by the manufacturer. Alcohol-impregnated wipes are a popular way to clean the skin using a disinfectant such as isopropyl alcohol.

An **antiseptic** prevents the multiplication of microorganisms. It has a limited action and does not kill all microorganisms.

All sterilization/disinfection techniques must be carried out safely and effectively following the manufacturer's instructions for correct use:

1. Select the appropriate method of sterilization or disinfectant for the object. ***Always*** follow the manufacturer's guidelines on the use of the sterilizing or disinfecting unit or agent.
2. Clean the object in clean water and detergent to remove dirt and grease. (Dirt left on the object might prevent effective sterilization or disinfection.)
3. Dry it thoroughly with a clean, disposable paper towel.
4. Sterilize or disinfect the object, allowing sufficient time for the process to be completed.
5. Following disinfection/sterilization handle the object with clean tongs or protective gloves. Place objects that have been sterilized or disinfected in a clean, covered container, ideally labelled. After 24 hours the object will be clean but not disinfected.

HEALTH & SAFETY

Using an autoclave

- The autoclave should only be used by those trained to do so.
- Not all objects can safely be placed in the autoclave. Before using this method, check whether the items you wish to sterilize can withstand this heating process.
- All objects should be cleaned, using an effective cleaning agent, e.g. surgical spirit, to remove surface dirt and debris before placing in the autoclave.
- To avoid damaging the autoclave, always use distilled de-ionized water that is purified to remove impurities.
- To avoid rusting, metal objects placed in the sterilizing unit must be of good-quality stainless steel.
- Never overload the autoclave. Follow manufacturer's instructions in its use.

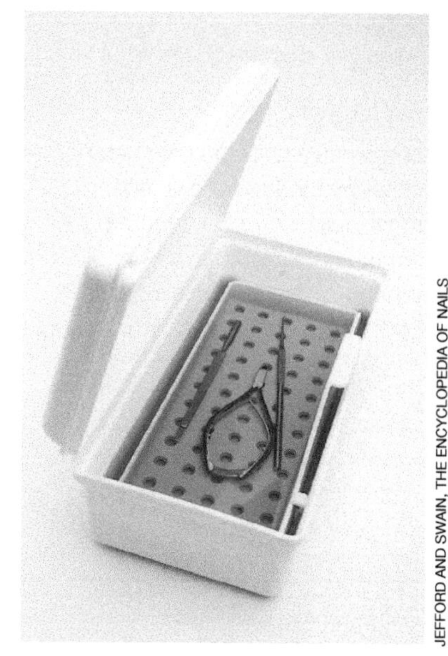

JEFFORD AND SWAIN, THE ENCYCLOPEDIA OF NAILS

A disinfection tray with liquid

Keep several sets of the tools you use regularly, so that you can carry out effective sterilization and disinfection.

HEALTH & SAFETY

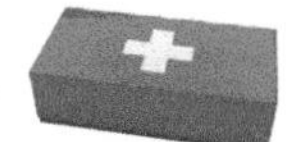

Using disinfectant

Disinfectant solutions should be changed as necessary to ensure their effectiveness. After removing the object from the disinfectant, rinse it in clean water to remove traces of the solution. (These might otherwise cause an allergic reaction on the client's skin.)

ALWAYS REMEMBER

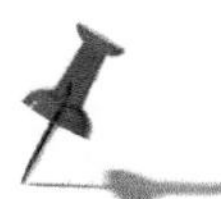

Before sterilization, surgical spirit applied with clean cotton wool may be used to clean the surface of small objects.

HEALTH & SAFETY

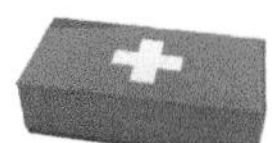

Damaged equipment

Any equipment in poor repair must be repaired or disposed of. Such equipment may be dangerous and may harbour germs.

Using chemical agents

Always wear protective gloves when using cleaning materials to prevent drying and irritation of the skin, which could lead to the skin disorder dermatitis.

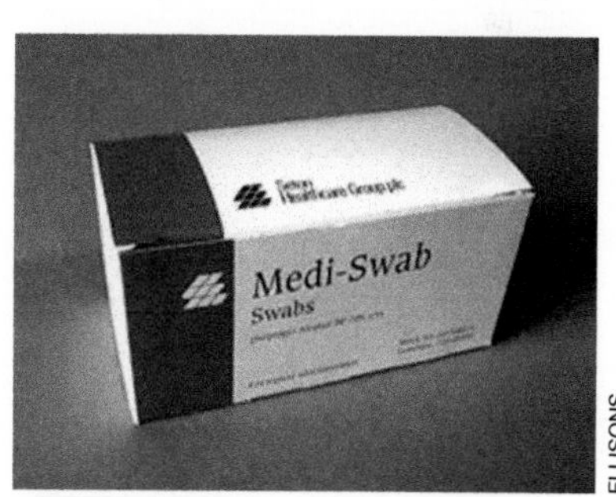

ELLISONS

Medi-swabs (sterile isopropyl tissues)

TOP TIP

HSE advice on cleaning

Advice on cleaning work surfaces and equipment can be found on the COSHH Essentials website: www .coshh-essentials.org.uk.

Workplace policies Each workplace should have its own workplace policy to identify hygiene rules.

- *Health and safety* Follow the health and safety policies for the workplace.
- *Personal hygiene* Maintain a high standard of personal hygiene. Wash your hands with a detergent containing **chlorhexidine gluconate** which protects against a wide range of bacteria. The addition of isopropyl alcohol provides a stronger hand disinfectant removing surface bacteria and fungi.

HEALTH & SAFETY

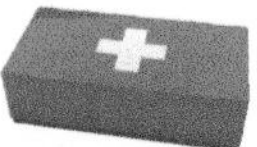

Cuts on the hands
Open, uncovered cuts provide an easy entry for harmful bacteria, and may lead to infection. Always cover cuts.

Misuse of Drugs Act (1971)
This Act places drugs into classes dependant upon their strength and effects on the body A is the most dangerous and C the least harmful. It also details the penalties for those caught possessing them. Therefore, you could be acting illegally.

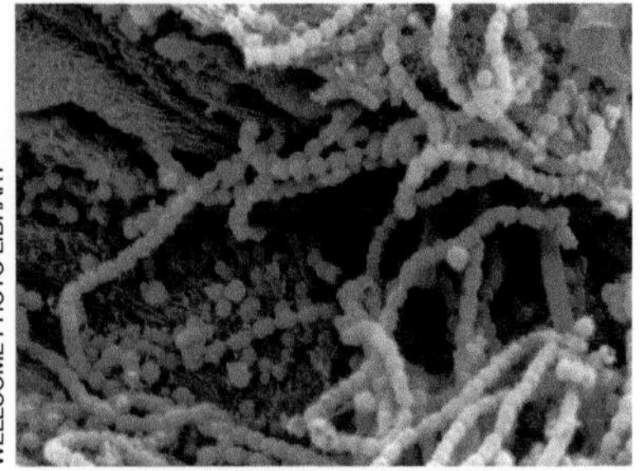

WELLCOME PHOTO LIBRARY

Example of a microscopic bacteria – streptococcus bacteria on the tongue

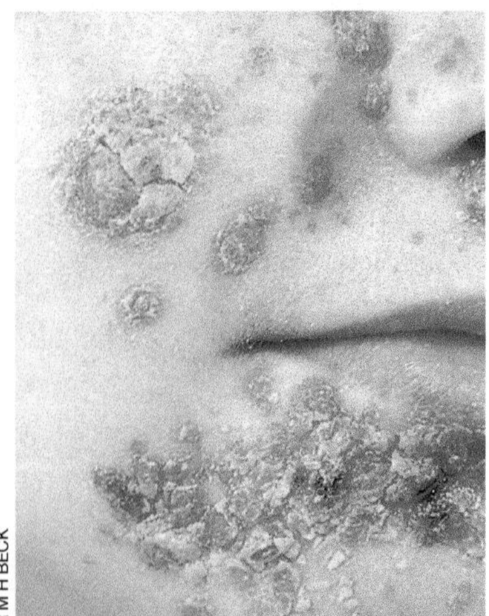

DR M H BECK

Impetigo

- *Cuts on the hands* Always cover any cuts on your hands with a protective dressing.
- *Cross-infection* Take great care to avoid cross-infection in the salon. *Never* treat a client who has a contagious skin disease or disorder, or any other **contra-indication**. Refer the client tactfully to their general practitioner (GP).
- *Use hygienic tools* Never use an implement unless it has been effectively sterilized or disinfected, as appropriate.
- *Disposable applicators* Wherever possible, use disposable applicators.
- *Working surfaces* Disinfect all working surfaces (such as trolleys and couches) with a chlorine preparation, diluted to the manufacturer's instructions. Cover all working surfaces with clean, disposable paper tissue.
- *Gowns and towels* Clean gowns and towels must be provided for each client. Towels should be laundered at a temperate of 60°C.
- *Laundry* Dirty laundry should be placed in a covered container.
- *Waste* including clinical waste and non-contaminated waste, must be disposed of following the COSHH procedures and guidelines provided by the local authority and training by the employer. For contaminated waste comply with the Controlled Waste Regulations (1992). Put waste in a suitable container lined with a disposable waste bag. A yellow **'sharps' container** or heavy duty yellow bag, should be available for clinical waste contaminated with blood or tissue fluid. Protective gloves should be worn to avoid risk of contamination.
- *Eating and drinking* Never eat or drink in the service area of the salon. Not only is it unprofessional, but harmful chemicals may also be ingested.
- *Drugs and alcohol* Never carry out services in the workplace under the influence of drugs or alcohol. Your competence will be affected putting yourself, clients and possibly colleagues at risk. Any accident as a result would be termed careless and you would be responsible.

Ensure that your behaviour at work meets your **workplace policies** and doesn't endanger yourself or others.

Skin diseases and disorders

The beauty therapist must be able to recognise the difference between healthy skin and one suffering from a skin disease or disorder. Certain skin disorders and diseases **contra-indicate** a beauty service: the service would put the beauty therapist and other clients to the risk of cross-infection. It is therefore essential that you are familiar with the skin diseases and disorders which you might come into contact with in the workplace. It is important to establish those that are a risk to you and those that are not, as well as the correct action to take. Related skin diseases and disorders are also discussed in Chapters 6, 7 and 8. If preparing a record card you may recognise a skin disease or disorder with potential to cause harm – a hazard. You will learn more about the characteristics of their appearance and how they are treated when you progress to level 2.

HEALTH & SAFETY

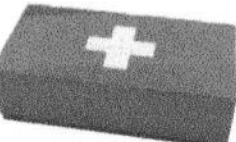

Skin problems
Before starting any service always check the client's suitability. The senior therapist will confirm with you if a service can go ahead, you are not qualified to make such decisions.

Bacterial infections

Bacteria are minute single-celled organisms of varied shapes. Large numbers of bacteria live on the surface of the skin and are harmless referred to as **non-pathogenic**; indeed some play an important positive role in the health of the skin. Others, however, are harmful referred to as **pathogenic** and can cause disease.

Impetigo An inflammatory disease of the surface of the skin, usually appearing on areas that can be seen.

Site: The commonly affected areas are the nose, the mouth and the ears, but impetigo can occur on the scalp or the limbs.
Diagnoses: Infectious

Conjunctivitis or pink eye Inflammation of an area of the eye called the mucous membrane that covers the eye and lines the eyelids.
Site: The eyes, either one or both, may be infected.
Diagnoses: Infectious

Hordeola or styes Infection of the sebaceous glands, oil glands, of eyelash hair follicles. It can be an effect of an eye condition blepharitis (inflammation of the eyelids).
Site: The inner rim of the eyelid.
Diagnoses: Infectious

Furuncles or boils Red, painful lumps, developing deeply into the skin.
Site: The back of the neck, the armpits and buttocks and thighs are common areas, but furuncles can occur anywhere.
Diagnoses: Infectious

Carbuncles Infection of numerous (more than one) hair follicles.
Site: In particular where there is friction, such as the back of the neck, or on the thighs. However, they can occur anywhere.
Diagnoses: Infectious

Paronychia Infection of the skin tissue surrounding the nail (the nail fold). If left untreated, the nail bed may become infected.
Site: The skin surrounding the nail plate.
Diagnoses: Infectious

Infectious Viral infections

Viruses are minute things, too small to see even under an ordinary microscope. They are considered to be **parasites**, as they require living tissue in order to survive. Viruses attack healthy body cells and multiply within the cell: eventually the cell walls break down, releasing the new virus to attack further cells, and so the infection spreads.

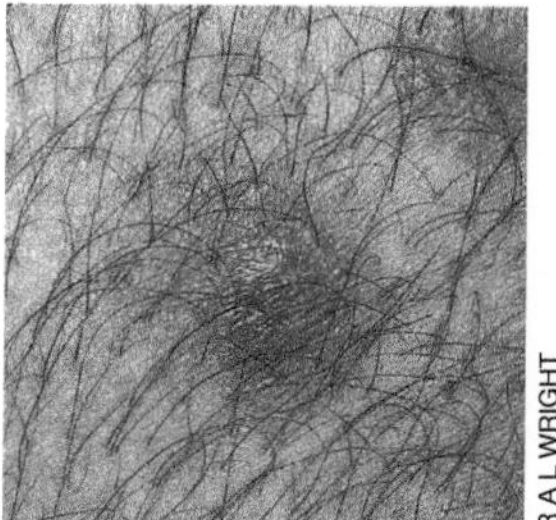

DR A L WRIGHT

Furuncle or boil

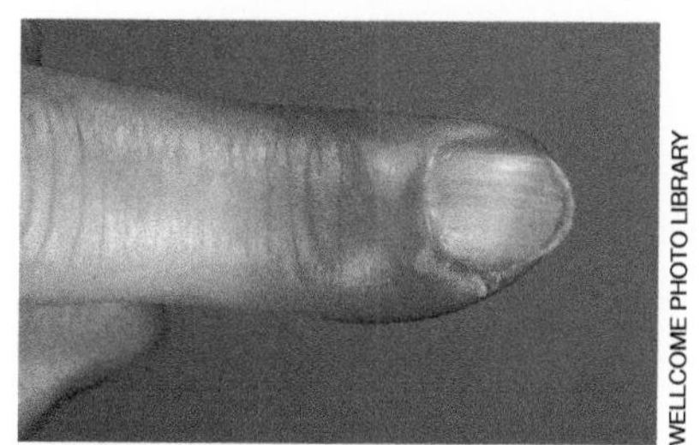

WELLCOME PHOTO LIBRARY

Paronychia

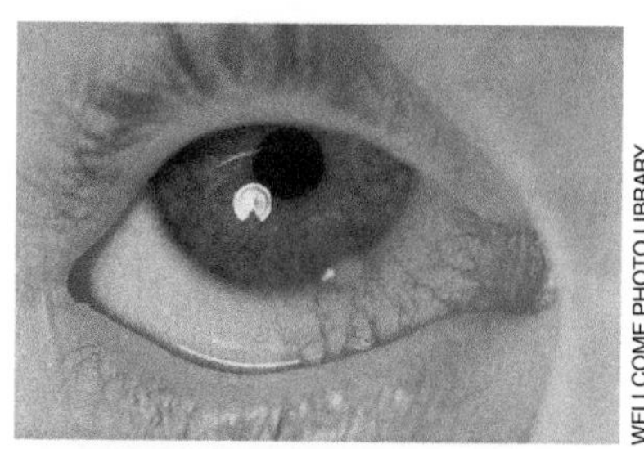

WELLCOME PHOTO LIBRARY

Conjunctivitis or pink eye

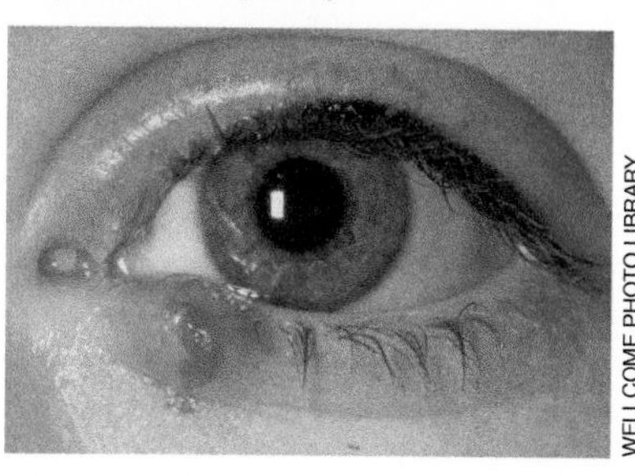

WELLCOME PHOTO LIBRARY

Hordeola or styes

HEALTH & SAFETY

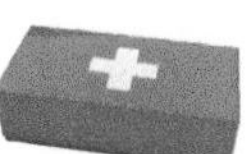

Boils

Boils occurring on the upper lip or in the nose should be referred immediately to a GP. Boils can be dangerous when located near to the eyes or brain.

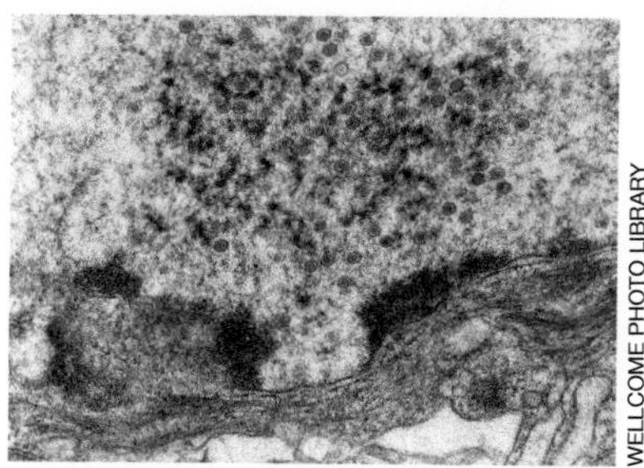

WELLCOME PHOTO LIBRARY

Example of a microscopic virus – herpes simplex virus (orange) in the centre of an epithelial cell-one which lines the surface of structures in the body

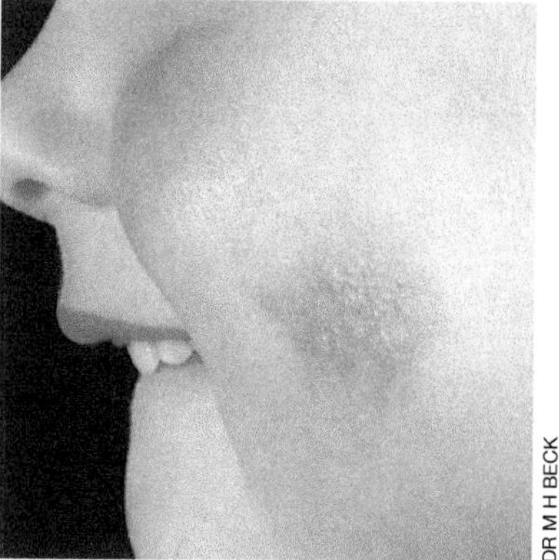

DR M H BECK

Herpes simplex

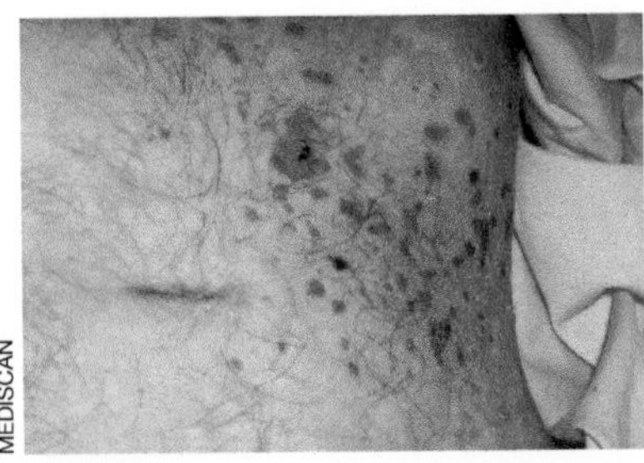
MEDISCAN
Shingles

Herpes simplex This is commonly referred to as a cold sore and is a skin condition that can return, appearing at times when the skin's resistance is lowered through ill-health or stress. It may also be caused by exposure of the skin to extremes of temperature or to UV light.
Site: The mucous membranes of the nose or lips; herpes can also occur on the skin generally.
Diagnoses: Infectious

Herpes zoster or shingles In this painful disease from the virus that causes chicken pox, the virus attacks nerve endings and is thought to lie inactive in the body and is triggered becoming active again when the body's defences are low.
Site: Commonly the chest and the abdomen.
Diagnoses: Infectious

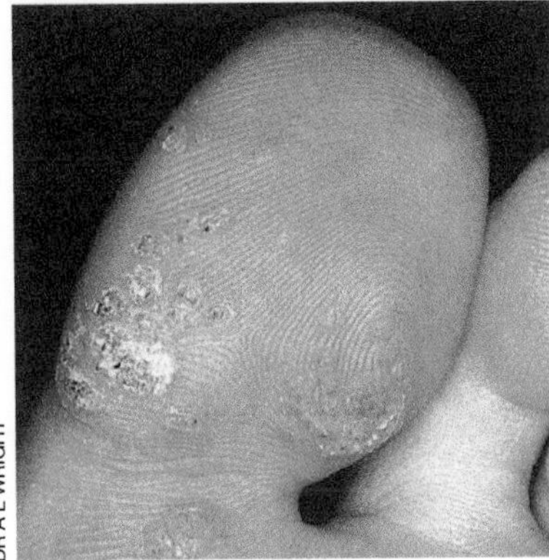
DR A L WRIGHT
plantar wart - verruca

Verrucae or warts Small epidermal skin growths. Warts can be raised or flat, depending upon their position. There are several types of wart: plane, common, plantar and mosaic.
Site:

- plane wart (flat wart): the fingers, either surface of the hand, face and legs
- common wart (verruca vulgaris): the hands, elbows and knees
- plantar wart (verruca): the sole of the foot and toes
- mosaic (palmar warts): hands and feet

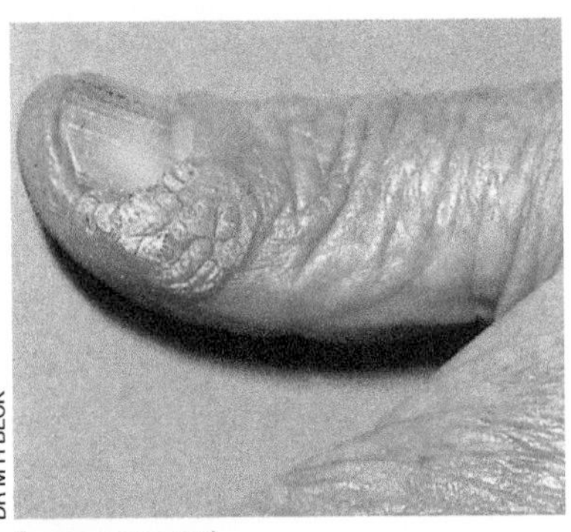
DR M H BECK
A common wart

Infectious Infestations

Scabies or itch mites (sarcoptes scabiei) A condition in which an **infestation** of a tiny mite parasite burrows beneath the skin and invades the hair follicles. The mite feeds on skin tissue and fluid as it burrows into the skin.
Site: Usually seen in warm areas of loose skin, such as the webs of the fingers, under the fingernails and the creases of the elbows.
Diagnoses: Infectious

Pediculosis capitis or head lice A condition in which small lice parasites crawl in scalp hair.
Site: The hair of the scalp.
Diagnoses: Infectious

Pediculosis pubis or pubic lice A condition in which small lice parasites crawl in body hair.
Site: Pubic hair, eyebrows and eyelashes.

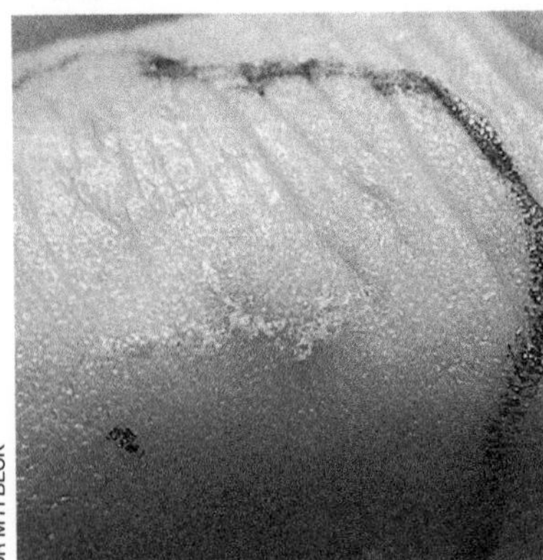
DR M H BECK
A scabies burrow

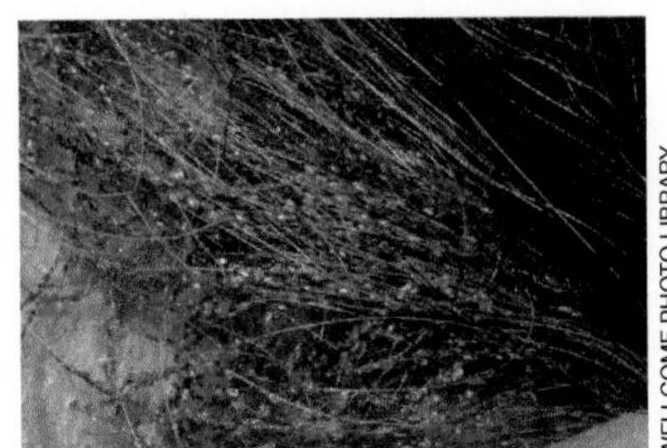
WELLCOME PHOTO LIBRARY
Example of a pediculosis capitis or head lice clinging to the hair

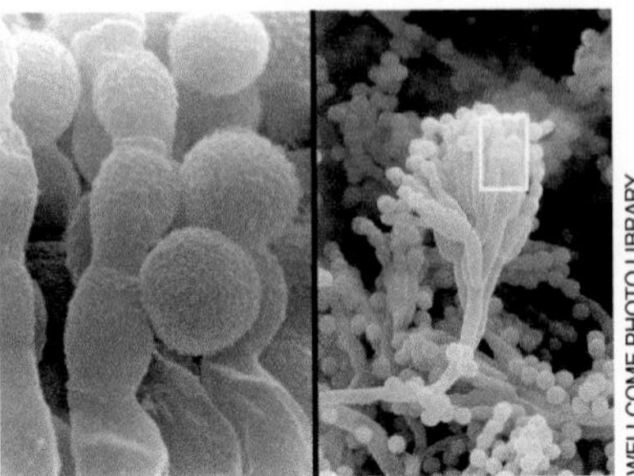
WELLCOME PHOTO LIBRARY
Example of a microscopic fungi – penicillium mould producing spores, plus very close-up view of spore formation

Pediculosis corporis or body lice A condition in which small parasites live and feed on body skin.

Site: Body hair.

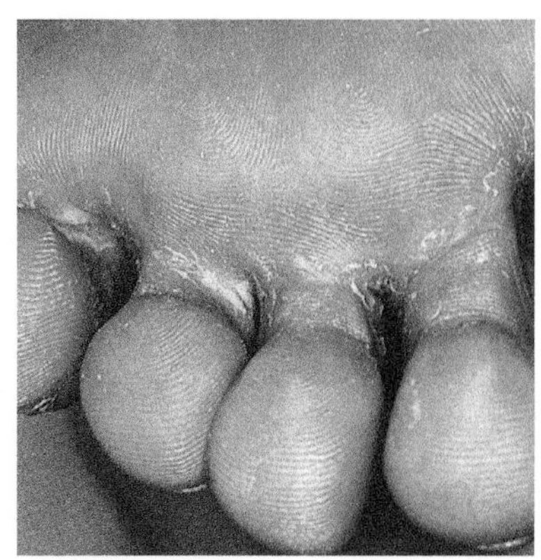

Tinea pedis or athlete's foot

Fungal diseases

Fungi are microscopic (minute) plants. They are parasites, dependent upon a host to live off. Fungal diseases of the skin feed off the waste products of the skin. Some fungi are found on the skin's surface; others attack the deeper tissues. Reproduction of fungi is by means of simple cell division or by the production of spores, reproductive structures. All listed fungal diseases are infectious

Tinea pedis or athlete's foot A common fungal foot infection.

Site: Commonly affects the webs of skin between the toes.

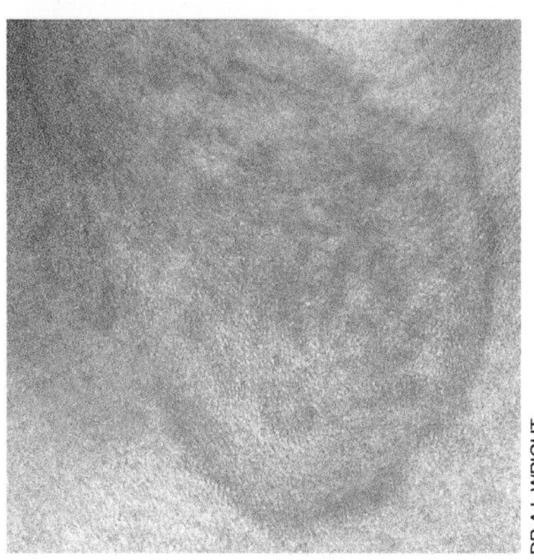

Tinea corporis or body ringworm

Tinea corporis or body ringworm A fungal infection of the skin.

Site: The trunk of the body, the limbs and the face.

Tinea unguium or onychomycosis Ringworm infection of the fingernails.

Site: The nail plate.

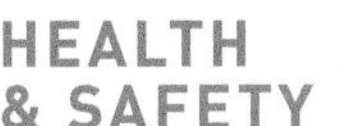
HEALTH & SAFETY
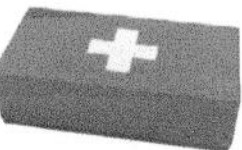

Artificial nails
Artificial nails can increase the risk of developing infection due to the natural nail plate being roughened and if not maintained correctly moisture can collect between the artificial nail and the natural nail plate which provides ideal growth for fungi.

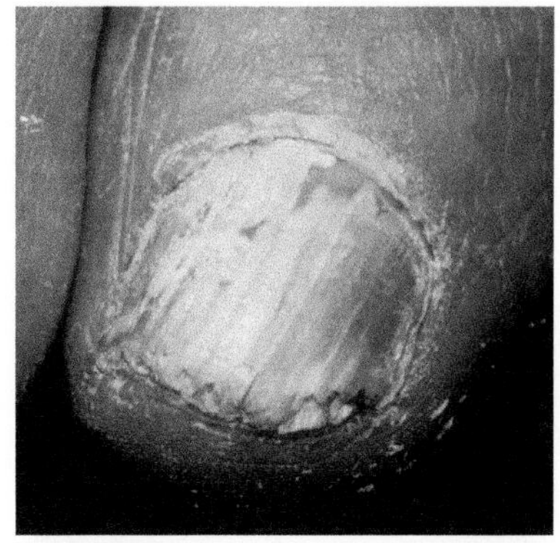

Tinea unguium

Sebaceous (oil) gland disorders

Milia Keratinization, hardening, of the skin over the hair follicle occurs, causing sebum to collect in the hair follicle. This condition is usually found on a dry skin type.

Site: The upper face or close to the eyes.

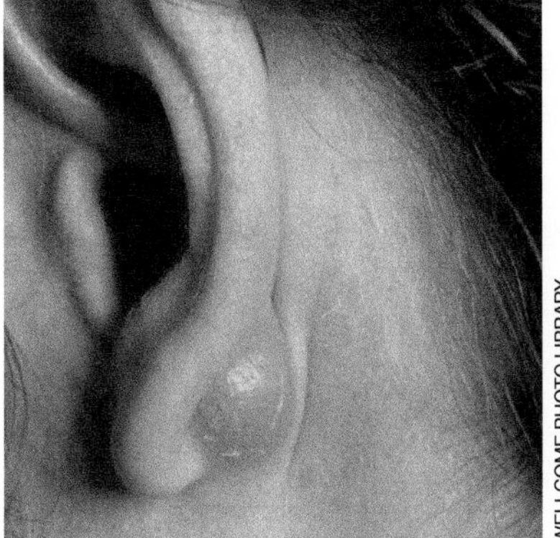

Non-infectious sebaceous cyst

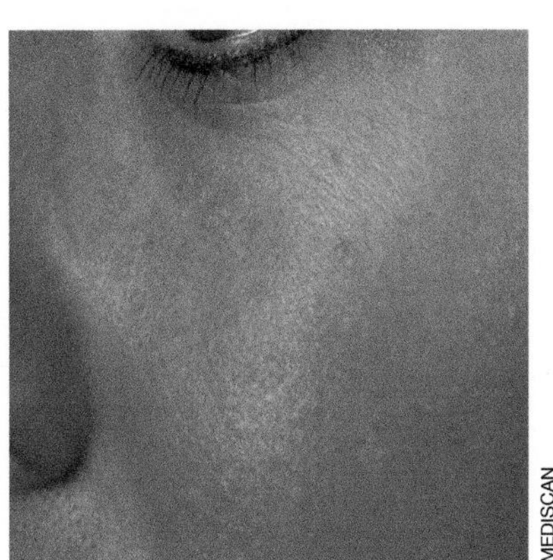

Seborrhoeic skin

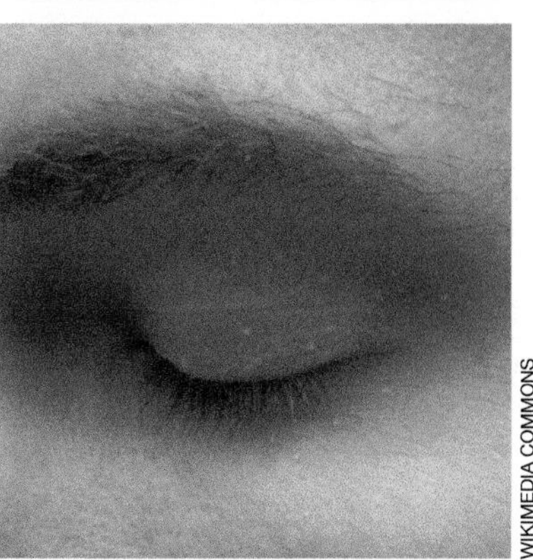

Milia on the eyelid

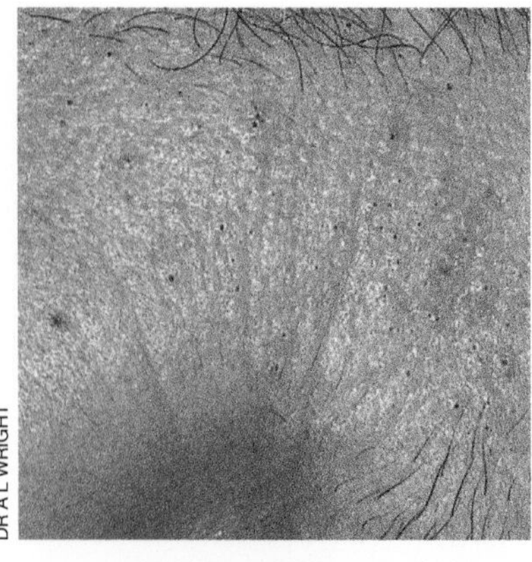
DR A L WRIGHT

Comedones or blackheads

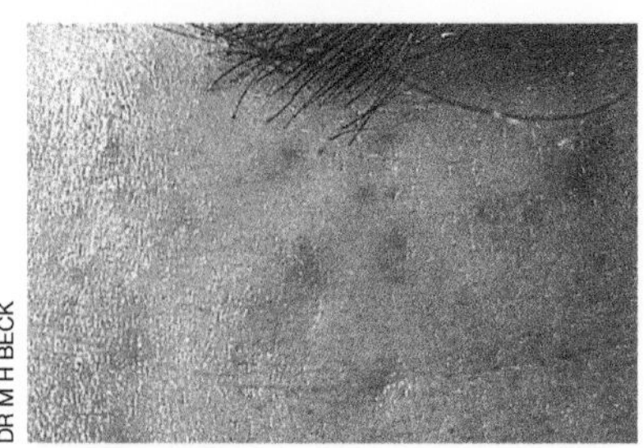
DR M H BECK

Acne vulgaris

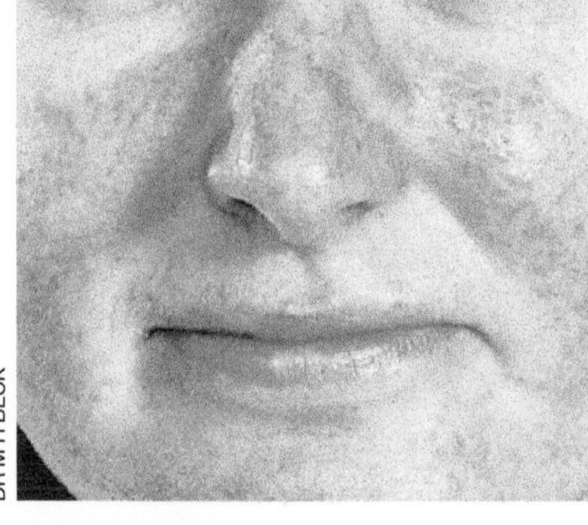
DR M H BECK

Rosacea

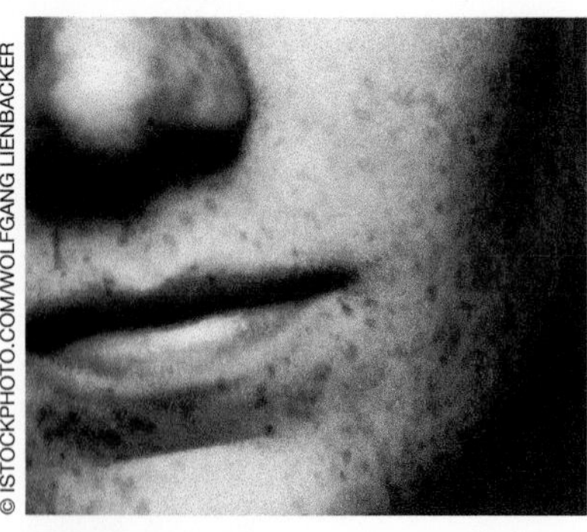
© ISTOCKPHOTO.COM/WOLFGANG LIENBACKER

Ephelides or freckles

TOP TIP

Hypo-pigmentation
Hypo-pigmentation may result from certain skin injuries, disorders or diseases.

Comedones or blackheads Too much sebum and keratinized cells block the opening of the hair follicle.
Site: The face (the chin, nose and forehead), the upper back and chest.
Diagnoses: Non-infectious

Seborrhoea Over secretion of sebum from the sebaceous gland. This usually occurs during puberty, as a result of hormonal changes in the body.
Site: The face and scalp. Seborrhoea may also affect the back and the chest.
Diagnoses: Non-infectious

Steatomas, sebaceous cysts or wens Localized sacs of sebum, which form in hair follicles or the sebaceous glands in the skin. The sebum becomes blocked, the sebaceous gland becomes enlarged and a lump forms.
Site: If the cyst appears on the upper eyelid, it is known as a **chalazion** or **meibomian cyst**.
Diagnoses: Non-infectious

Acne vulgaris Hormone imbalance in the body at puberty affects the activity of the sebaceous gland, causing an increased production of sebum. The sebum may be come blocked within the sebaceous gland openings onto the skins surface, causing congestion and bacterial infection of the surrounding tissues.
Site: Commonly on the face, the nose, the chin and the forehead. Acne may also occur on the chest and back.
Diagnoses: Non-infectious

Rosacea Too much sebum secretion combined with a constant inflammatory condition, caused by widening or dilation of the blood capillaries.

Non-infectious Pigmentation disorders

Pigmentation color of the skin varies, according to the person's genetic characteristics. In general, the darker the skin, the more pigment (melanin) is present, but some abnormal changes in skin pigmentation can occur.

- **Hyper-pigmentation** – increased pigment production
- **Hypo-pigmentation** – loss of pigmentation in the skin

Ephelides or freckles Multiple, small hyper-pigmented areas of the skin. Exposure to UV light (as in sunlight) stimulates the production of melanin, intensifying their appearance.
Site: Commonly the nose and cheeks of fair-skinned people. Freckles may also occur on the shoulders, arms, hands and back.
Diagnoses: Non-infectious

Lentigo (plural, lentigines) Hyper-pigmented areas of skin, slightly larger than freckles. Lentigo simplex occur in childhood. Actinic (solar) lentigines occur in middle age as a result of sun exposure.
Site: The face, hands and shoulders.

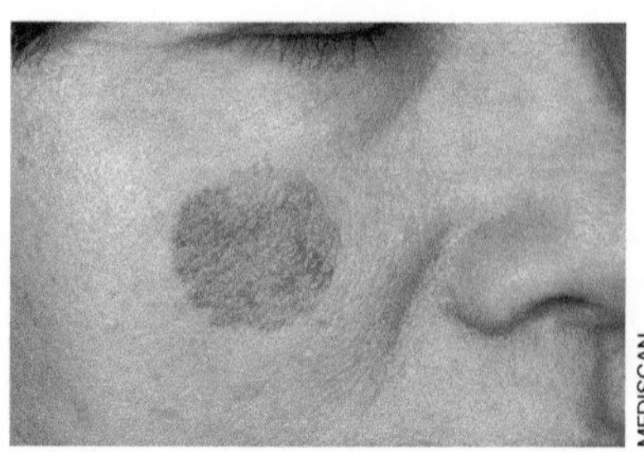
MEDISCAN

Lentigo

Chloasmata or liver spots Hyper-pigmentation in specific areas, stimulated by a skin irritant such as UV light, usually affecting women and darkly pigmented skins. The condition often occurs during pregnancy and usually disappears soon after the birth of the baby. It may also occur as a result of taking the oral contraceptive pill. The female hormone oestrogen is thought to stimulate melanin production.
Site: The back of the hands, the forearms, the upper part of the chest, the temples and the forehead.
Diagnoses: Non-infectious

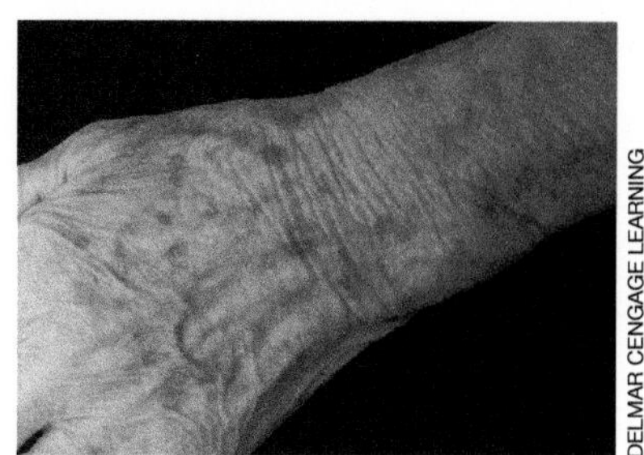

DELMAR CENGAGE LEARNING

Chloasmata or liver spots

Dermatosis papulosa nigra Often called flesh moles, these are recognised by multiple benign (non-cancerous), small brown to black hyper-pigmented papules, common among dark-skinned people.
Site: Usually seen on the cheeks and forehead, although they may appear on the neck, upper chest and back.
Diagnoses: Non-infectious

Vitiligo or leucoderma Patches of completely white skin which have lost their pigment, or which were never pigmented.
Site: The face, the neck, the hands, the lower abdomen and the thighs. If vitiligo occurs over the eyebrows, the hairs in the area will also lose their pigment.
Diagnoses: Non-infectious

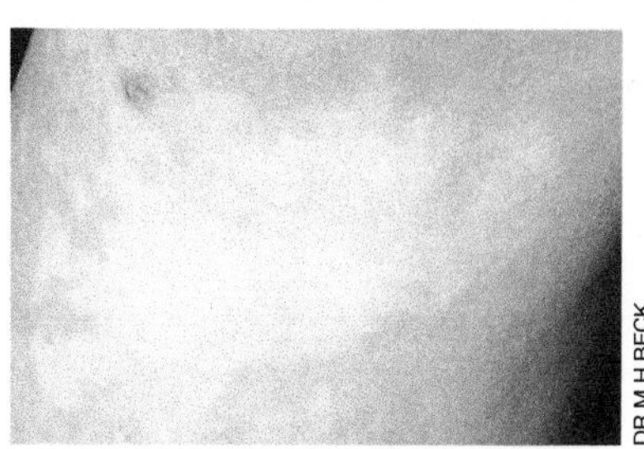

DR M H BECK

Vitiligo or leucoderma

Albinism The skin is unable to produce the melanin pigment and the skin, hair and eyes lack colour.
Site: The entire skin.
Diagnoses: Non-infectious

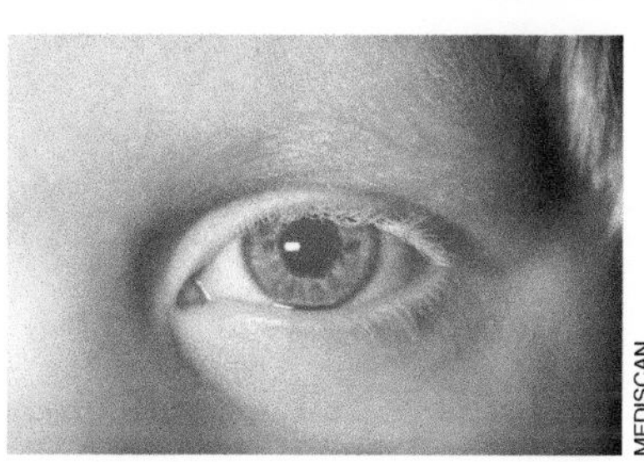

MEDISCAN

Albinism

Vascular naevi There are two types of naevus of concern to beauty therapists: vascular and cellular. **Vascular naevi** are skin conditions in which small or large areas of skin pigmentation are caused by the permanent dilation of blood capillaries.

Erythema An area of skin in which blood capillaries have dilated, due either to injury or inflammation.
Site: Erythema may affect one area (locally) or all of the skin (generally).

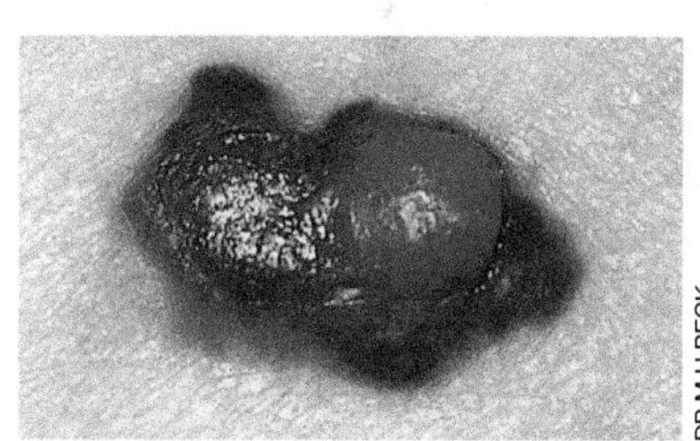

DR M H BECK

Malignant melanoma

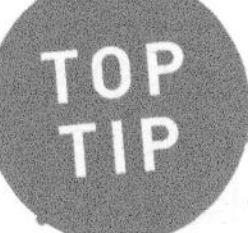

Vascular disorders

If there is a vascular skin disorder, avoid over-stimulating the skin or the problem will become more noticeable and the service may even cause further damage.

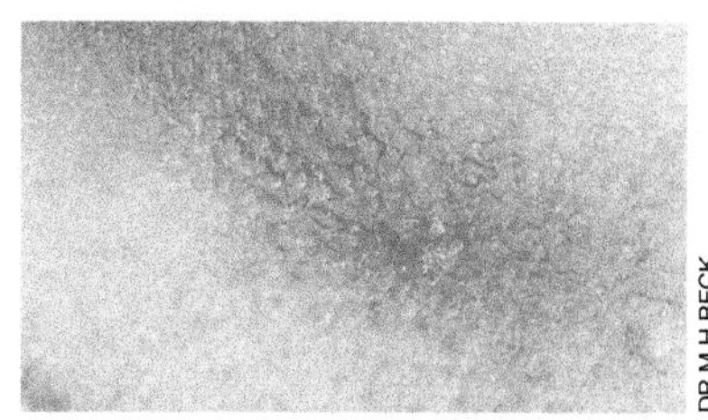

DR M H BECK

Spider naevi or stellate haemangiomas

HEALTH & SAFETY

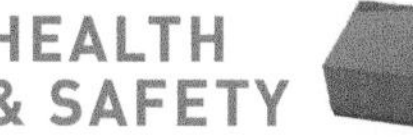

Moles

If moles change in shape or size, if they bleed or form crusts, seek medical attention.

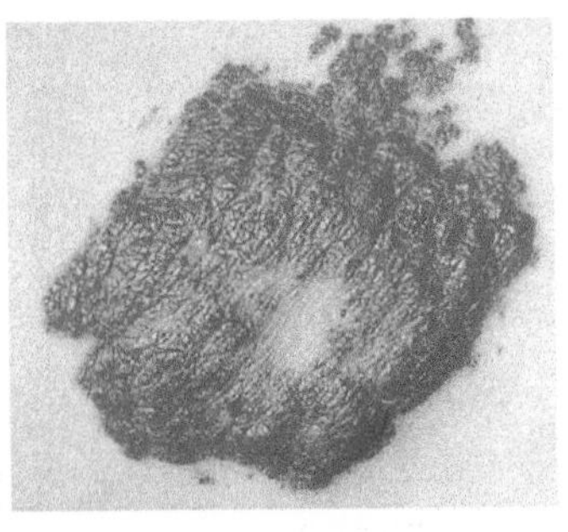
DR M H BECK

Naevi vasculosis or strawberry marks

Dilated capillaries Capillaries near the surface of the skin that are permanently dilated.
Site: Areas where the skin is neglected, dry or fine, such as the cheek area.
Diagnoses: Non-infectious

Spider naevi or stellate haemangiomas Dilated blood vessels, with smaller dilated capillaries radiating from them.
Site: Commonly the cheek area, but may occur on the upper body, the arms and the neck. Spider naevi are usually caused by an injury to the skin.
Diagnoses: Non-infectious

Naevi vasculosis or strawberry marks Red or purplish raised marks which appear on the skin at birth.
Site: Any area of the skin.
Diagnoses: Non-infectious

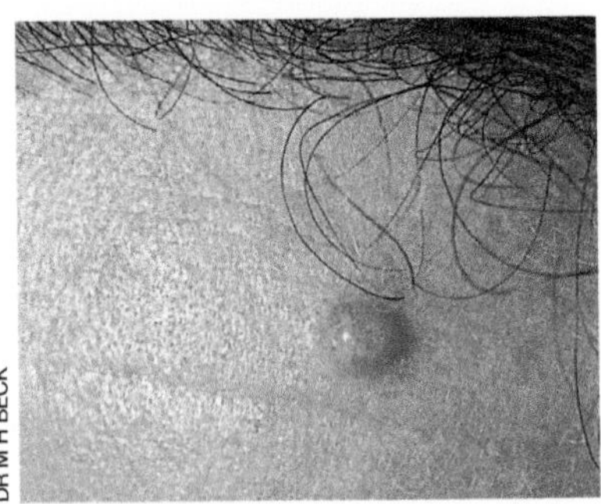
DR M H BECK

Benign naevus

Capillary naevi or port-wine stains Large areas of dilated capillaries that contrast noticeably with the surrounding areas.
Site: Some 75 per cent occur on the head; they are probably formed at the foetal stage. Naevi may also be found on the neck and face.
Diagnoses: Non-infectious

Cellular naevi or moles **Cellular naevi** are skin conditions in which changes in the cells of the skin result in skin irregularities.

Malignant melanomas or malignant moles Rapidly growing skin cancers, usually occurring in adults.
Site: Usually the lower abdomen, legs or feet.
Diagnoses: Non-infectious

TOP TIP

Naevi numbers and skin colour
Caucasian skin normally has up to four times as many naevi than black skin.

HEALTH & SAFETY

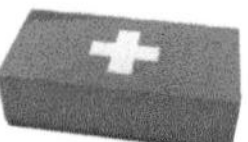

Malignant melanoma risk
The risk of melanoma increases as the number of naevi increases. Therefore clients with lots of naevi or moles are at highest risk.

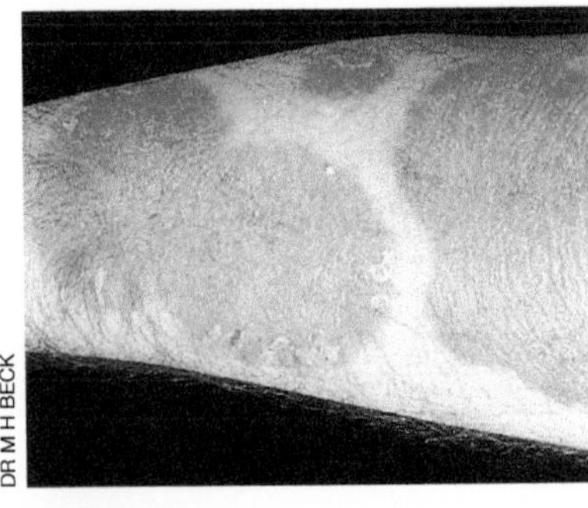
DR M H BECK

Psoriasis

Junction naevi Localized collections of naevoid cells that arise from the mass production locally of pigment-forming cells (melanocytes).
Site: Any area.

Dermal naevi Localized collections of naevoid cells.
Site: Usually the face.
Diagnoses: Non-infectious

Hairy naevi Moles exhibiting coarse hairs from their surface.
Site: Anywhere on the skin.
Diagnoses: Non-infectious

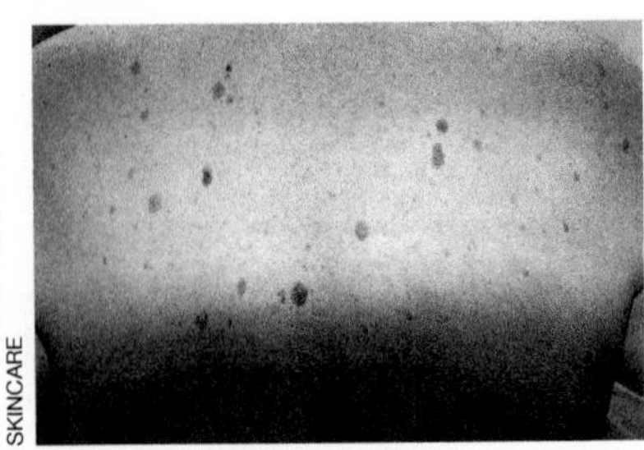
DR JOHN GRAY, THE WORLD OF SKINCARE

Seborrhoeic or senile warts

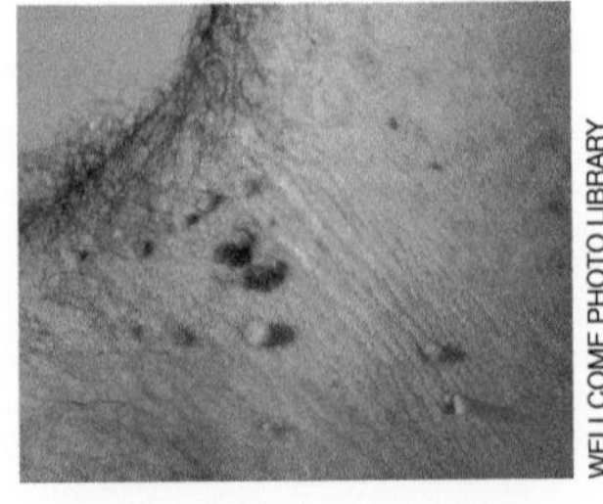
WELLCOME PHOTO LIBRARY

Verrucae filliformis or skin tags

Skin disorders involving abnormal growth

Psoriasis Patches of itchy, red, flaky skin, the cause of which is unknown.
Site: The elbows, the knees, the lower back and the scalp.
Diagnoses: Non-infectious

Seborrhoeic or senile warts: Raised, pigmented, benign tumours occurring in middle age.
Site: The trunk, the scalp and the temples.

Verrucae filliformis or skin tags These verrucae appear as threads growing from the skin surface.
Site: Mainly seen on the neck and the eyelids, but may occur in other areas such as under the arms.
Diagnoses: Non-infectious

Xanthomas Small yellow growths appearing upon the surface of the skin made up of cholesterol (a fatty substance carried in the blood) deposits.
Site: Common on the eyelids, but can appear anywhere on the body.
Diagnoses: Non-infectious

Keloids Keloids occur following skin injury and are overgrown abnormal scar tissue which spreads, recognised by excess deposits of collagen (a fibre found in the dermis part of the skin that helps gives it its strength). To avoid skin discoloration the keloid must be protected from UV exposure.
Site: Located over the site of a previous wound or other lesion skin injury or disorder.

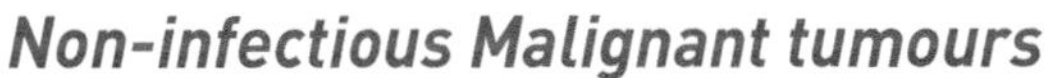

Non-infectious Malignant tumours

Squamous cell carcinomas or prickle-cell cancers Malignant growths originating in the epidermis.
Site: Anywhere on the skin.
Diagnoses: Non-infectious

Basal cell carcinomas or rodent ulcers Slow-growing malignant tumours, occurring in middle age.
Site: Usually on the face.

Non-infectious Skin allergies

The skin can protect itself to some degree from damage or invasion. Specialized cells called **mast cells** detect damage to the skin; if damage occurs, the mast cells burst, releasing the chemical **histamine** into the tissues. Histamine causes the blood capillaries to

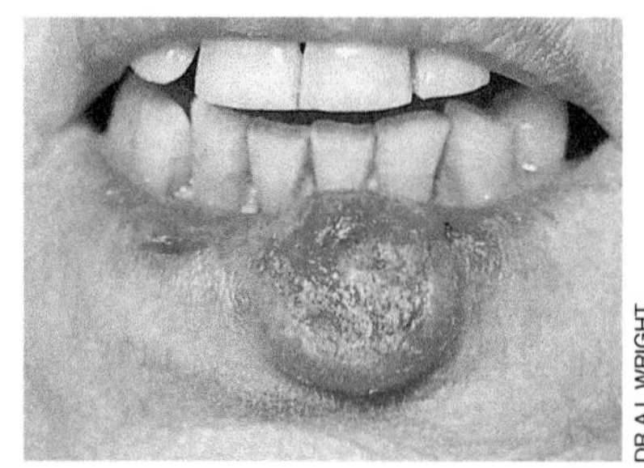

Squamous cell carcinoma

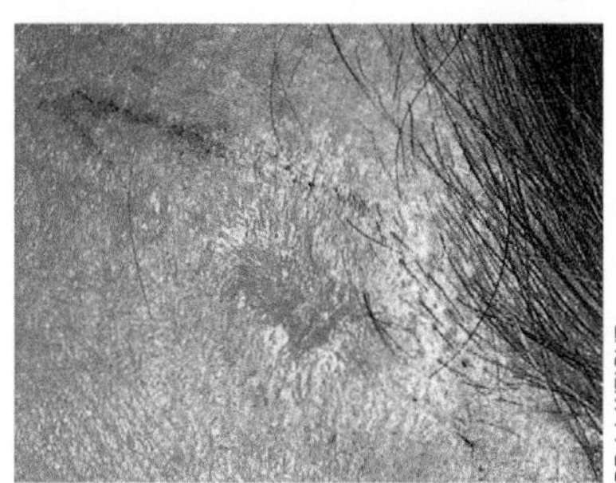

Basal cell carcinomas

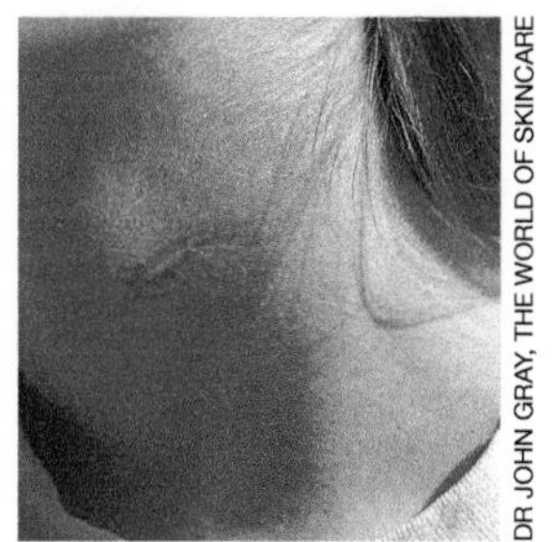

Keloids

HEALTH & SAFETY

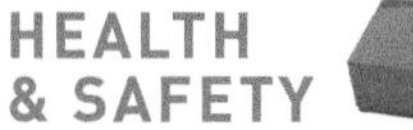

Record any known allergies
When completing the client record card, always ask whether your client has any known allergies.

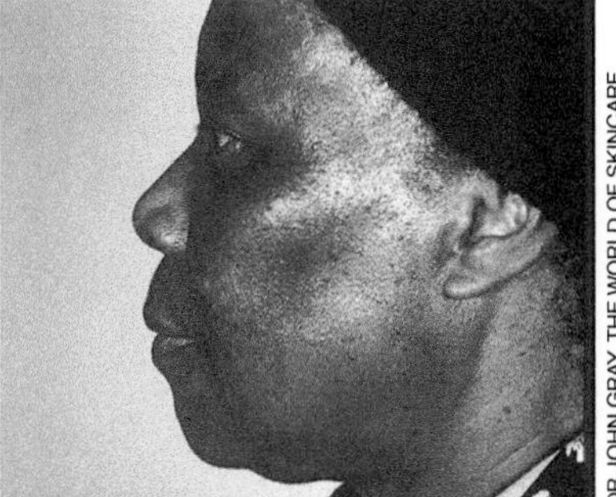

Allergic reaction to an ingredient in hair dye

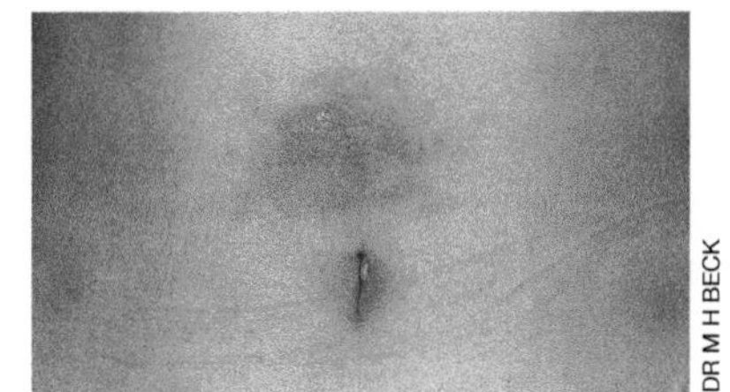

Allergic reaction to a nickel button

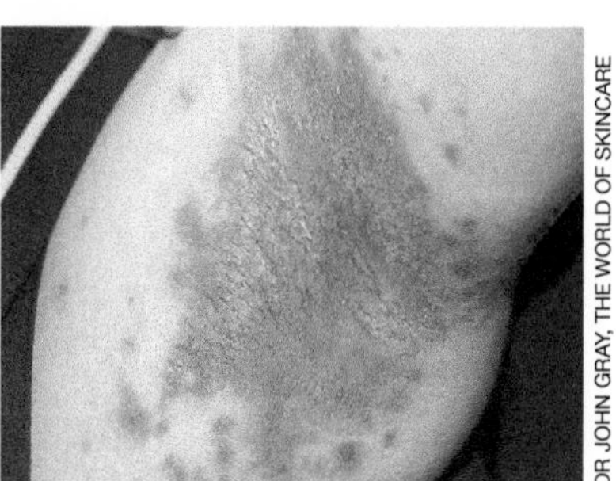

Allergic reaction to an antiperspirant

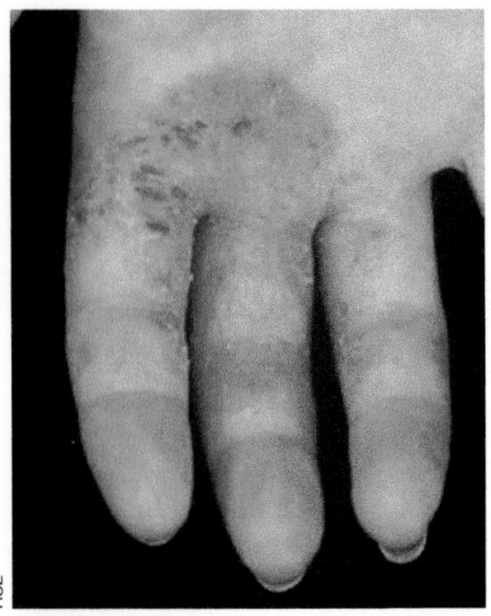
HSE
Contact dermatitis

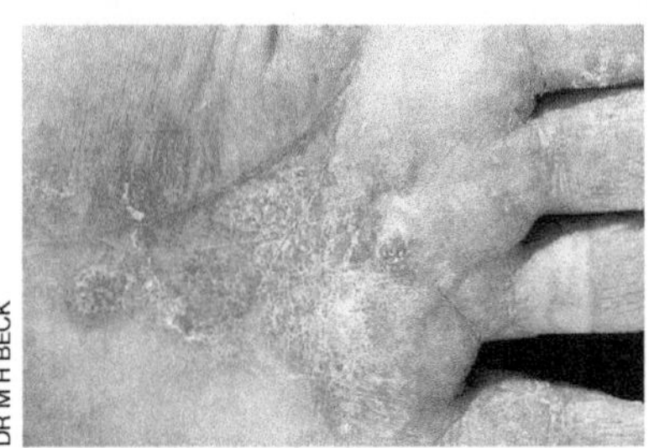
DR M H BECK
Eczema

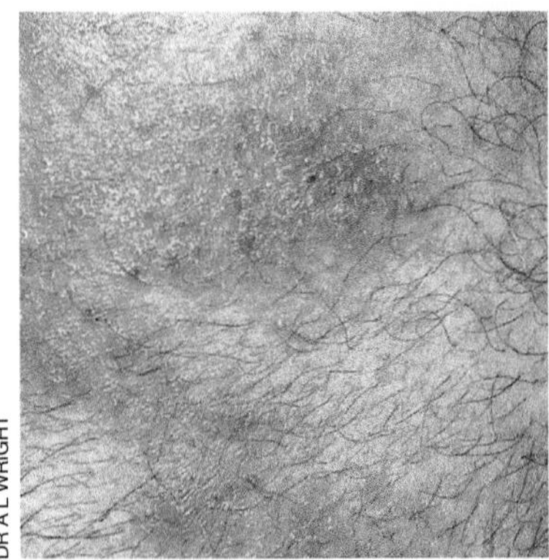
DR A L WRIGHT
Urticaria (nettle rash) or hives

DR M H BECK
Urticaria (nettle rash) or hives

widen, giving the reddening we call 'erythema'. The increased blood flow carries materials in blood which tend to limit the damage and begin repair.

If the skin is sensitive to and becomes inflamed on contact with a particular substance, this substance is called an **allergen**. Allergens may be animal, chemical or vegetable substances, and they can be inhaled, eaten or absorbed following contact with the skin. An **allergic skin reaction** appears as irritation, itching and discomfort, with reddening and swelling (as with nettle rash). If the allergen is removed, the allergic reaction subsides.

Each individual has different tolerances to the various substances we encounter in daily life. What causes an allergic reaction in one individual may be perfectly harmless to another.

Here are just a few examples of allergens known to cause allergic skin reactions in some people:

- metal objects containing nickel
- sticking plaster
- rubber
- lipstick containing eosin dye
- nail polish containing formaldehyde resin
- hair and eyelash dyes
- lanolin, the skin moisturising agent
- detergents that dry the skin
- foods – well-known examples are peanuts, cow's milk, lobster, shellfish and strawberries
- plants such as tulips and chrysanthemums.

Dermatitis An inflammatory skin disorder in which the skin becomes red, itchy and swollen. There are two types of dermatitis. In *primary dermatitis* the skin is irritated by the action of a substance on the skin, and this leads to skin inflammation. In *allergic contact dermatitis*, the problem is caused by intolerance of the skin to a particular substance or groups of substances. On exposure to the substance the skin quickly becomes irritated and an allergic reaction occurs.
Site: If the skin reacts to a skin irritant outside the body, the reaction is localized. Repeated contact with the allergen will lead to a general hypersensitivity. If the irritant gains entry to the body it will be transported in the bloodstream and may cause a general allergic skin reaction.
Diagnoses: Non-infectious

Eczema Inflammation of the skin caused by contact, internally or externally, with an irritant.
Site: The face, the neck and the skin, particularly at the inner creases of the elbows and behind the knees.
Diagnoses: Non-infectious

Urticaria (nettle rash) or hives A minor skin disorder caused by contact with an allergen, either internally (food or drugs) or externally (insect bites).
Site: At the point of contact.
Diagnoses: Non-infectious

ALWAYS REMEMBER

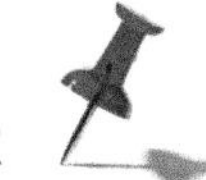

To avoid potential hazards and risks in the workplace you should:

- be aware of the workplace health and safety policy and your role in its implementation
- ensure your personal presentation and conduct at work meets health and safety and legislative requirements in line with your workplace policies
- follow the most recent workplace policies for your job role and manufacturers' instructions for the safe use of resources
- follow the latest health and safety legislation related to your work
- know who is responsible for health and safety in your workplace. Pass on any suggestions immediately for reducing health and safety risks within your job role
- report or deal immediately with any risk which could be a hazard within your responsibility, meeting workplace policies and legal requirements
- be aware of first-aid arrangements in the event of an accident or illness occuring
- know the workplace fire evacuation advice and procedure
- ensure your working practice minimizes the possible spread of infection or disease.

HEALTH & SAFETY

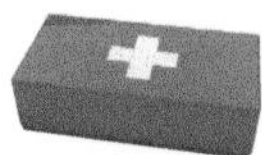

Hypoallergenic products
The use of hypoallergenic products minimizes the risk of skin contact with likely irritants.

Allergies
You may suddenly become allergic to a substance that has previously been perfectly harmless. Equally, you may over time cease to be allergic to something.

Infection following allergy
Following an allergic skin reaction in which the skin's surface has become itchy and broken, scratching may cause the skin to become infected with bacteria.

GLOSSARY OF KEY WORDS

Accident book a written record of any accident in the workplace. Incidents in the accident book should be reviewed to see where improvements to safe working practice could be made.

Accident form a detailed report form to be completed following any accident in the workplace.

Antiseptic a chemical agent that prevents the multiplication of microorganisms. It has limited action and does not kill all microorganisms.

Aseptic the methods used to eliminate bacteria when performing a service procedure from British standards. Glossary of terms relating to disinfectants.

Autoclave an effective method of sterilization, suitable for small-metal objects and beauty therapy tools. Water is boiled under increased pressure and reaches temperatures of 121–134°C.

Bacteria minute, single-celled organisms of various shapes. Large numbers live on the skin's surface and are not harmful (they are non-pathogenic); others, however, are harmful (pathogenic) and can cause disease.

Contra-indication a problematic symptom that indicates the service may not proceed.

Control risk the means by which risks identified are removed or reduced to acceptable levels.

Control of Substances Hazardous to Health (COSHH) Regulations (2002) these regulations require employers to identify hazardous substances used in the workplace and state how they should be correctly stored and handled.

Controlled Waste (Amendment) Regulations (1993) categorizes waste types. The Local Authority provides advice on how to dispose of waste types in compliance with the law.

Cosmetic Products (Safety) Regulations (2008) part of consumer protection legislation that requires that cosmetics and toiletries are safe in their formulation and are safe for use for their intended purpose as a cosmetic and comply with labelling requirements.

Cross-infection the transfer of contagious microorganisms.

Disinfectant a chemical agent that destroys most microorganisms.

Electricity at Work Regulations (1989) these regulations state that electrical equipment in the workplace should be tested every 12 months, by a qualified electrician. The employer must keep records of the equipment tested and the date it was checked.

Employers' Liability (Compulsory Insurance) Act (1969) this provides financial compensation to an employee should they be injured as a result of an accident in the workplace. A certificate indicating that a policy of insurance has been purchased should be displayed.

Environmental conditions this includes heating, lighting, ventilation and general comfort requirements for the workplace or service.

Fire Precautions Act (1971) legislation that states that all staff must be familiar with, and trained in fire, and emergency evacuation procedures for their workplace.

Fungi microscopic plants. Fungal diseases of the skin feed off the waste products of the skin. They are found on the skin's surface or they can attack deeper tissues.

Hazard a hazard is something with potential to cause harm.

Health and Safety at Work Act (1974) legislation that lays down the minimum standards of health safety and welfare requirements in all workplaces.

Health and Safety (Display Screen Equipment) Regulations (1992) these regulations cover the use of visual display units (VDUs) and computer screens. They specify acceptable levels of radiation that is given off from the screen and identify correct posture, seating position, permitted working heights and rest periods.

Health and Safety (First Aid) Regulations (1981) legislation that states that workplaces must have appropriate and adequate first-aid provision.

Health and safety policy each employer of more than five employees must have a written health and safety policy issued to their employees outlining their health and safety responsibilities.

Hygiene requirements the expected standards as required by law, industry codes of practice or written procedures specified by the workplace.

Infestation a condition where animal parasites live off and invade a host.

Legislation laws affecting the beauty therapy business relating to products and services, the business premises and environmental conditions, working practices and those employed.

Local Government (Miscellaneous Provisions) Act (1982) legislation that requires that salons offering any form of skin piercing be registered with the local health authority. This registration includes both the operators who will be carrying out the service and the salon premises where the service will be carried out.

Management of Health and Safety at Work Regulations (1999) this legislation provides the employer with an approved code of practice for maintaining a safe, secure working environment.

Manual Handling Operations Regulations (1992) legislation that requires the employer to carry out a risk assessment of all activities undertaken which involve manual handling (lifting and moving objects).

Personal Protective Equipment (PPE) at Work Regulations (2002) this legislation requires employers to identify through risk assessment those activities that require special protective equipment to be worn.

Posture the position of the body, which varies from person to person. Good posture is when the body is in alignment. Correct posture enables you to work longer without becoming tired; it prevents muscle fatigue (tiredness) and stiff joints.

Provision and Use of Work Equipment Regulations (PUWER) (1998) this regulation lays down important health and safety controls on the provision and use of equipment.

Public Liability Insurance protects employers and employees against the consequences of death or injury to a third party while on the premises.

Reporting of Injuries, Diseases and Dangerous Occurrences Regulations (RIDDOR) (1995) these regulations require the employer to notify the local enforcement officer in writing, in cases where employees or trainees suffer personal injury at work.

Regulatory Reform (Fire Safety) Order (2005) this legislation requires that the employer or designated 'responsible person' must carry out a risk assessment for the premises in relation to fire evacuation practice and procedures.

Responsible persons this term is used in the health and safety unit to mean the person or persons at work to whom you should report any issues, problems or hazards. This could be a supervisor, line manager or your employer.

Risk the likelihood of a hazard's potential being recognized.

Secondary infection bacterial penetration into the skin causing infection.

Sterilization the total destruction of all microorganisms in metal tools and equipment.

Viruses the smallest living bodies, too small to see under an ordinary microscope. Viruses invade healthy body cells and multiply within the cell. Eventually the cell walls break down and the virus particles are freed to attack further cells.

Workplace (Health Safety and Welfare) Regulations (1992) these regulations provide the employer with an approved code of practice for maintaining a safe, secure working environment.

Workplace policies this covers the documentation prepared by your employer on the procedures to be followed in your workplace. Examples are your employer's safety policy statement, or general health and safety statements and written safety procedures covering aspects of the workplace that should be drawn to the employees' (and 'other persons' ') attention, pricing policies and customer service policies.

Workplace practices any activities, procedures, use of materials or equipment and working techniques used in carrying out your job. Lifting techniques and maintaining good posture while working are also included.

ASSESSMENT OF KNOWLEDGE AND UNDERSTANDING

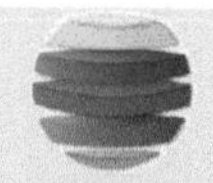

FUNCTIONAL SKILLS

Having covered the learning objectives for **make sure your own actions reduce risks to Health and Safety**, test what you need to know and understand by answering the following short questions below.

The information covers:

- actions to avoid health and safety risks
- dealing with significant risks in your workplace
- taking the right action in the event of a danger.

Actions to avoid health and safety risks

1 What are your main legal responsibilities under the Health and Safety at Work Act (1974)?

2 Name **four** different pieces of legislation relating to health and safety in the workplace.

3 What is the purpose of a salon health and safety policy? What sort of information does it include?

4 Give **five** examples of good personal presentation in maintaining health and safety in the salon.

5 Name a piece of equipment in the workplace used for sterilization and disinfection.

6 Why must you always be aware and look for hazards in the workplace?

7 What do you understand by good posture, and why is it important for you to consider when working?

8 What do you understand by the following terms:
- sterilization?
- disinfection?
- cross-infection?
- secondary infection?

9 It is a heavy box but you will be able to lift it. How should a large box be lifted from the floor level to be placed on the work surface?

Dealing with significant risks in your workplace

1 What hazards may exist in the beauty therapy workplace?

2 Why must you always be aware of possible hazards?

3 In your role in the salon, describe four potential hazards and what precautions you would take to prevent them becoming a risk?

4 While preparing thermal mitts for a specialized nail service you notice that the wires in the lead are exposed. What action should you take?

5 If you were unable to deal with a risk because it was outside of your responsibility, what action would you take?

6 What does the abbreviation COSHH stand for? Why is it important to follow suppliers' and manufacturers' instructions for the safe use of materials and products?

7 When cleaning the area after a wax depilation service, what personal protective equipment (PPE) should you wear and how should this waste be disposed of?

Taking the right action in the event of a danger

1 What is the procedure for dealing with an accident in the workplace?

2 What is a fire drill? What is the fire evacuation procedure in your salon? How often should this be carried out?

3 In the event of a real fire, after having safely evacuated the building, how would you contact the appropriate emergency service?

4 What action should be taken in the event of a suspected gas leak?

5 What actions can be taken to follow environmentally friendly working practices?

6 The air conditioning system in the salon has broken. Who should you inform to deal with this? What is the possible risk of inadequate ventilation?

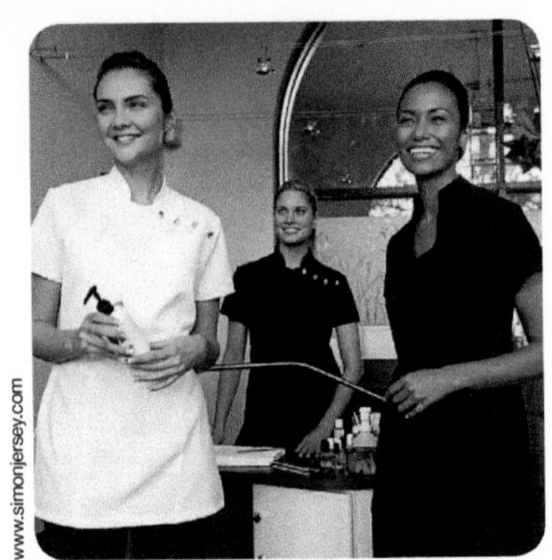
www.simonjersey.com

3 Developing positive working relationships

Learning Objectives

This chapter covers the **Contribute to the development of effective working relationships** unit. The way you carry out your duties and the way you conduct yourself and support other staff, called colleagues, can make a big difference to the success of the business. It is essential for any beauty therapy business to be a success that staff work together to provide the best possible service to all its clients – this requires good teamwork. As a Level 1 beauty therapist you can learn from every situation, observe how they are handled by senior staff and this will help you to gain experience and develop within your job role.

There are **three** learning outcomes which you must achieve competently:

1 **Develop effective working relationships with clients**
2 **Develop effective working relationships with colleagues**
3 **Develop yourself within the job role**

Your assessor will observe your performance on **at least three occasions, two** of which will cover your contact and communication with clients, called interaction and **one** of which will cover your interaction with colleagues.

From the **range** statement, you must show that you have:

- Taken part (participated) in all types of learning opportunities shown below.
  - active participation in training and development activities
  - active participation in salon activities
  - watching technical activities (practical application of beauty therapy skills).

(continued on the next page)

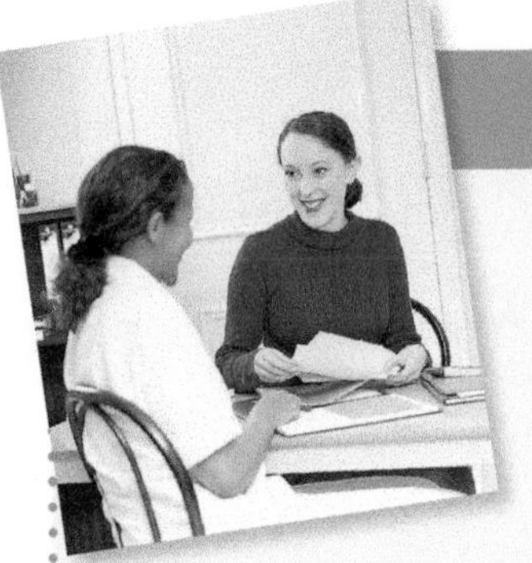

ROLE MODEL

Joanne Mackinnon

Key Skills Programme Manager at The London College of Beauty Therapy

"After completing a combined hairdressing and beauty therapy course in Gloucestershire, I worked for several years in salons in South West London while completing teacher training and teaching evening classes in manicure.

I joined The London College of Beauty Therapy as a trainee lecturer in 1999; since then I've been a lecturer, assessor and internal verifier for beauty therapy courses and programme manager for Key Skills and Additional Learning Support. I have also had the opportunity to train new lecturers and assessors, many of whom join us directly from the beauty industry.

(continued)

- To develop yourself within your work role you need to collect evidence to prove that you have participated in staff development activities over a period of time.

When contributing to the development of effective working relationships it is important to use the skills you have learnt in the following units:

Health and Safety

Prepare and maintain the salon service work area

Good **working practices** and working relationships in the **workplace** are essential, with both clients and colleagues. These are developed through having good 'people skills' which help you to work with and support others at all times. These are workplace skills that you can develop which will enable you to be successful in your beauty therapy career.

Developing effective working relationships with clients

Clients want to enjoy their visit to the workplace and remember they are paying for their service. Their service includes the whole experience from when they walk through the door to when they leave. Some clients may be lost even before an appointment is made. Related to poor communication skills or systems and procedures when enquiring about a service, which may be by telephone, face to face or on-line booking systems. All clients should feel satisfied that their needs have been met and hopefully exceeded, because remember, they have choices where they receive the service and may choose to go elsewhere in the future if dissatisfied.

A client will form an initial impression of the workplace and its employees though their communication skills and by their appearances and you must always remember first impressions count. A client will gain confidence in you by your professional image. It demonstrates to the client immediately that you are clean and hygienic and that if you have respect and high standards for yourself you will probably have high standards and respect when dealing with others.

There are expected standards with regard to your appearance which were discussed in chapter 2, Health and Safety and there are also expected standards for behavior. Always do your best to meet your salon's standards and **salon requirements** for appearance and behaviour. These expectations will be discussed when you start your training at the induction.

Outcome 1: Develop effective working relationships with clients

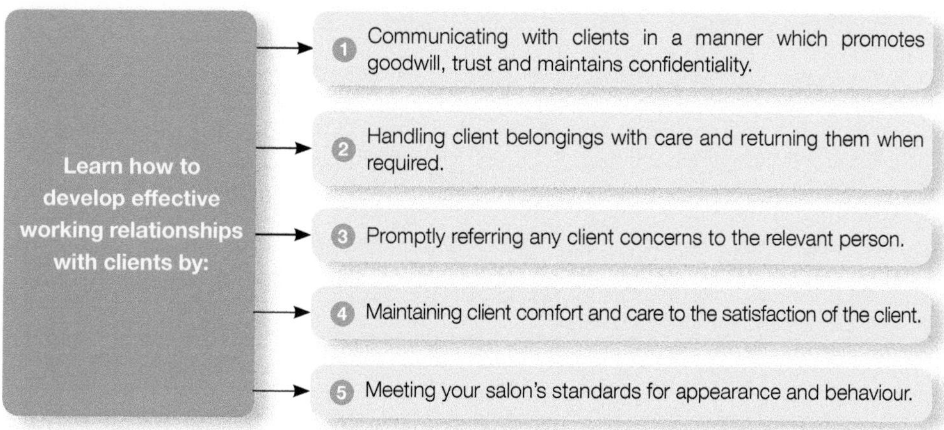

Standards for workplace appearance

- At all times have a smart, professional, **personal appearance** and follow the expected dress code for your workplace. This creates the impression of the quality of service that can be expected.
- Always have high standards of personal hygiene.
- Never eat, drink (water may be permitted) or chew gum in front of a client.
- Care for your skin using the correct skincare products and wear an attractive, light day make-up. A healthy skin is a good advertisement for the salon.

BEST PRACTICE

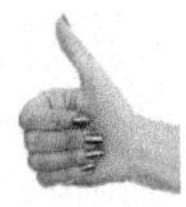

Personal appearance

Habia explains personal appearance requires the following:

- **Hair** should be taken away from the face so that it does not interfere with the service.

  If you had to touch your hair to move it out of the way this could lead to cross-infection and would not be hygienic and off-putting to the client.
- **Nails** must be clean, a suitable length and free of nail polish.

  Nails if not clean would cause cross-infection and again would be off-putting to the client. Long nails could scratch the client and collect germs under the nail. Nail polish can cause an allergic reaction in some clients and if chipped would look poor.
- **Jewellery** should be minimal

  Jewellery is restricted to a wedding band and small, stud earrings. Large jewellery could affect service application becoming a health and safety hazard, e.g. long neck chains.
- **Shoes** should be clean; low heeled and fit the foot.

  Ill-fitting shoes will cause discomfort leading to foot disorders over a period of time. The shoes should protect the feet from hazardous work substances that may be spilt on the feet, the sole should be non-slip. Low-heeled shoes prevent postural aches and pains to the back, foot and leg.
- **Workwear uniforms** should be freshly laundered.

  You will work closely next to clients so a clean overall should be worn every day to remove any stale odours and to present a clean, smart image. Remember to protect your overall with an apron when performing messy jobs.

ACTIVITY

Personal presentation

1. What is your workplace dress code?
2. How can you ensure that you always have a high standard of hygiene at the start of the day and throughout the day?
3. What type of foods could you have during the day to provide you with energy and to maintain fresh breath? What foods and drinks should you avoid?
4. What make-up products would you wear for every day in the salon? What make-up looks may be unsuitable and why?

BEST PRACTICE

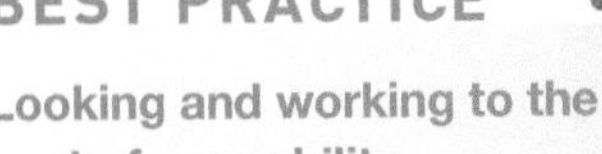

Looking and working to the best of your ability

Set the alarm clock to ensure you have enough time to arrive to work looking smart and fresh. If you do not get enough sleep this can leave you feeling tired and irritable, this is not an excuse for poor appearance and attitude.

Plan ahead, do you need to wash your overall ready for the next day or prepare a healthy lunch? Allow enough time to carry out any necessary tasks the night before.

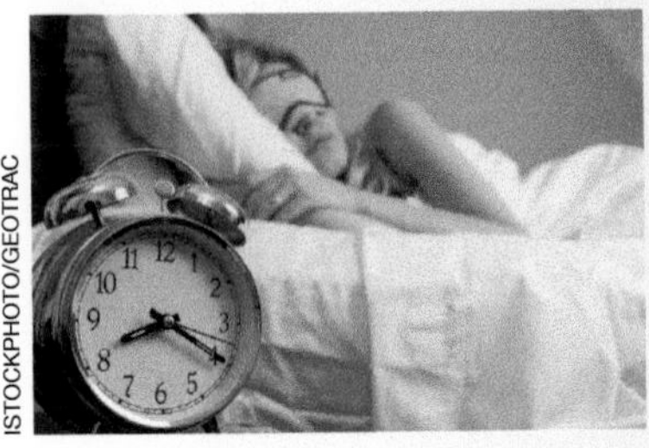

ISTOCKPHOTO/GEOTRAC

ALWAYS REMEMBER

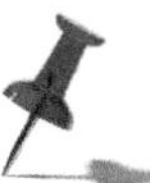

Fashion v professional image

Beauty therapy is a fashion-related industry where there will be new season make-up colours and application techniques for example. However, workwear including your overall and footwear should conform to the standards of dress code which is smart and business-like – not necessarily fashionable!

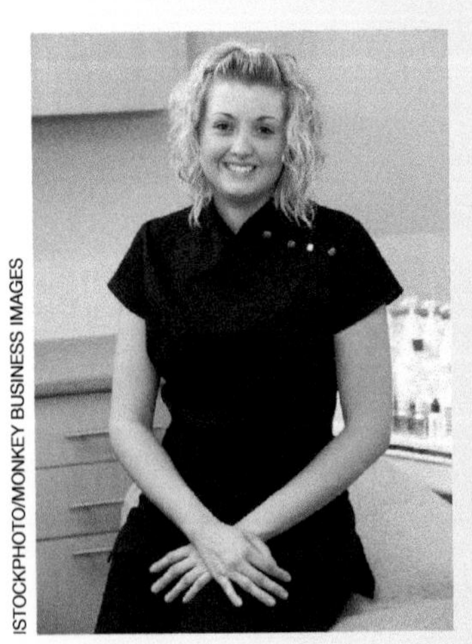

ISTOCKPHOTO/MONKEY BUSINESS IMAGES

> **Good presentation makes a great first impression**
> Both you and your working area should be of a high standard at all times. Neatness, hygiene and good organization will gain client confidence allowing them to relax and enjoy their service.
>
> **Joanne Mackinnon**

ACTIVITY

Collect suitable images for the workplace of:

- different overalls
- footwear
- hairstyles
- hair coverings (if worn)

You look the part but remember your behaviour is just as important to the client for them to make a judgement.

Standards for workplace behaviour

- Meet your salon standards for conduct and behaviour.
- Meet your **workplace policies** and **organizational requirements** for time-keeping and attendance.
- Be polite and courteous at all times to both clients and colleagues.
- Never lose your temper, discuss others or swear in front of a client.
- Engage in appropriate conversation with clients and also with your colleagues in front of clients.
- Avoid controversial topics and avoid passing on your opinion on things.
- Communicate clearly – avoid being too loud.
- Be friendly and helpful.
- If you have personal issues with a colleague or client remember this is the workplace and any **grievance** (complaint) should be settled as quickly as possible to ensure a happy, friendly workplace atmosphere.

BEST PRACTICE

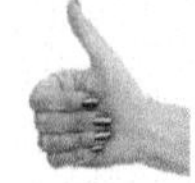

Service standards
Many organizations have a service standard that states the standards of service a client can expect. The team should be committed to delivering this standard at all times – consistently.

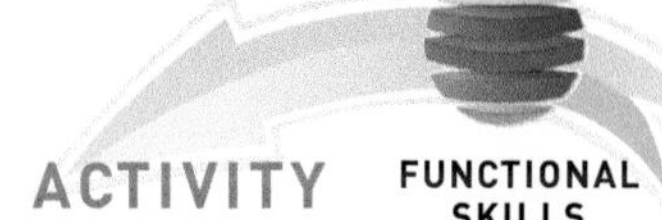

ACTIVITY FUNCTIONAL SKILLS

Service standards
What would be your workplace standard for delivering a facial which would ensure client comfort and satisfaction throughout? List how would this be achieved.

Communicating with clients

Remember that we are all individuals and as such are all unique. This affects the way we see things and as we age our life experiences affect this further. When communicating we must consider this at all times. We will have different values and opinions but that does not mean they are right. Always treat clients with respect and as individuals.

> **Treat each client as an individual**
> A beauty therapist must be skilled, knowledgeable and professional, with the ability to adapt the service and advice provided to suit each client's individual needs. A thorough consultation is required to ensure this happens.
>
> **Joanne Mackinnon**

Communication can be both verbal and non-verbal and by the written word. It is the way we exchange information and develop understanding between each other.

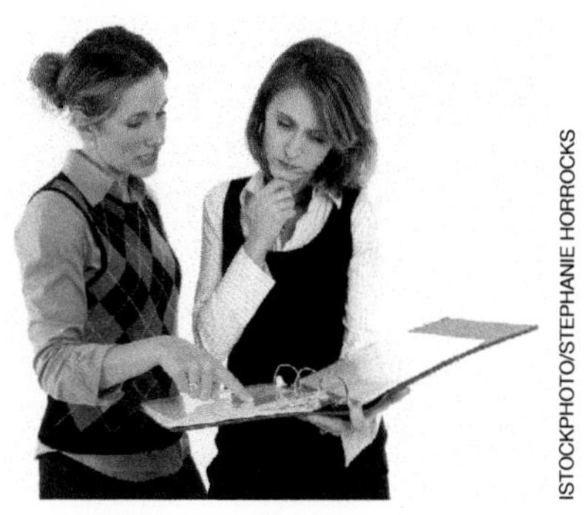

ISTOCKPHOTO/STEPHANIE HORROCKS

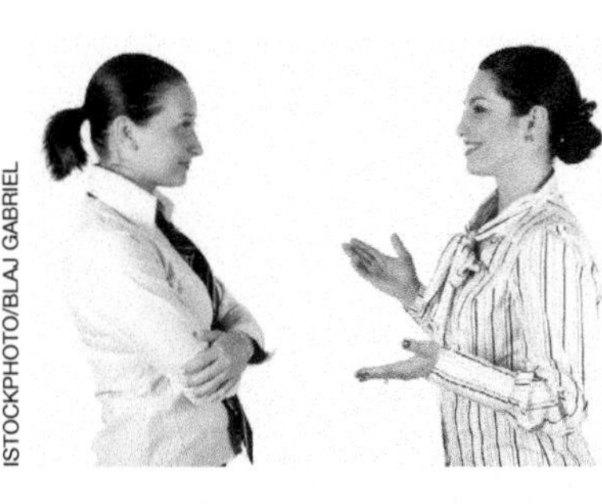
ISTOCKPHOTO/BLAJ GABRIEL

Good communication will:

- gain client confidence
- quickly develop a professional relationship
- aid clients understanding about products and services
- resolve any misunderstandings, ensuring client satisfaction

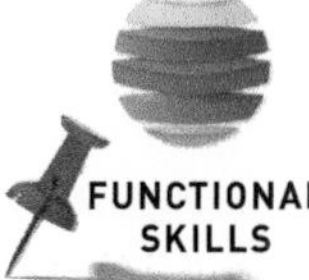

ALWAYS REMEMBER

Communicating using the written word

Increasingly correspondence is by email as it is quick and convenient as clients can receive messages by their mobile phone if they have this facility. Any communication should be well written, easily understood and spellchecked as it is a professional, business communication not a communication with friends. If unsure ask a senior member of staff to check before you send.

When taking messages or making handwritten appointments write neatly and record information accurately.

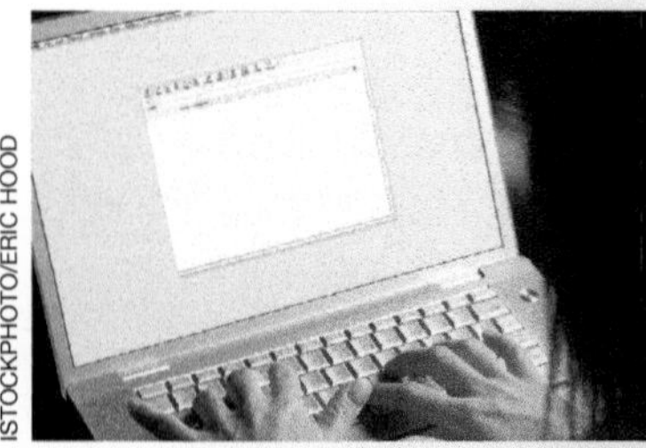
ISTOCKPHOTO/ERIC HOOD

Communication using Email

Verbal communication is when you talk directly to another person. This may be directly face-to-face or indirectly using the telephone.

Non-verbal **body language** is also referred to as communication using the body.

When communicating with a client it should be in a manner which develops friendliness and trust. The client will be possibly sharing personal, private information and she must feel confident in your professionalism and capability. Consider your pace (how fast you speak), especially if explaining something new to the client. Speak clearly and precisely and avoid slang.

Check client understanding before you move the conversation forward, allowing the client to ask questions.

If a client is confused about any information you have given them, find out which part they are unsure about. Repeat the information in stages, checking understanding at each stage. Allow time for the client to consider what you have told them and provide further information as necessary. Check client understanding and that they are clear and satisfied with what you have explained. Explanation should be adapted to suit the situation.

It is important to listen to your clients for effective communication. Pay attention to what the client is saying, do not interrupt – you can listen with your ears and if face to face with your eyes too!

Consider your own body language, be relaxed and attentive, nod and shake your head and smile in agreement. Use relaxed, gentle hand movements.

Good communication will enable you to understand the needs of the client and try hard to ensure they are met.

When a relationship is developed with your client, value it, be discreet, never gossip or share your client confidences.

Finding out more information

When you need to find out more information from the client this requires you to use questioning and listening skills. Questions need to be used which are termed as 'open questions', those that encourage the other person to talk and cannot be answered with yes or no (these are called closed questions). Open questions start with 'how', 'why', 'what', 'when' and 'which'. An example of an open question when making a client appointment for a service is 'when would you like your leg wax?'. A closed question would be 'would you like a leg wax?'.

Brush up on your basic skills

Whether or not you enjoyed Maths, English and ICT at school, remember that employers need beauty therapists with the skills to meet industry timings, carry out stock checks, book accurate appointments, keep client records and even prepare promotional materials. The time to ask for help is while you are training as this will help your progression.

Joanne Mackinnon

Having the knowledge now to build a good relationship with the client what would you do if you had a dissatisfied client?

Dealing with client dissatisfaction

If a client was dissatisfied you would be aware of this by their communication with you. Remember this may be verbal directly (face to face) or indirectly (telephone) or non-verbal communication body language and the written word. If a client is dissatisfied they may be angry and complain or they may not complain saying nothing but leave the salon never to return. It is therefore important to improve any feelings of dissatisfaction immediately.

When dealing with a client who you know or think is dissatisfied the following actions will help:

- Do not make the situation personal, remember the client is usually not angry with you but about the situation.
- Ask the client if they have been satisfied with their service? If not, listen to what they have been unhappy with, remember do not interrupt – listen. This will let the client voice their opinion and they will usually then calm down.
- Note and go over with the client verbally the facts and take appropriate action within your responsibility, this may be to refer the complaint on.
- Refer any concerns immediately to the **relevant person** in the workplace.
- Inform the client of your actions at all times.
- Stay calm and be patient.
- Always remain courteous, professional, continuing to create a positive impression.
- You may have a complaints procedure so you should understand how and when this is to be used.

Client dissatisfaction can usually be resolved through good customer care and communication.

Avoiding client dissatisfaction

- All staff to work together to deliver the agreed services standards
- Ensure a client has a thorough consultation before any service by a colleague with the appropriate technical expertise so that the clients expectations are met.
- Regularly check client satisfaction. If you have any concerns about a client inform a senior member of staff immediately.
- Inform the client about any disruption to a service, e.g. a beauty therapist running late affecting service delivery. Politely inform them of the situation and the choices they have.
- Resolve problems immediately, leaving the client satisfied.

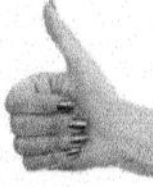

BEST PRACTICE

Know your client
Learn your client's likes and dislikes! This will improve their experience. Avoid all controversial topics of conversation such as sex, religion and politics! Never be judgmental.

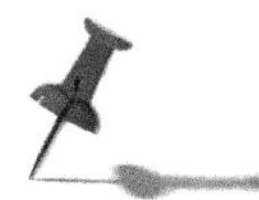

ALWAYS REMEMBER

Poor communication
Your communication can influence a person's mood for good and bad. Think of when you have been at the receiving end of poor manners, how did it make you feel?

The way you handle a client either face to face or on the telephone could leave her feeling satisfied or dissatisfied.

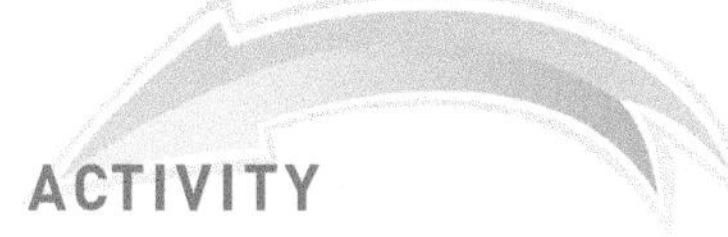

ACTIVITY

Recognizing non-verbal communication
What does this girl's facial expression communicate to you?

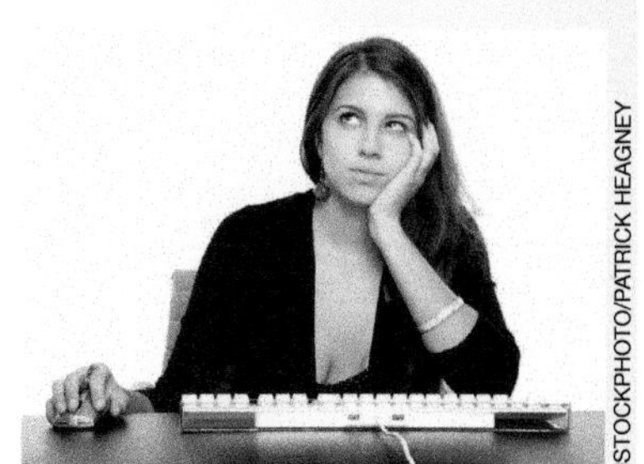

ISTOCKPHOTO/PATRICK HEAGNEY

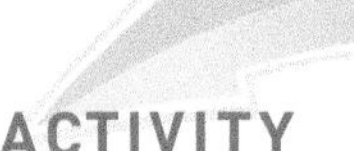

ACTIVITY

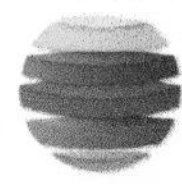

Examples of reasons for client dissatisfaction

Think of five reasons why a client may be dissatisfied with her experience when visiting the salon, an example has been provided.

Reason for client dissatisfaction	How could this situation be avoided?
1. A beauty therapist rushing her service because she is running late.	Knowing that she is running late the beauty therapist could ask another beauty therapist to prepare for and start her next service (with agreement from the client). In this way the next client will start on time, the beauty therapist will catch up and the client she is working on will not need to be rushed.
2.	
3.	
4.	
5.	

Customer care is essential: clients provide the salon's income and your wages. The success of the business depends upon satisfied clients. Clients will assess how well they think you deliver your services, your customer care.

Client care

- Greet the client on their arrival and ask how they would like to be addressed, i.e. formally Mrs Smith or informally by their first name, e.g. Jenny.
- Introduce yourself and your role in the client's service that day.
- Do not discuss confidential information with a client in front of other clients, find a private area.
- Confirm their appointment and update them of any things that may affect their appointment, e.g. the beauty therapist is running late.
- Apologize if the client has experienced any delay.
- Offer to take their outer coat and for all other personal belongings. Place the client's belongings in the appropriate area for storage as per your workplace policy. These must be returned to the client immediately at the end of the service.
- Offer hospitality, i.e. refreshments such as tea/coffee and magazines.
- Be attentive at all times.
- If the client is new, explain all stages of client preparation within your area of responsibility as this will help them feel more relaxed.
- Invite the client to ask questions while in your care and if you cannot answer them as it lies outside your responsibility, refer on.

- Ask the client if they are happy with the service provided directly, i.e. 'are you happy with your nails?' You may invite the client to fill in a customer satisfaction card if your workplace uses them.
- Compliment the client appropriately on their service, e.g. 'your skin looks bright and fresh' following a facial. This must be adapted to suit the situation as it would become repetitive if you passed on the same compliment every time!

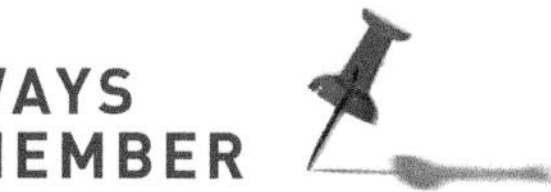

ALWAYS REMEMBER

Treat all clients as you would expect to be treated yourself.

There is no place for poor working relationships in the workplace. A great deal of time is spent in the workplace working alongside your colleagues and it will:

- become stressful
- have a negative effect on your performance if you are unhappy
- affect the client's experience as it will affect the workplace atmosphere
- affect the spirit of the team working together for the success of the business.

Outcome 2: Develop effective working relationships with colleagues

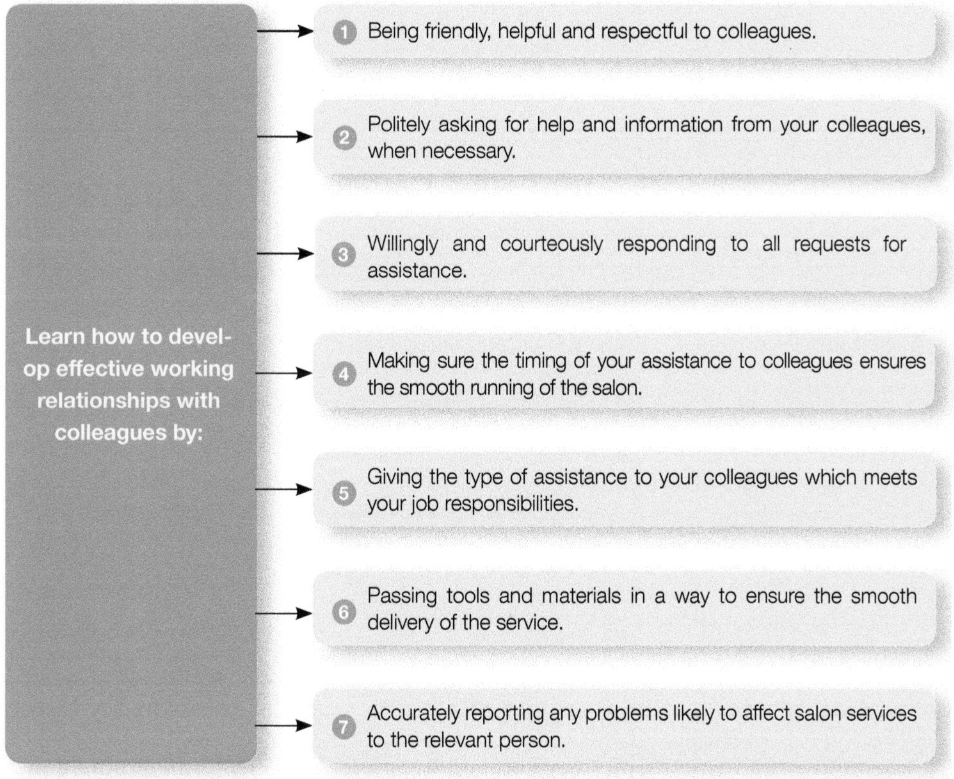

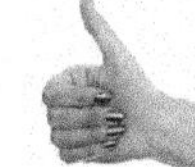

BEST PRACTICE

Teamwork

The team should meet regularly to ensure that it remains focused on its targets and to ensure that communication within the team is good. It is also an ideal time to share ideas and raise any concerns. Together as a team you should be able to openly share ideas to solve any problem.

Each member of staff should have a **job description**. This states:

- job title
- job role
- duties and responsibilities
- work locations (the place you will work)
- any other circumstances which will affect duties and responsibilities such as attending staff training events

The job role of a level 1 beauty therapist is to assist junior and senior beauty therapists in preparing and maintaining their work area. You will need to understand and anticipate when you are required to assist. This may also include assisting with salon reception duties, facial skincare services, day make-up and nail services. You must always ensure that your actions reduce risks to health and safety at all times.

TOP TIP

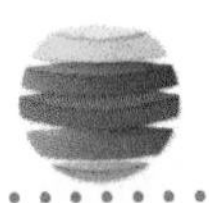

FUNCTIONAL SKILLS

Using the job description to measure your performance

Your job description forms the basis of your performance review where your ability to meet the required standards will be discussed. If these are not met it is important to identify the problem to correct any area of unsatisfactory or poor performance. Know what it says and measure your performance against it.

TOP TIP

Hygiene is a responsibility for all

When preparing and maintaining the beauty therapy work area ensure the highest standard of hygienic, cleanliness and tidiness at all times. Clean as required, do not wait to be asked, e.g. a waste bin is full and requires emptying. If you can see this, so can clients!

Never take short cuts with hygiene and protect yourself wearing appropriate PPE at all times as you may come into contact with strong chemicals and contaminated waste.

Support and guidance should only be requested when needed. It is important to use your initiative – if something needs doing and you have the **opportunity** and authority to do it, complete the task. It is important that you know who to refer to if unsure of any request that is asked of you and to know the **limits of your own authority**. There should be a staffing structure so that you know who is responsible for what and who you should approach in different situations.

It is important that you only work within your job role for reasons of safety and effectiveness. Performing additional roles outside your job description may mean you are not meeting the requirements of the beauty therapy **National Occupational Standards (NOS)**. These standards state the skills required to complete things competently. The result could cause harm to yourself or others and you could be held responsible.

Be friendly, helpful and respectful with colleagues when responding to requests for **assistance**. Accurately, courteously and immediately respond to their needs.

Do not cause unnecessary disruption to a service or create a hazard. When assisting, place tools and materials in a way that enables the smooth delivery of the service. Have a low profile presence, for example if a client had an allergic reaction to a product and the beauty therapist required assistance from you to provide a certain product this should be done calmly without causing concern to the client.

If it is not possible to respond immediately explain when you will be able to. This is important in busy trading conditions such as Christmas – you need to always be ready to expect the unexpected.

Never ignore any problem that may affect the delivery of services – always report these to the relevant person, examples include faulty equipment, low stock levels, double appointment bookings, etc.

HEALTH & SAFETY

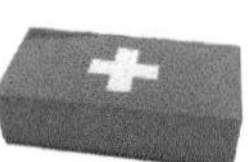

Operating outside your job role means that you are not complying with the Health and Safety at Work Act (1974) and are breaking the law!

Look after your tools and your tools will look after you

Check your tools and equipment are of good quality before use. Ensure they are thoroughly sterilized or disinfected, using a suitable method, between services and stored correctly so that they are not damaged.

Joanne Mackinnon

ACTIVITY

Requests for assistance

What are the common requests for assistance? Add to the list:

- Switching on the wax heater at the beginning of the day and checking it is at the correct temperature.

TOP TIP

Working under pressure

When the salon is busy it is expected you will be too. Put yourself in the right frame of mind, stay calm – slow, deep breathing can help when under pressure.

Make the most of your time
Use any time available between your clients to help busier colleagues, check that there is enough stock or ensure the salon is looking its best by cleaning, preparing and maintaining work areas.

Joanne Mackinnon

TOP TIP

Use your time effectively
If you are not busy you may ask to observe your colleagues, taking the opportunity to increase your knowledge and experience of different services.

Appeal and grievance procedure

If you felt you were being treated unfairly or have a disagreement or complaint with a colleague that you cannot sort out, this grievance or complaint should be reported to the relevant person in the workplace, usually the person who supports and reviews your personal development. Each workplace is different so it must be reported to the correct person, moaning to the wrong person could make things worse. You should be aware of the appeals and grievance procedure and what action to take if necessary.

The appeals and grievance procedure should make sure that the complaint is fully investigated (looked into) and the correct action takes place following this. Sometimes disciplinary action may occur with staff. This is then checked regularly to check it does not occur again.

For a team to work effectively any problem should be fixed as quickly as possible so that good working relationships can be rebuilt.

ALWAYS REMEMBER

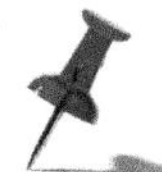

Client observations

Clients will notice non-verbal communication so never show irritation. If you are unhappy about something, or even being treated unfairly, there is a correct time and place for this to be discussed.

Outcome 3: Develop yourself within the job role

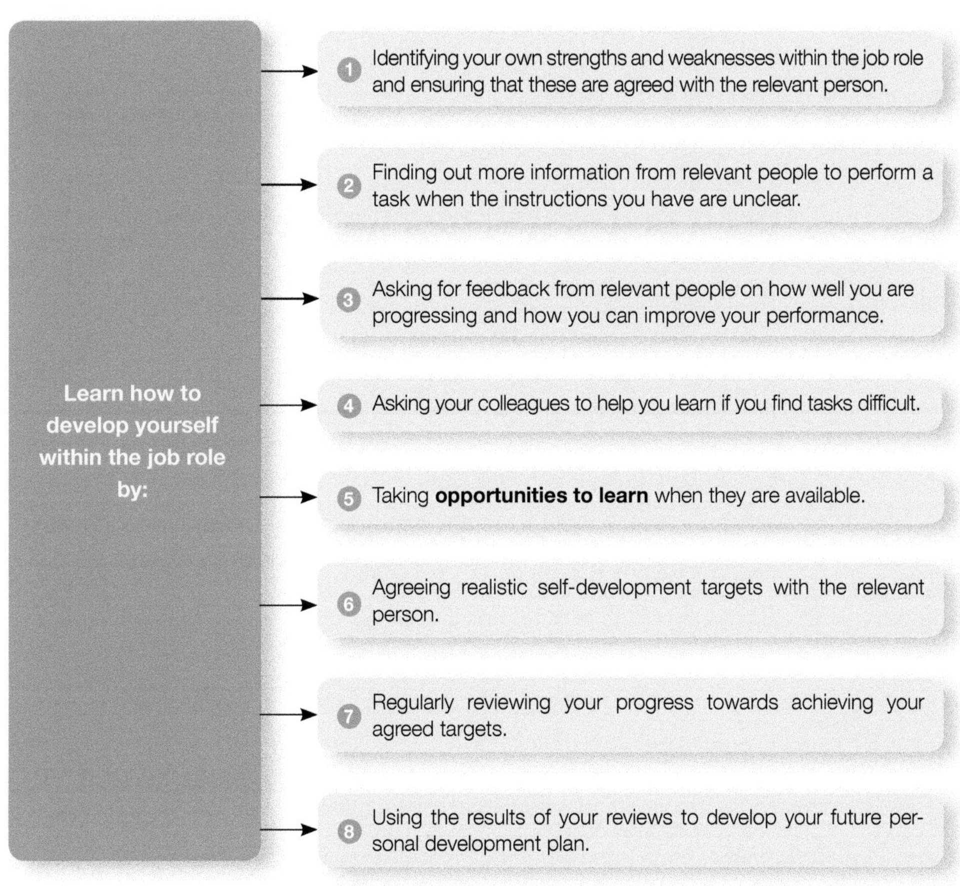

The ability to meet the expected standards as stated in your job description is referred to as your personal effectiveness. You need to take responsibility, 'ownership' of meeting the personal targets set and required of you.

Standards that your performance is reviewed against include:

- your job description
- beauty therapy NOS at Level 1
- expected workplace standards (remember appearance and behaviour)
- personal targets – these are identified in your own personal development plan
- productivity targets, i.e. with regard to retail sales (only if these have been set for you).

It is important that your personal targets are achieved as this means that you are achieving what is required and expected of you.

Targets should be **S M A R T**

Specific This means you will know exactly what you have to do.

Example Target: **Complete the Assist with day make-up unit.**

You must achieve competence on at least **three** occasions, each involving a **different** client.

These clients must each have a **different skin type: dry**, **oily** and **combination**.

Measurable Evidence is recorded in your candidate log book as each skin type is completed, your achievement of the target can be measured. Also, when the target is completed you will have the skills and experience of applying make-up to suit different skin types, this will be measured by the fact you can carry out more skills.

Achievable The target must be possible to achieve. You must have received the necessary training, experience and opportunities in order to complete the target by the date set. The personal development you require to achieve this must be recorded in your development plan.

Realistic The target should be relevant to the role you are currently undertaking. It may be, for example, you will not be able to complete the target because of busy trading conditions over the Christmas period. This may require you to prioritize and use other skills such as preparing and maintaining the beauty therapy work areas and assisting with reception. In this case the target should be re-negotiated. A new date for completion is set.

Timed When should the task be done by? This should be sufficient time to allow you to complete the target set, meeting the required standard.

Targets set must be agreed between yourself and the person responsible for setting them.

Once set you must ensure that you take responsibility for meeting the targets.

The following should be planned:

- What training is required and when will this take place?
- What tasks need to be completed to achieve the targets?

- What standards are expected to be reached?
- When is assessment expected to take place?
- When is a review of progress towards these agreed targets to take place?
- The NOS help you to identify your development needs because when reading what you need to do and know you will be able to immediately see if you are confident with this or if you need to learn or practice more in any area.

Opportunities to learn

Make a good impression on potential employers by making the most of any opportunities you have for further training by attending additional courses and work placements. Going to trade exhibitions and updating your knowledge by reading textbooks, journals and websites will help you.

Joanne Mackinnon

TOP TIP

Meeting the standard

If you only have applied make-up to dry and combination skin types you will need to identify how and when you will gain skills working on an oily skin type in order to be competent across the skin type range.

TOP TIP

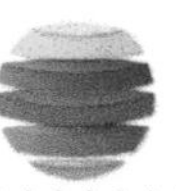

FUNCTIONAL SKILLS

Accessing the National Occupational Standards (NOS) and qualifications relevant to your job role

Visit www.habia.org – and the awarding body for your qualification, i.e. www.cityandguilds.com, www.edexcel.com, www.itecworld.co.uk, www.vtct.org.uk to find out more about your qualification, the standards required and opportunities for progression.

ALWAYS REMEMBER

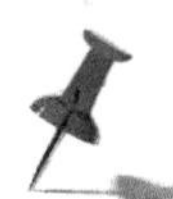

Take responsibility

For non-completion of targets take responsibility for yourself where you know you can improve – do not make excuses and blame others.

Taking responsibility and having initiative is a requirement at level 2. Develop these employability skills as you prepare to progress.

- It is important to meet targets set as this enables you to achieve your qualification, take on more responsibility and progress your training to the next level.
- Some targets you may exceed and these are your 'strengths' while other targets you may not achieve as quickly for a variety of reasons and these may be your 'weaknesses'.
- It is important to be aware of your strengths and weaknesses within your job role.

Performance review or appraisal

The performance review looks at your progress and will identify if there is a problem and what additional actions need to take place to improve your performance and prevent unsatisfactory performance or non-achievement of the targets set.

An updated action plan can then be written up with a new date for review.

Sometimes you may feel that you are progressing well but there are still recommendations, these are not criticisms, be positive and not defensive when receiving feedback. If you feel your training needs are not being met, speak up but not in a way that is aggressive. But remember, if unhappy with your review there is a grievance or appeals procedure.

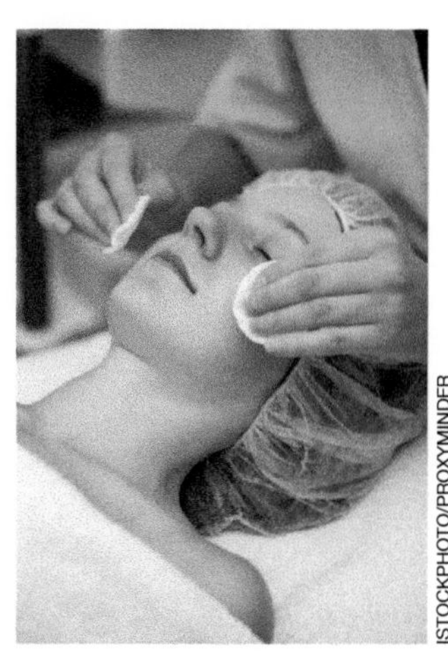

ISTOCKPHOTO/PROXYMINDER

A beauty therapist demonstrating facial skills

Every day you can learn something new just by observing experienced staff performing their everyday duties.

Opportunities to learn include:

- taking part in salon training activities
- observing technical skills you will be learning when you progress to the next level
- reading professional trade magazines
- attending trade seminars where you will see new developments in beauty therapy that your workplace may introduce
- undertaking **Continuous Professional Development (CPD)** activities to develop your technical skills and keep up-to-date with new techniques.

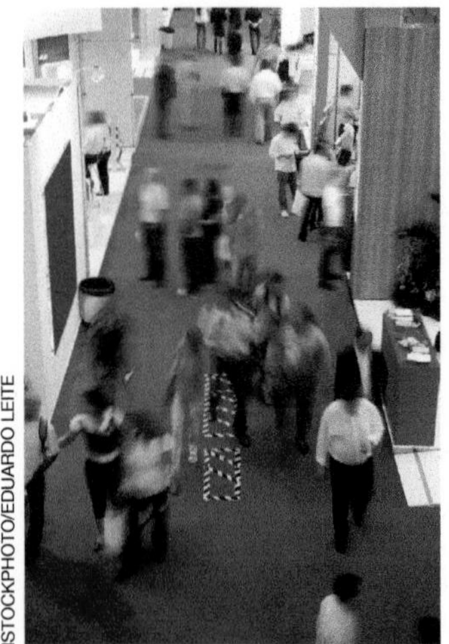

ISTOCKPHOTO/EDUARDO LEITE

A trade fair

ACTIVITY

Continuous Professional Development (CPD)
Keep examples of how you have kept yourself professionally updated and place the evidence in your portfolio, e.g. a ticket to a trade show. You can use this as evidence for this unit on how you have taken part in opportunities to learn.

GLOSSARY OF KEY WORDS

Assistance providing help and support.

Body language communication involving the body.

Communication the exchange of information and understanding between people.

Continuous Professional Development (CPD) activities undertaken to develop technical skills to ensure current, professional experience.

Grievance a cause for concern or complaint.

Job Description written details of a person's work role, duties and responsibilities.

Limits of your own authority your level of responsibility as written in your own job description and workplace policies.

National Occupational Standards (NOS) standards set to support performance in beauty therapy. These can be obtained from the Hairdressing and Beauty Industry Authority (Habia) website: www.habia.org.uk.

Opportunity a situation that makes it possible to do something that you have to do or want to do.

Organizational requirements beauty therapy procedures or work rules provided by the workplace management.

Personal appearance expected standards of workplace appearance.

Relevant person an individual responsible for supervising you during a given task or service, or the person whom you are required to report things to.

Salon requirements any salon procedures or work rules issued by the workplace management.

Target a goal to achieve usually within a timescale.

Verbal communication occurs when you talk directly to another person either face to face, directly or indirectly, or over the telephone.

Working practices any activities, procedures, use of materials or equipment and working techniques used in carrying out your job.

Workplace this word is used to describe the place in which you carry out your work. Normally, this will be your salon.

Workplace policies this covers the documentation prepared by your employer on the procedures to be followed in your workplace.

ASSESSMENT OF KNOWLEDGE AND UNDERSTANDING

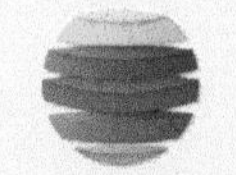

FUNCTIONAL SKILLS

Having covered the learning objectives for **contribute to the development of effective working relationships** answer the following short questions below.

The information covers:

- salon and legal requirements
- communication
- procedures and targets
- improving your performance.

Salon and legal requirements

1 Why is it important to only carry out tasks that are within your job responsibility?

2 List **five** examples of good standards of behaviour that are expected of you when working in the workplace?

3 What is client care and why is good client care important?

4 What does personal presentation mean? What are your salon standards for personal presentation?

5 If you were unsure how to carry out a particular task asked of you what would you do?

Communication

1 How can you gain client confidence in you when communicating?

2 What are 'open' and 'closed' questions and when would you choose to use each? Write an example of an open and a closed question.

3 What is non-verbal communication?

4 If a client was angry because her service would be delayed what action would you take?

5 Why is it valuable to listen to a client and not interrupt them when they are speaking?

Procedures and targets

1 If you were unhappy with an assessment decision what would be the correct action to take?

2 What are personal development targets?

3 What is the importance of meeting your personal targets?

4 How do you know the standards that are expected of you when completing your work responsibilities?

5 Who would you ask for feedback on progress towards meeting your personal targets?

Improving your performance

1 What is Continuous Professional Development (CPD)?

2 Why is it important to be familiar with the National Occupational Standards for your qualification?

3 Why should you keep checking and updating your progress for your personal development plan?

4 Why is it important to have good working relationships with your colleagues?

5 If you had difficulties working with another beauty therapist and it could not be resolved, what action should you take?

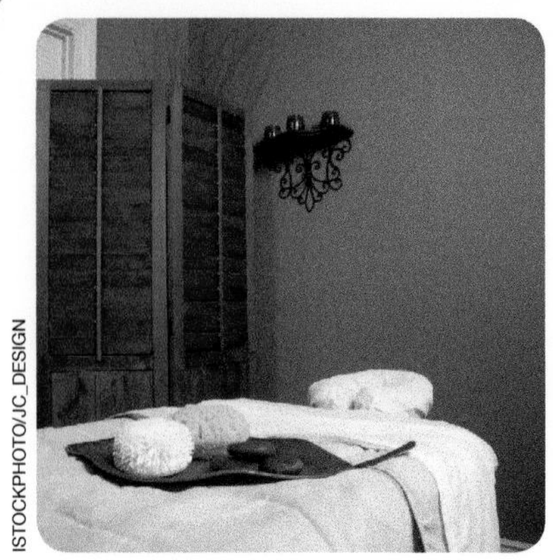
ISTOCKPHOTO/JC_DESIGN

4 Preparing and maintaining the salon treatment work area

Learning Objectives

This chapter covers the **Preparing and maintaining the salon treatment work area** unit.

This unit is all about the skills you will need to prepare and maintain (look after) the beauty therapy work area for waxing, eye services, facial, make-up services and nail services. It will help you to learn about the materials and equipment that are needed for each service and how to maintain the work area so it is always ready and of the correct standard for the next client.

You will also have a responsibility to handle and store the client's records

There are **two** learning outcomes which you must achieve competently:

1 **Prepare the treatment work areas**

2 **Maintain the treatment work areas**

Your assessor will observe your performance on **at least three occasions** which will be recorded.

From the **range** statement, you must show that you have:

- prepared and maintained work areas for **six** out of the ***eight** services
- have prepared all types of environmental conditions.

*However, you must prove to your assessor that you have the necessary knowledge, understanding and skills to be

(continued on the next page)

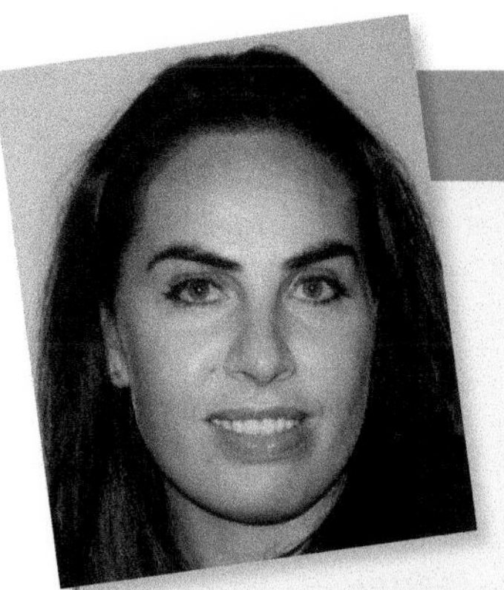

ROLE MODEL

Vicky Ann Kennedy

Spa Operations Manager, The Sanctuary Spa

"I have been the principal owner of a very successful beauty clinic since 1991. I knew the career path I wanted to take by the age of 12, but had to wait until the age of 19 before it became a reality. I trained at Bolton College under Lorraine Nordmann, and became Student of the Year when I left. I have carried on striving to achieve every day since.

Before starting my own business, I had not worked in many other places, but I already knew how I wanted things to be done and how standards should be followed.

I think that if your heart is in it, working in the beauty industry is very rewarding and a beauty salon is a lovely, happy place to work. I have no regrets and after nearly 20 years, still enjoy every day.

(continued)

able to perform competently for all eight services, these are:

- waxing
- eye services
- make-up
- facial
- manicure
- pedicure
- nail art
- nail enhancements.

When preparing and maintaining the salon treatment areas it is important to use the skills you have learnt in the following units:

Health and Safety

Developing positive working relationships

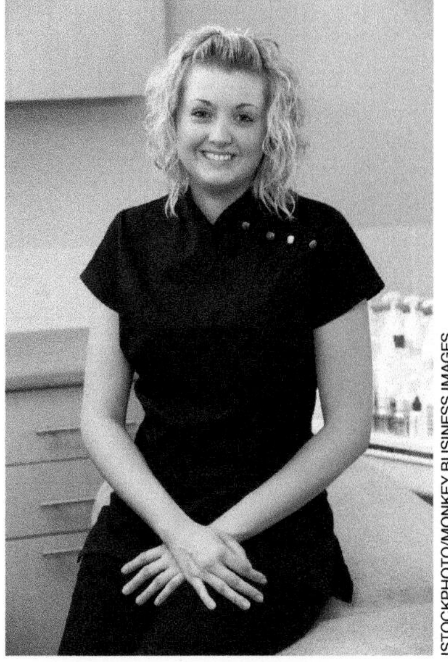

ISTOCKPHOTO/MONKEY BUSINESS IMAGES

Everything you do reflects on the salon

Practical skills, knowledge and understanding

This table will help you to check your progress in gaining the necessary practical skills, knowledge and understanding for **Preparing and maintaining the salon treatment work area**. Tick (✓), when you feel you have gained the practical skills, knowledge and understanding in the following areas:

	Practical skills, knowledge and understanding checklist	✓
1	The correct environmental conditions needed for each service, including: • lighting • heating • ventilation • general comfort.	
2	Contamination control – selecting and using the correct method of disinfection/sterilization for tools and equipment necessary for each service.	
3	Preparing the treatment area for **waxing** services following all health and safety requirements.	
4	Preparing the treatment area for **eye** services following all health and safety requirements.	
5	Preparing the treatment area for **make-up** services following all health and safety requirements.	

Keep aware when working
Using your skills in communication always check during service that your client is comfortable and not feeling any discomfort.

Vicky Ann Kennedy

TOP TIP

Habia Codes of Practice
When preparing the areas refer to the following good practice codes

- Code of practice for nail services
- Code of practice for waxing
- Heath and safety pocket guide

6	Preparing the treatment area for **manicure** services following all health and safety requirements.
7	Preparing the treatment area for **pedicure** services following all health and safety requirements.
8	Preparing the treatment area for **nail art** services following all health and safety requirements.
9	Preparing the treatment area for **nail enhancement** services following all health and safety requirements.
10	Preparing the treatment area for **facial** services following all health and safety requirements.
11	Personal presentation and hygiene meets the required industry and workplace standard at all times.
12	Good communication skills verbal and non-verbal are used with clients and colleagues which consider their needs.
13	Client's records are made available for the start of each client service.
14	Correct methods of waste removal and disposal are followed for each service.
15	Manufacturers' guidelines for the care and maintenance of equipment are followed.
16	Cleaning and preparation of the treatment area is well organized, ensuring it is ready for further services.
17	Correct storage of client record card takes place following each service, meeting the legislation needs of the Data Protection Act (1998).

Keep your standards up Always make sure that you keep your standards high, especially when dealing with hygiene and avoiding cross-infection. Remember the good practices that you learnt when training and always use them.

Vicky Ann Kennedy

When you have ticked all the areas you can, ask your assessor to assess you on **Preparing and maintaining the salon treatment work area.** After practical assessment, your assessor might decide that you need more practice to improve your skills. If so, your assessor will tell you how and where you need to improve to gain competence.

After assessment of what you need to know and understand there may be 'gaps' that require you to study further. Your assessor will tell you what you need to study further to achieve the required level of understanding.

Preparing and maintaining the salon treatment work areas

As a Level 1 beauty therapist it is a requirement that you support your colleagues by providing assistance with services carried out on clients. This will ensure the smooth running of the appointment schedule, helping to ensure client satisfaction as delays will where possible be avoided. One of your roles is to prepare and maintain the working areas for the following Level 2 beauty therapy services:

- waxing
- eye services

- make-up service
- facial
- manicure service
- pedicure service
- nail art
- nail enhancements.

ALWAYS REMEMBER

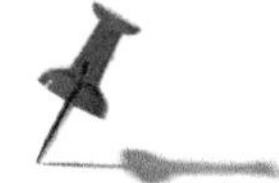

Environment conditions
These include heating, lighting, ventilation and general comfort of all in the workplace. These conditions must be suitable for each service to be carried out correctly and safely.

Preparing and maintaining the beauty therapy salon treatment work area requires you to carry out the following responsibilities:

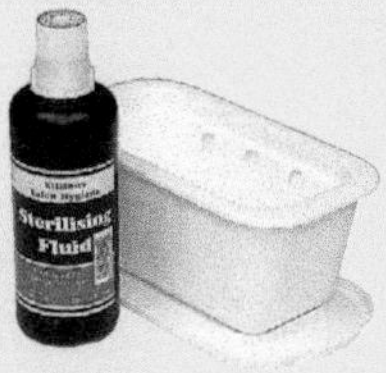

ELLISONS

Steriliize/disinfect equipment before service

↓

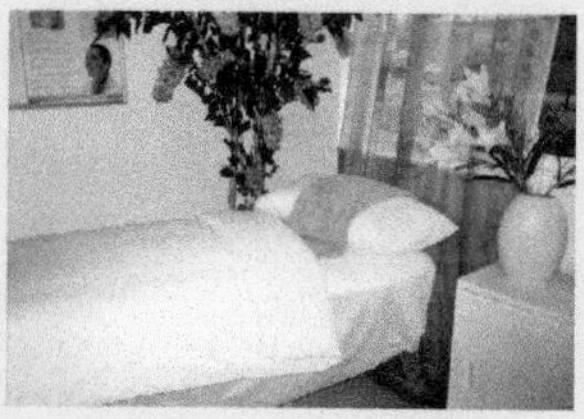

ELLISONS

Make sure the environmental conditions are correct for the service

↓

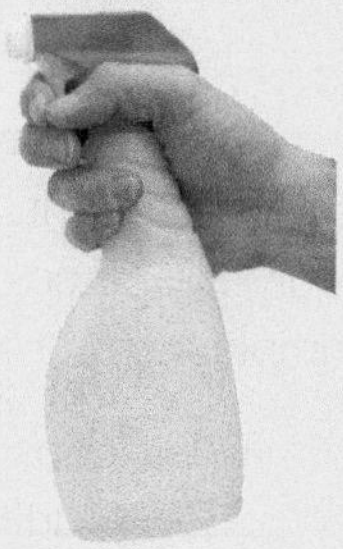

Disinfect work surfaces to be used

↓

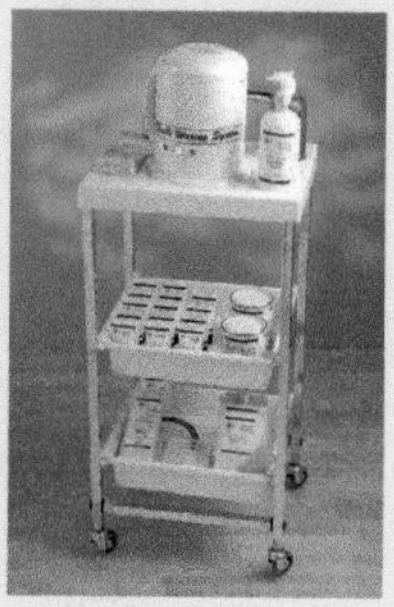

ELLISONS

Prepare treatment area
Ensuring all the required equipment and materials are available and ready to use

↓

ALWAYS REMEMBER

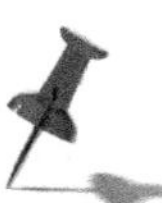

Manufacturers' guidelines

Each product will by law have instructions provided with it to say how it should be safely used. If you are preparing the work area and you notice the product is different than normal, check the instructions for safe use within your responsibility for handling it. Report it, if you think there is a quality issue to the responsible person.

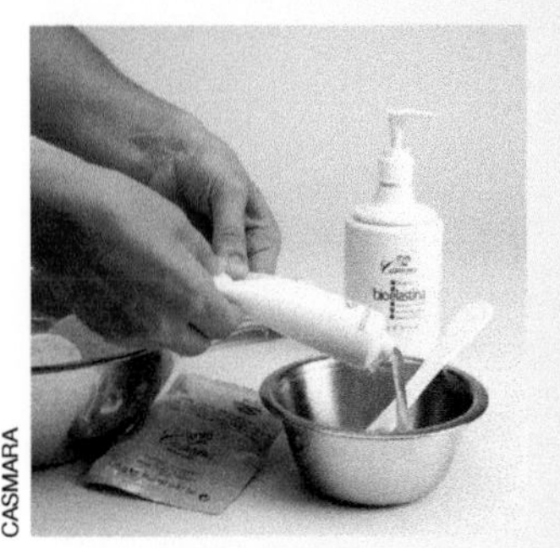
CASMARA

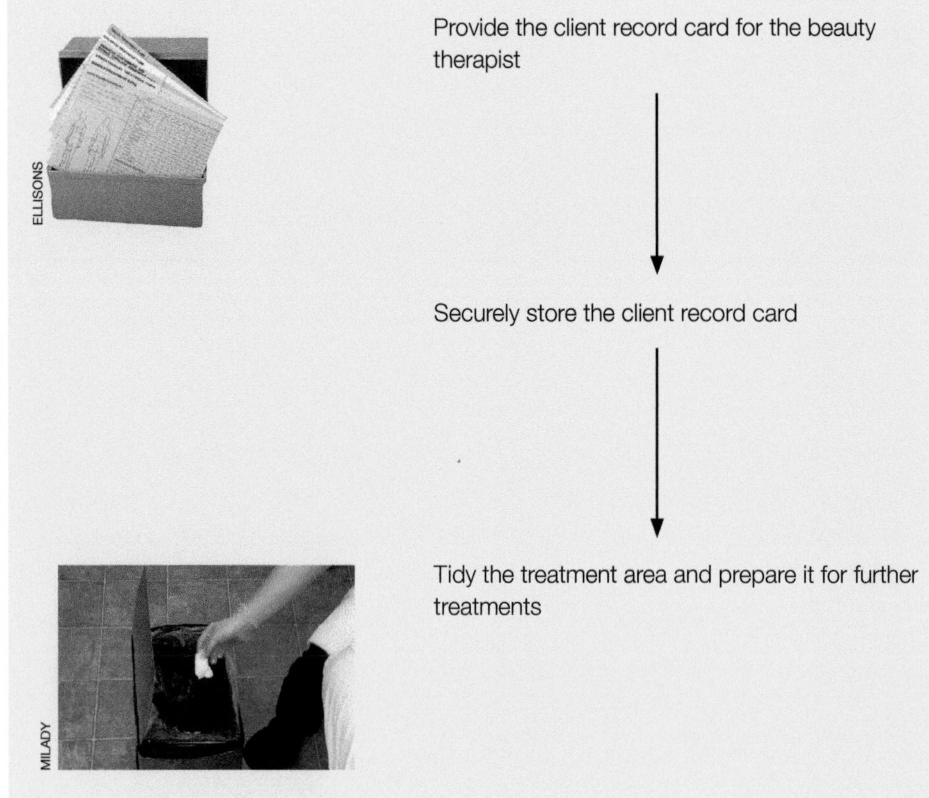

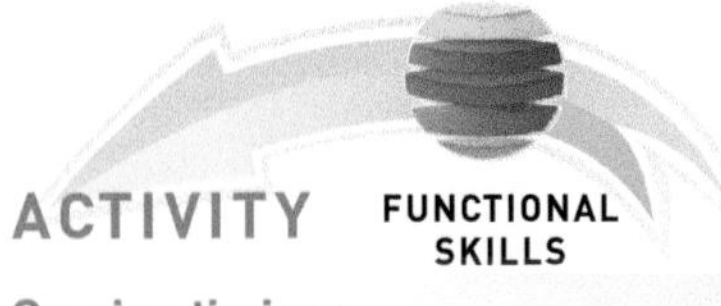

ACTIVITY FUNCTIONAL SKILLS

Service timings

Sometimes more than one area of waxing is required. Using the service timings table shown, how long would you allow for a client receiving:

- half leg, bikini and underarm wax?
- full leg, bikini and underarm wax?
- eyebrow and facial wax?

Reception

The reception is an important area to refer to when planning what services you need to prepare for.

Check your appointment schedule regularly as changes can occur during the day.

You need to allow sufficient time to prepare the work area for each service. Check the appointment schedule regularly to see what service is next.

To prepare the work area, allow at least 10 minutes to make sure you have all the equipment, materials and products necessary for the service. Certain pieces of equipment might have preparation requirements. For example, wax must be heated before use. Allow enough time for this, so that the equipment is available for use as required.

It is important to know how long each service takes so that you are available to tidy the service area when it has finished, preparing it for the next client.

Service timings

Service	**Maximum service time allowed (minutes)*	*Service*	**Maximum service time allowed (minutes)*
Eyebrow shape	15 mins	Make-up (evening/special occasion)	45 mins
Eyelash tint	20 mins	Day make-up	30 mins
Facial	60 mins	Manicure	45 mins

Service	*Maximum service time allowed (minutes)	Service	*Maximum service time allowed (minutes)
Eyebrow wax	15 mins	Pedicure	50 mins
Underarm wax	15 mins	Facial including lash tint and eyebrow shape	80 mins
Half-leg wax	30 mins	Eyebrow shape and eyelash tint	30 mins
Bikini line wax	15 mins	Eyebrow tint	10 mins
Arm wax	30 mins	Eyebrow tint, shape and lash tint	30 mins
Full leg	45 mins	Facial and make-up	90 mins
Half leg, bikini and underarm wax	60 mins	Nail art	5–10 mins (per nail)
Full leg, bikini and underarm wax	75 mins	Nail enhancements (This will vary dependant on the system used and service requirement.)	120 mins
		Artificial lashes (flares)	20 mins
		Partial lashes (flares)	10 mins
		Artificial lashes (strips)	10 mins
		Partial lashes (strips)	10 mins

*Specialist services may require longer following manufacturers' instructions.

In addition to the service timings listed above you are required to practically assist, performing facial, make-up and nail services as part of your Level 1 qualification, allow the following times for these services:

facial service	30 minutes
nail service	30 minutes
make-up service	30 minutes

Health and safety

For each service it is important that hygienic practice is considered before preparing the beauty therapy work area and during its maintenance. This will help prevent **cross-infection** – the transfer of harmful bacteria/microorganisms from one person to another.

> **Sterilize your tools**
> Never use tools that are not completely sterile. Use disposable products where possible.
> **Vicky Ann Kennedy**

ALWAYS REMEMBER

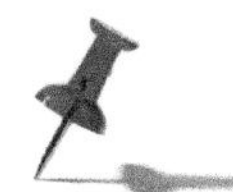

Client record card

- You are responsible for collecting the client record card before each service and for storing it again afterwards.
- The client's personal details are confidential. It is important that you comply with the Data Protection Act (1998): all information relating to a client should be stored securely and only those staff with agreement to do so should be able to look at it. So, as soon as all service details have been recorded on the record card it should be put back into secure storage.
- Do not leave client record cards lying about! The information held is confidential.

Depending on the tools and equipment required for each beauty therapy service, they can be prepared hygienically either by disinfection or by sterilization methods:

- **Sterilization** destroys all living microorganisms
- **Disinfection** destroys some, but not all, microorganisms and slows down their growth.

Sometimes the tool or equipment cannot be hygienically cleaned and is thrown away or disposed of. This is called a **consumable**.

You should select the correct method to hygienically prepare your work area – sterilization or disinfection – to ensure a safe working environment is provided.

Codes of practice are available from Habia showing best and also essential health and safety working practices approved by industry and health and safety advisors.

An autoclave is used when small tools or pieces of equipment need to be **sterilized**. This heats water to a temperature of 121–134°C. Metal objects and some sponge materials can be sterilized in an autoclave.

Disinfection is achieved by placing tools or small pieces of equipment – often plastic, which is unsuitable for the high temperatures achieved in the autoclave (as they would melt) – in a chemical disinfectant or in an UV cabinet.

For further information on **hygiene** practice in the workplace, refer to Chapter 2 p. 29.

ELLISONS

An autoclave

ACTIVITY

Identify **five** items of tools or equipment you may have to prepare for services in.
Using the table headings shown below tick what method you would use to ensure good health and safety practice for those chosen. An example is shown:

Tool/Equipment	Sterilization	Disinfection	Consumable (disposed of immediately after use)
Example *Lip brush* ****If a non-disposable lip brush was used as shown below this would be disinfected.*** ELLISONS Lip brush			✓
1			
2			
3			
4			
5			

Hygiene checks

- Ensure that all tools and equipment are clean, disinfected/sterile, before every use.
- Disinfect work surfaces after every client.
- Use disposable items whenever possible. Discard immediately after use in a covered, lined waste container. Dispose of waste from the waste container often following your workplace waste disposal procedures.
- Follow hygienic codes and practices at all times.
- Maintain a high standard of personal hygiene at all times.
- Wear PPE to avoid skin irritation, which could lead to the skin disease dermatitis.

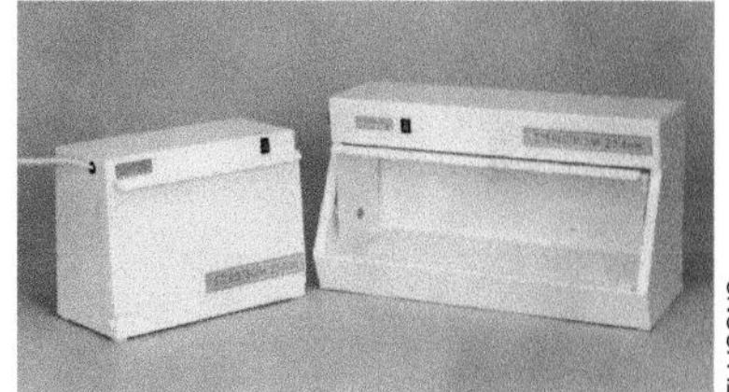
ELLISONS

UV light cabinets

Outcome 1: Prepare the treatment work areas

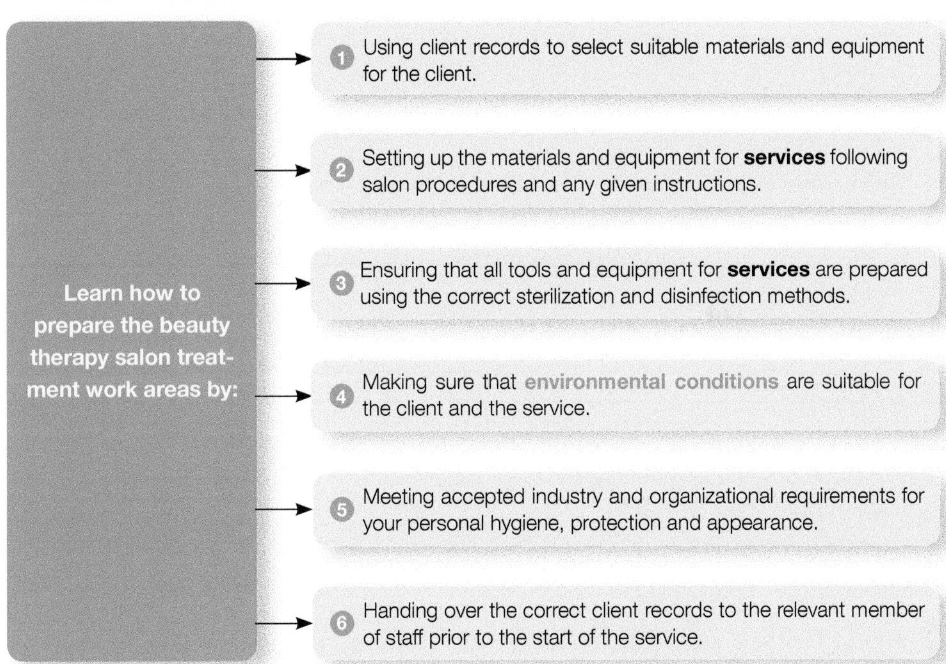

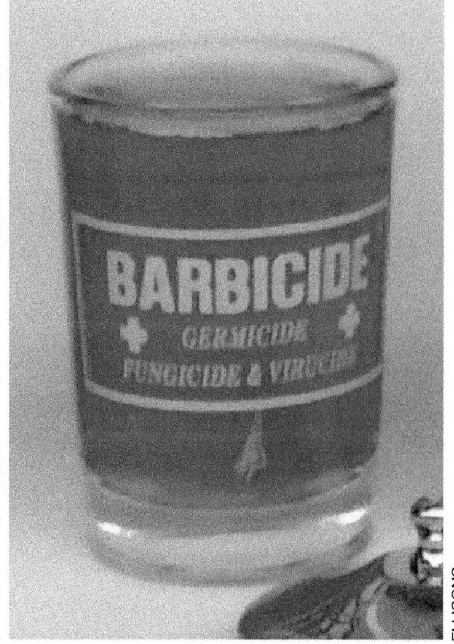

ELLISONS

Chemical disinfectant for the storage of small tools and equipment

BEST PRACTICE

Preparing the beauty therapy salon treatment work area

1 Ensure all equipment, products and consumables for service are available for the service for the beauty therapist to select from.
2 Ensure there is adequate hygiene in the service area.
3 Wash your hands before preparing the beauty therapy work area. Wear PPE i.e. apron and gloves to avoid contact with cleaning chemicals.
4 Ensure your personal appearance and hygiene meets industry and organizational standards.
5 Ensure that the service area is adequately lit, is of a comfortable temperature and is suitably ventilated. Poor environmental conditions can affect the quality of the service and comfort of the client and beauty therapist.
6 Prepare the work environment tools and equipment to meet all health and safety legislation requirements.
7 Obtain the client record card to obtain related personal information service details.

Outcome 2: Maintain the treatment work area

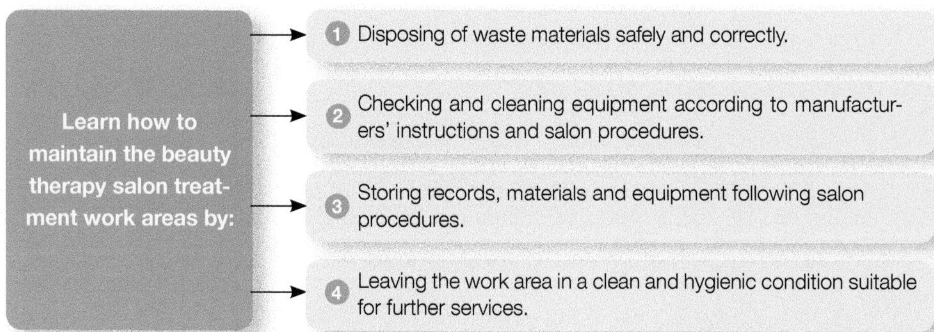

BEST PRACTICE

Maintaining the beauty therapy salon treatment work area

1 Clean and prepare equipment and materials for the next client following health and safety procedures and manufacturing guidelines.
2 Dispose of all waste materials following the service following industry and organizational, legislative requirements.
3 Store clients' records securely in the designated area following the service, complying with the Data Protection Act (1998).
4 Clean all work surfaces to minimize cross-infection between each client and the beauty therapist.
5 Prepare the service area for further services.
6 Check the appointment book to plan time effectively to prepare the service area for the next client.

A description of each service follows, with explanations of how to prepare and maintain each salon work area.

Preparing and maintaining the salon treatment work area for waxing service

Wax service involves using wax to remove hairs temporarily from the face and body. Waxing removes both the visible hair – the hair shaft (seen above the skin's surface) – and the root (the part of the hair inside the skin), so when the hair re-grows it is completely new hair. It will be usually 4–6 weeks before the client requires the waxing service again.

Waxing service applied to the eyebrows

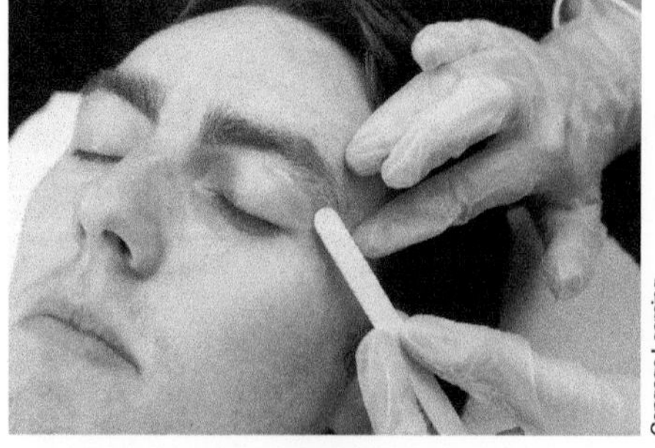

Warm wax is applied to the eyebrow hair using a disposable spatula

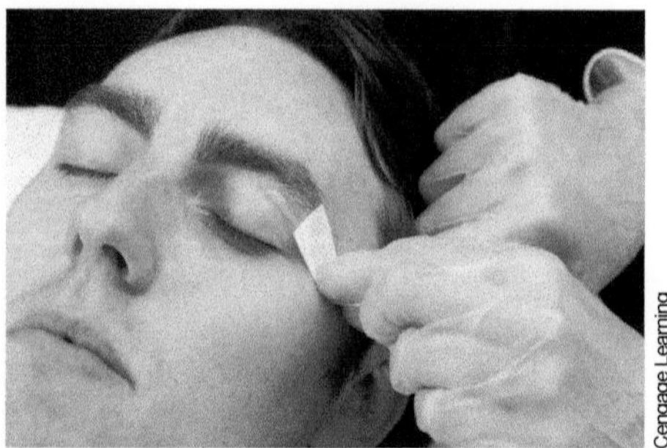

Removing the unwanted hair using a wax strip

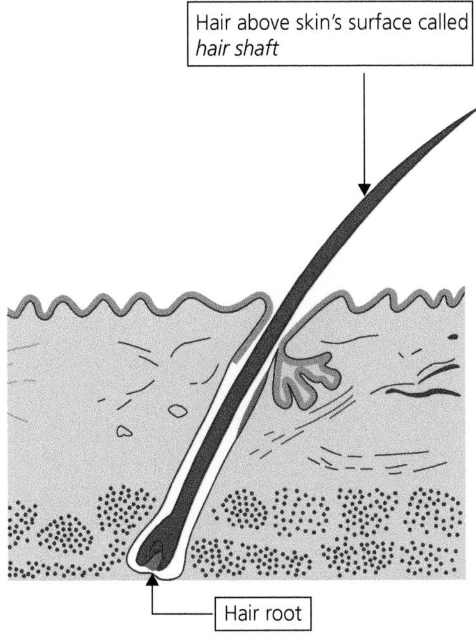

Hair follicle

ALWAYS REMEMBER

Waxing removes the whole hair, so a completely new hair must grow before the client requires the service again.

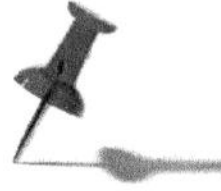

ALWAYS REMEMBER

There are different types of wax. The most suitable for your client and their service is chosen.

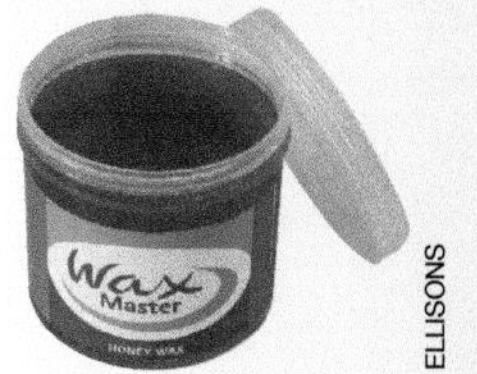

Honey warm wax

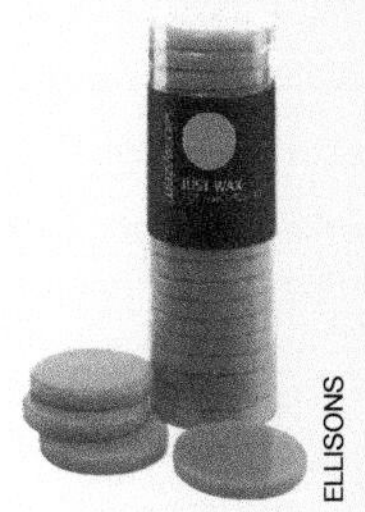

Hot wax discs

There are different wax types and systems available for use. Your salon might use only one, or more than one type/system. Select and prepare the choice of wax as guided by the beauty therapist who will be performing the service:

- **Warm wax** is heated in a special, low-temperature heater to around 43°C, when it becomes runny. Warm waxes are frequently made of mixtures of glucose syrup, resin to help the wax stick, oil to help removal, water and fragrances. Zinc oxide is added to cream wax providing an opaque colour. Warm wax is available in cartridge/tubes with either a disposable applicator or roller applicator. The wax containers are heated to the correct working temperature. A disposable applicator head is provided for each. Always follow the waxing manufacturers' instructions on correct, hygienic preparation for use.
- **Hot wax** is applied at a higher temperature than warm wax – around 50°C. Blocks or pellets of solid wax are heated in a special heater until a thickish, runny consistency is achieved. This wax requires longer to heat than warm wax.
- **Sugaring** is an ancient and popular method of hair removal. A mixture of sugar, lemon and water is applied as a paste, called sugar paste, or as a traditional warm wax called strip sugar.

Refer to the equipment and materials checklist on p. 68 to make sure you have everything that is needed for the waxing service.

HEALTH & SAFETY

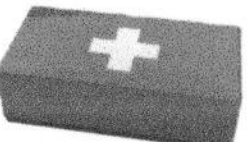

Personal Protective Equipment (PPE) at Work Regulations (1992)

There is a risk of contact with body fluids during waxing. It is recommended that special protective equipment is worn when handling cleaning chemicals and contaminated equipment and waste.

It is the employer's responsibility to make PPE available to employees; it is the employee's responsibility to use it.

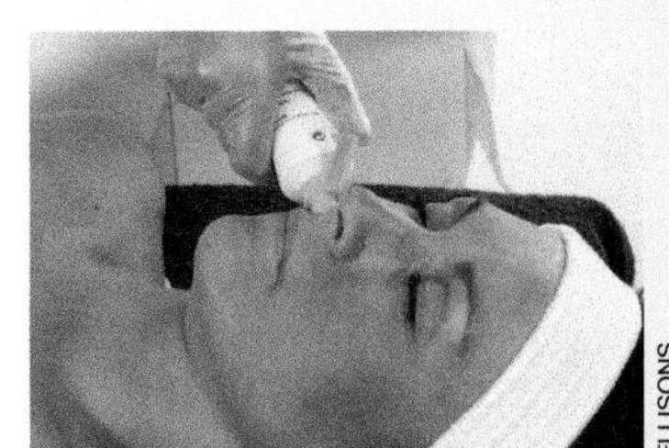

Service image of wax application to the upper lip using a disposable applicator head on a warm wax tube system. PPE gloves are worn.

Sterilization and disinfection

- Small metal tools should be sterilized after use. First they should be cleaned with surgical spirit and clean cotton wool to remove surface dirt, debris and wax before they are sterilized in the autoclave. They should be stored in the UV cabinet after sterilization to keep them sterile and ready for use. Alternatively store in a clean lined covered container.
- Towels should be boil washed at 60°C to destroy harmful microorganisms and prevent cross-infection.
- Wash your hands before handling clean equipment.

HEALTH & SAFETY

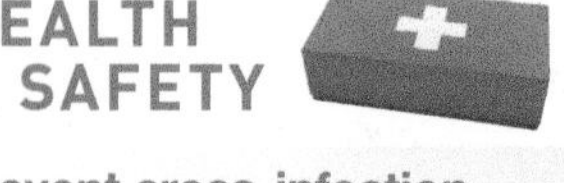

Prevent cross-infection
If you have a cut on your hand you should wear a protective sterile dressing to prevent cross-infection and secondary infection to yourself.

Keeping your appointments on time Clients like to be seen promptly so try not to run behind with your appointments. Always keep the service area tidy and clean as you work so it can be quickly prepared ready for the next client.

Vicky Ann Kennedy

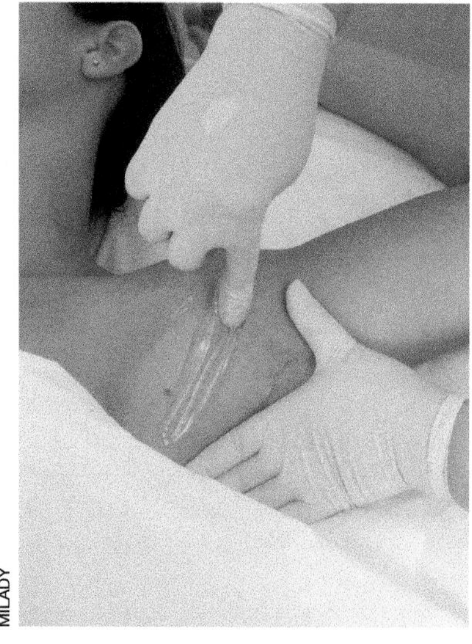
MILADY

Sugar paste applied to the underarm hair

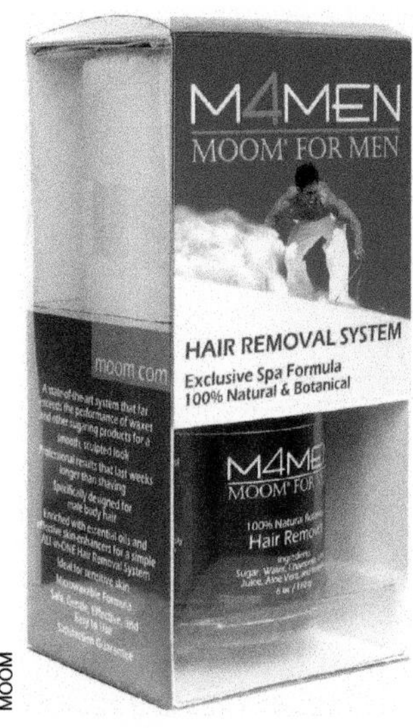

MOOM

Wax formulated for men's hair removal

Refer to the equipment and materials checklist below to make sure that you have all that is required to perform waxing services.

EQUIPMENT AND MATERIALS CHECKLIST FOR WAXING SERVICE

		WARM WAX	*HOT WAX*	*CARTRIDGE/TUBE WAX SYSTEM*	*STRIP SUGAR*	*SUGAR PASTE*
SORISA	Couch – with sit-up and lie-down positions and an easy-to-clean surface	☐	☐	☐	☐	☐
SORISA	Trolley – to hold all the necessary equipment and materials	☐	☐	☐	☐	☐
	Protective plastic couch cover	☐	☐	☐	☐	☐

		WARM WAX	HOT WAX	CARTRIDGE/TUBE WAX SYSTEM	STRIP SUGAR	SUGAR PASTE
ELLISONS	Disposable tissue roll to cover the trolley surface and couch	☐	☐	☐	☐	☐
ELLISONS	Disposable wooden spatulas – a selection of different sizes used for application of wax or petroleum jelly to different body parts	☐	☐		☐	
	Wax removal strips (bonded fibre or fabric) cut to size for the waxing service	☐	☐	☐	☐	
	Talcum powder (purified) to prevent the wax from sticking to the skin, assist the wax application technique chosen where necessary and to make fair hair more visible		☐			☐
ELLISONS	Cotton wool pads, to cleanse and apply products soothing aftercare to the skin	☐	☐	☐	☐	☐
ELLISONS	Facial tissues, to protect client's clothing and to blot the skin dry after cleansing and after wax application	☐	☐	☐	☐	☐
	Skin cleanser (pre-wax lotion) to hygienically remove surface dirt, cosmetic products, dead skin and body oils	☐	☐	☐	☐	☐
ELLISONS	Surgical spirit or a commercial cleaner designed to clean equipment	☐	☐	☐	☐	☐

		WARM WAX	*HOT WAX*	*CARTRIDGE/TUBE WAX SYSTEM*	*STRIP SUGAR*	*SUGAR PASTE*
SORISA	Towels for protecting the client's clothing and for modesty when clothing has been removed	☐	☐	☐	☐	☐
ELLISONS	Small stainless steel scissors for trimming long hairs before waxing	☐	☐	☐	☐	☐
ELLISONS	A jar of disinfecting solution to hold small metal tools, e.g. tweezers and scissors	☐	☐	☐	☐	☐
SORISA	Tweezers for removing stray, very short hairs following waxing	☐	☐	☐	☐	☐
BEAUTY EXPRESS LTD	Petroleum jelly to cover areas that must not be waxed over, e.g. moles	☐	☐	☐	☐	☐
	Wax	*Prepare according to the workplace waxing system used and the beauty therapist's chosen system for the client* *Wax heater, set at recommended temperature (as appropriate)*				
ELLISONS	After wax lotion with soothing, healing and cooling properties, to be applied to the area after hair removal	☐	☐	☐	☐	☐
ELLISONS	Mirror (clean) – for facial waxing to discuss and agree the service plan and show the client the results to confirm satisfaction	☐	☐	☐	☐	☐

		WARM WAX	*HOT WAX*	*CARTRIDGE/TUBE WAX SYSTEM*	*STRIP SUGAR*	*SUGAR PASTE*
ELLISONS	Apron for hygiene and to protect workwear from wax spillages	☐	☐	☐	☐	☐
ELLISONS	Disposable gloves – used when waxing the under-arm and bikini areas where 'spot' bleeding commonly can occur	☐	☐	☐	☐	☐
ELLISONS	Bin (swing top) – lined with a heavy duty disposable polythene bin liner	☐	☐	☐	☐	☐
ELLISONS	Client record card – so that the client's details can be recorded before and after the service	☐	☐	☐	☐	☐
ELLISONS	Aftercare leaflets – to provide guidance notes for the client to follow after the service	☐	☐	☐	☐	☐

HEALTH & SAFETY

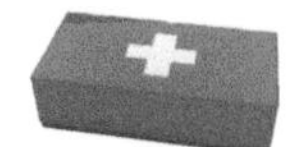

Storing liquids

To prevent damage to the electrical equipment and electric shock to the beauty therapist, liquids must not be stored next to electrical equipment such as chemical disinfectant. Keep any liquids on another shelf on the trolley.

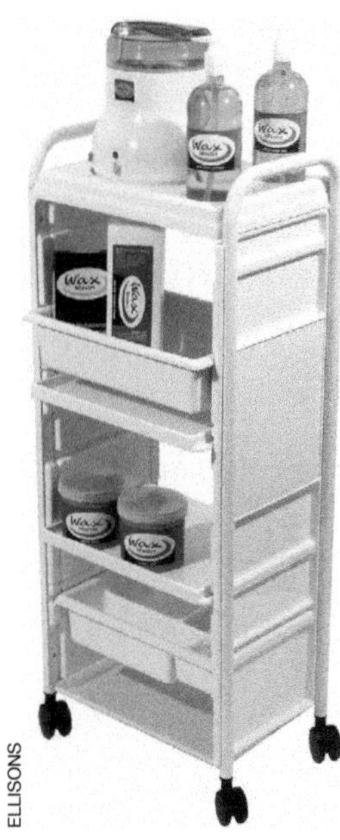

Waxing trolley

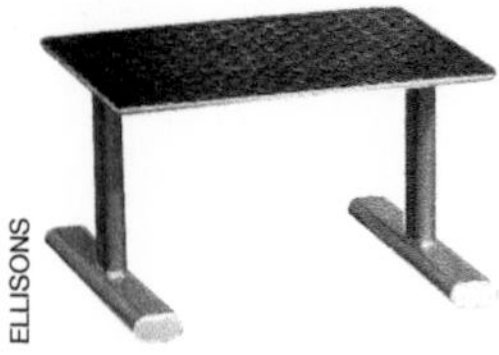

Client step

TOP TIP

Jobs for the day

One of your first tasks at the start of the day will be to switch on the wax heater so that it is ready for the first client. Forgetting to do this will cause unnecessary delay.

You may need to cut wax strips to size for different body parts. However, strips are available for purchase in different sizes.

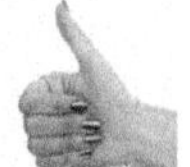

BEST PRACTICE

Code of practice waxing services

The code of practice is a guide for the minimum level of health and safety required for waxing services. It is important to be aware of current health and safety requirements when preparing and maintaining the area for waxing services.

Preparing the treatment work area

1 The area should be clean and tidy. The trolley should be stable and wires placed to avoid trips.

2 Check the temperature of the working area: the client must not be too warm or they will sweat, which will affect the success of the wax application to the skin. Increase ventilation in the service area as necessary to keep the temperature suitable for the service. This will vary dependent upon each salon some will have air conditioning or rely on natural air ventilation.

3 There should be a clean, empty covered bin in the service area, lined with a heavy duty polythene bin liner. Where contaminated waste is collected this bag is yellow to identify what it contains and how the waste should be disposed of.

4 Disinfect all work surfaces including the couch surface and cover them with clean, disposable paper tissue.

5 Prepare cotton wool: provide a selection of damp and dry cotton wool on the trolley, usually in small bowls which must be covered to keep clean and hygienic.

6 The couch should be covered with a clean plastic protective sheet. Disposable paper-tissue bedroll should be placed over the plastic sheet for additional protection and comfort.

7 Place a towel neatly on the couch to protect the client's clothing and to cover them when they have undressed.

8 Check the trolley to make sure it contains everything that is needed to carry out the service.

9 Collect metal tools, e.g. scissors and tweezers from the UV cabinet (having been previously sterilized) and put them into a disinfecting solution on the trolley.

10 The wax must be at a suitable temperature for use (heated as recommended by the manufacturer according to wax type and system, allow enough time for this):

- **warm wax** is heated in a wax heater to between 43°C and 48°C – when it should be warm and fluid in consistency. An individual cartridge/tube of warm **wax** is heated on a medium setting in a heating and storage compartment until it reaches a fluid consistency.
- **hot wax** is heated to 50°C
- **strip sugar** wax is heated to 43–48°C
- **sugar paste** is heated in the microwave or heater, following the manufacturer's guidelines, until it is soft.

11 If the client has a mobility issue then assistance should be provided to get onto the couch. This may be small steps or you may have a hydraulic bed which can be electronically raised and lowered.

12 Position the couch according to the part to be treated. The couch should be in the sit-up position, unless the client is only having their bikini line or underarm areas waxed, in which case it should be flat. The couch can be adjusted later for client comfort when preparing them for their waxing service.

13 Collect the client's record card and place on the service trolley.

14 Confirm that preparation of the work area meets with the senior beauty therapist's satisfaction.

Maintaining the treatment work area

Clean, tidy and leave the work area in a suitable condition for further services.

- Dispose of used wax materials after use.
- If the cartridge/tube warm wax system has been used, replace the disposable applicator or clean the roller applicator head if used according to manufacturer's instructions. So it is ready for the next client.
- Clean the wax heaters using equipment cleaner, thoroughly removing any wax spillages. Ensure this is used safely as it is highly flammable and must not enter the wax when cleaning the wax heater.
- Dispose of the paper-tissue bedroll.
- Wipe the plastic couch cover with surgical spirit and clean cotton wool to remove any wax spillages.
- Empty the bin that was used to collect waste in the service area. Replace the polythene bin liner with a new one.
- Remove used metal tools from the work area so that they can be sterilized in the autoclave. First wipe the surface of the tools with clean cotton wool and surgical spirit.
- Disinfect work surfaces.
- Disposable waste from waxing might have body fluids on it; potentially it is a health risk. It must be handled, collected and disposed of according to the COSHH procedures, Habia code of practice, training by the employer and local environment agency in accordance with the Controlled Waste Regulations (1992). Disposable protective gloves must be worn when cleaning up and disposing of waste products and materials after the service; they will help protect you from contact with body fluids and contamination.
- Protective towels should be removed from the service area and should be laundered.
- Return the client record card to the secure storage area for client data.

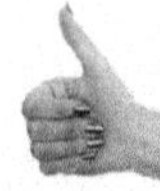

BEST PRACTICE

You may wish to use disposable gloves for hygiene and personal protection when carrying out maintenance of the waxing area.

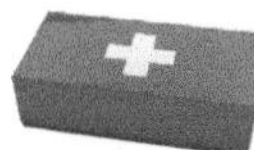

HEALTH & SAFETY

Contaminated waste
A yellow sharps container or heavy duty yellow sack should be available for waste contaminated with blood or tissue fluids.

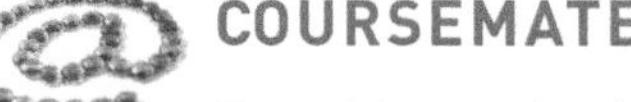

COURSEMATE

For a video on cleaning up, please see this book's accompanying CourseMate.

Ongoing maintenance

- Check the wax level in the different wax heaters regularly, and replenish with new wax as necessary. This should be done in advance of the next service application so that the wax is at the correct temperature and working consistency and there is enough wax to carry out at the next service.
- Check that there is enough stock i.e. wax, spatulas, strips, disposable gloves and apron and tell the relevant person if supplies seem low. So that replacement stock can be ordered.
- At the end of the working day, switch off the wax heater.

Preparing and maintaining the salon treatment work area for eye services

Eye services involve preparation for any of the following services:

- eyebrow shaping
- eyelash and eyebrow permanent tinting
- eyelash extension application, either strip lashes or individual flare lashes.

TOP TIP

Pointed tweezers are ideal for precisely applying individual flare lashes

Eyebrow shaping

Eyebrow shaping service involves removing the brow hair, to maintain a shape or create a new shape. Hairs are removed using small metal tools called tweezers. There are two types – manual and automatic:

- manual tweezers remove stray hairs and are used to define the brow shape
- automatic tweezers (as shown in the photos of tweezing below) are designed to remove the bulk of unwanted hair, they have a spring-loaded action.

Cengage Learning

Tweezing between the brows with automatic tweezers

Cengage Learning

Tweezing using manual tweezers to define the finished eyebrow shape

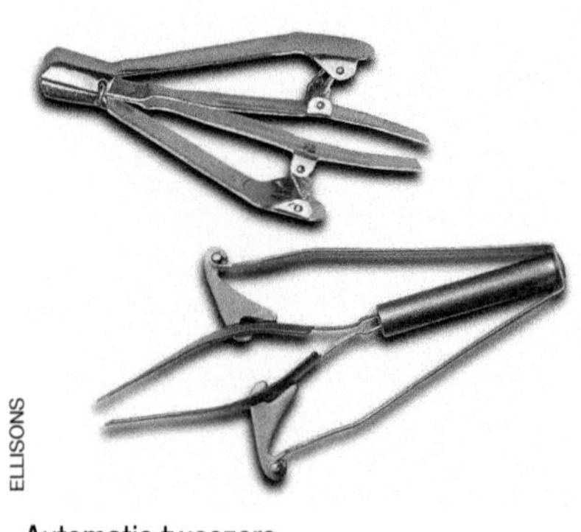

ELLISONS

Automatic tweezers

Eyelash and eyebrow tinting

In the **eyelash and eyebrow tinting service** the hairs of the eyelashes and eyebrows are permanently coloured using a dye to improve the appearance of the eye area making the hair more obvious. The tinting service can be performed on the eyelashes, the eyebrow area or to both.

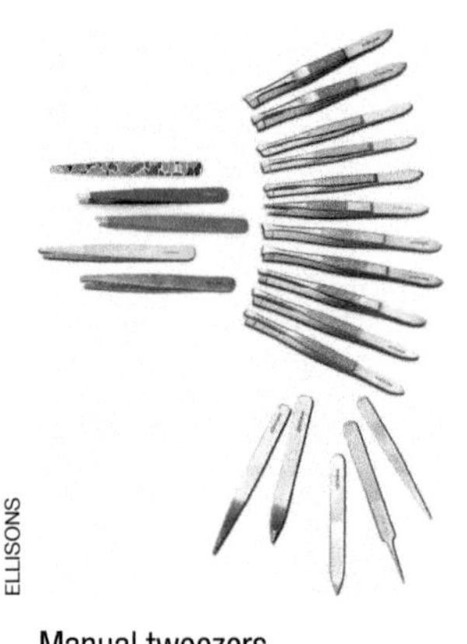

ELLISONS

Manual tweezers

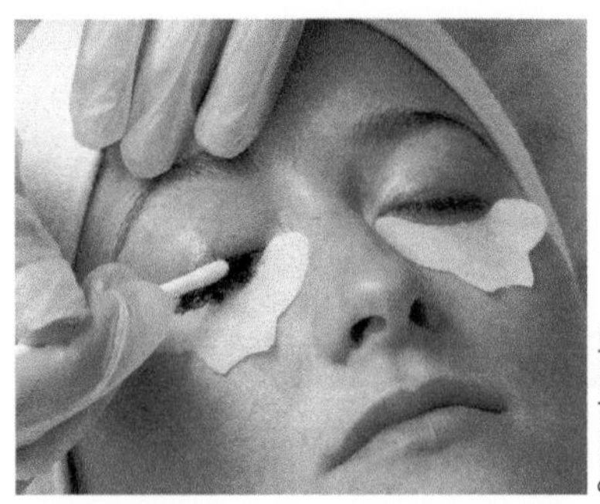

Cengage Learning

The eyelash tint applied which will darken the natural eyelashes

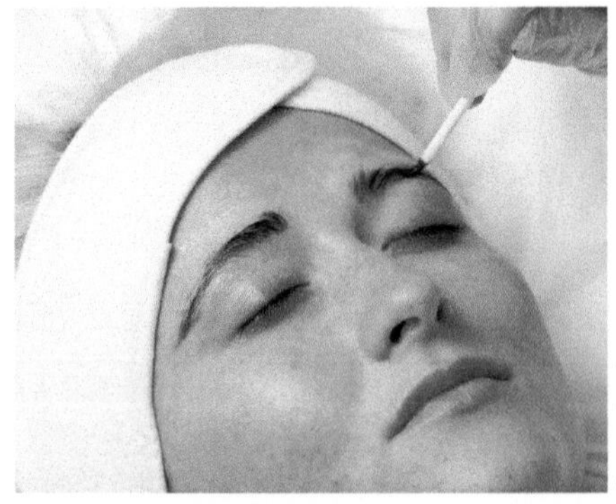

Cengage Learning

The eyebrow tint applied which will darken the natural eyebrows

The eyelashes will look longer and thicker after the service. The eyebrows will look thicker and darker as all hairs in the area are permanently coloured. The eyebrows can be shaped following colouring to the desired shape.

TOP TIP

Brow hairs

Brow hairs can be removed quickly using wax, which is basically mass tweezing.

Eyelash extensions

Eyelash extensions are threads of artificial hair which are attached to the client's natural lashes, imitating the natural eyelashes and making them appear longer and thicker.

There are three types – semi-permanent individual flare and single lashes and strip lashes:

- strip lashes, are designed to be worn for a short time period, e.g. a day
- individual flare and single lashes can be worn for up to 4 weeks. In-fill lashes may be required to replace lost lashes and maintain the look.

Positioning the strip lash to the upper lid lash hair following make-up application

Sterilization and disinfection

- Small metal tools such as tweezers and scissors (needed to trim long hair) should be sterilized after use. Clean them with surgical spirit and clean cotton wool and then sterilize them in the autoclave. Store them in the UV cabinet or clean, covered, lined container after sterilization, ready for use.
- Applicators for permanent tinting ideally should be disposable, and thrown away after use. If a non-disposable brush is used this must be cleaned with a professional brush cleaner and then placed in the UV cabinet to remove the majority of microorganisms.
- Disinfect bowl for mixing permanent tint before use.
- Towels and headbands should be boil washed to destroy harmful microorganisms and prevent cross-infection. Disposable headbands are ideal as these are thrown away after use.
- Wash your hands before handling clean equipment.

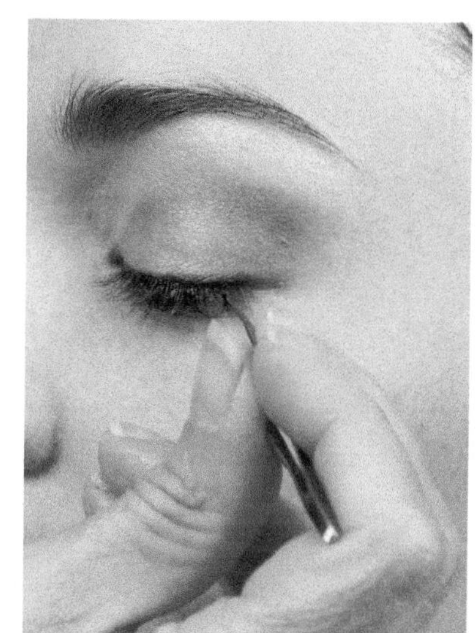

Applying an individual flare lash to the upper lid lash hair following make-up application

TOP TIP

Sterilized equipment

Always have more than one pair of sterilized tweezers and scissors available.

A clean, sterile pair will be required if the beauty therapist drops the tweezers they are using on the floor.

If using a non-disposable applicator brush for permanent tinting, several brushes will be required to allow for effective cleaning.

Refer to the equipment and materials checklist to make sure that you have all that is required to perform each eye service.

EQUIPMENT AND MATERIALS CHECKLIST FOR THE EYE SERVICES, EYEBROW SHAPING, PERMANENT TINTING AND EYELASH EXTENSIONS

		EYEBROW SHAPING	*PERMANENT TINTING*	*EYELASH EXTENSIONS*
ELLISONS	Couch – with sit-up and lie-down positions and an easy-to-clean surface	☐	☐	☐

		EYEBROW SHAPING	*PERMANENT TINTING*	*EYELASH EXTENSIONS*
SORISA	Trolley – to hold all the necessary equipment and materials	☐	☐	☐
ELLISONS	Medium-sized towels to protect the client's clothing	☐	☐	☐
ELLISONS	Disposable tissue roll to cover the trolley surface	☐	☐	☐
ELLISONS	Headband to protect the client's hair from any chemical services and to keep scalp hair away from the eye area	☐	☐	☐
	Non-oily eye make-up remover to cleanse the eye area (also to prevent it causing difficulty when carrying out tinting service as oil will cause a barrier)	☐	☐	☐
ELLISONS	Damp cotton wool for cleansing the service area, removing service products and to protect the skin	☐	☐	☐
ELLISONS	Facial tissues, for blotting dry the skin/eyelashes	☐	☐	☐
SORISA	Magnifier lamp (cold) to enlarge the appearance of the service area when performing eyebrow shaping making it easier to see the hair that needs to be removed	☐		
	Disposable spatulas to remove cosmetic products from containers		☐	

		EYEBROW SHAPING	*PERMANENT TINTING*	*EYELASH EXTENSIONS*
ELLISONS	Cotton buds to apply and remove products from the area	☐	☐	☐
ELLISONS	Tweezers – manual and automatic	☐		☐
ELLISONS	Disposable gloves; these may be worn when performing an eyebrow shape to avoid contact with body tissue fluids. They may also be worn to protect the hands against contact with chemicals that could cause skin irritation for a beauty therapist with allergies to the product ingredients	☐		
ELLISONS	A jar of disinfecting solution to hold small metal tools following sterilization	☐		☐
CLEAN+EASY	Antiseptic cleansing lotion to prepare and disinfect the area before eyebrow hair removal to reduce the possibility of infection	☐		
ELLISONS	Soothing antiseptic lotion or cream to reduce redness and assist skin healing following eyebrow hair removal	☐		
BEAUTY EXPRESS LTD	Coloured permanent tints, available in black, brown, blue and grey		☐	

		EYEBROW SHAPING	*PERMANENT TINTING*	*EYELASH EXTENSIONS*
SALON SYSTEMS	Hydrogen peroxide – 10 vol, 3% strength		☐	
BEAUTY EXPRESS LTD	Petroleum jelly, to protect the skin from staining during eyelash tinting		☐	
SALON SYSTEMS	Eye shields to protect from skin staining or chemical irritation		☐	☐
ELLISONS	Non-metallic bowl to mix the permanent tint and hydrogen peroxide		☐	
	Disposable brushes to apply the permanent tint		☐	
SALON SYSTEMS	Surgical spirit to wipe the points of the tweezers to remove eyelash extension adhesive and to clean them before sterilization	☐		☐
BEAUTY EXPRESS LTD	Eyelash extension adhesive for strip lashes. Eyelash extension adhesive for individual flare lashes			☐
ELLISONS	Strip eyelash lengths in a selection of colours and lengths. Individual flare lashes in a selection of colours and lengths			☐

	EYEBROW SHAPING	*PERMANENT TINTING*	*EYELASH EXTENSIONS*
Eyelash adhesive solvent for the removal of individual false lashes			☐
Scissors to trim the length of the strip lash or trim long brow hair	☐		☐
Sterilized small dish lined with foil to place the eyelash adhesive in during lash application			☐
Hand mirror (clean) to discuss and agree the service plan and show the client the results	☐	☐	☐
Bin (swing-top) lined with a disposable bin liner	☐	☐	☐
Client's record card so that the client's details can be recorded before and after the service	☐	☐	☐
Aftercare leaflets – to provide guidance notes for the client to follow after the service	☐	☐	☐

HEALTH & SAFETY

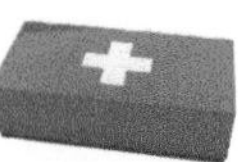

Storing chemicals safely

Do not put chemicals such as hydrogen peroxide near a wax heater on the trolley. The heat could affect the quality (and effectiveness) of the chemicals and they could even become dangerous if they are flammable.

Make sure you follow the COSHH (Control of Substances Hazardous to Health) guidelines on how equipment should be stored (see Chapter 2).

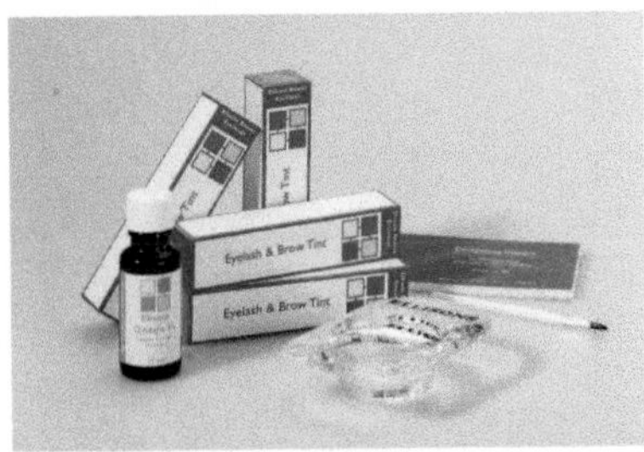

Eyelash tinting products

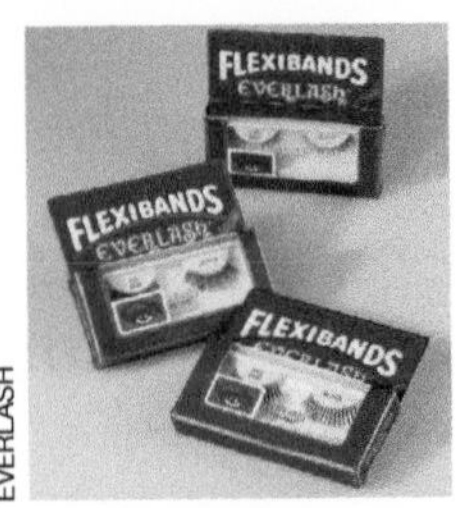

EVERLASH

Eyelash extensions

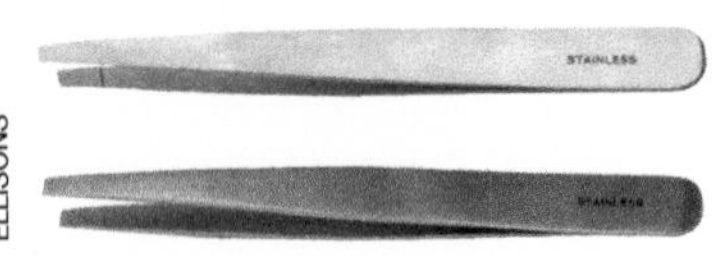

ELLISONS

Manual eyebrow shaping tweezers

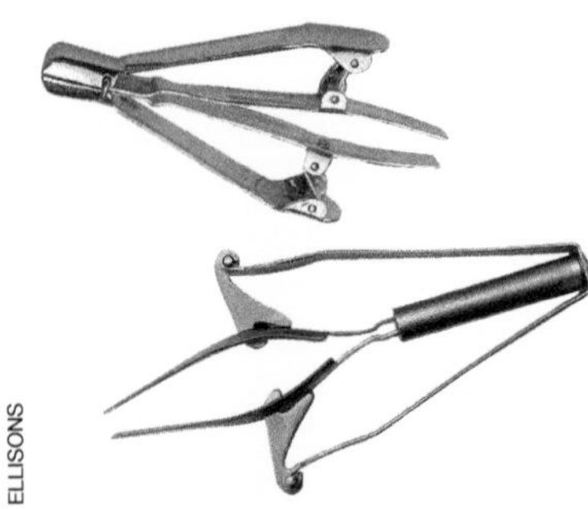

ELLISONS

Automatic eyebrow shaping tweezers

Preparing the work area

1. The area should be clean and tidy.
2. Check the temperature of the working area: the client must not be too warm. Increase ventilation as necessary.
3. There should be a clean, empty covered bin in the work area lined with a polythene bin liner.
4. Disinfect all work surfaces and cover with clean, disposable, paper tissue.
5. Check the trolley to make sure it contains everything that will be needed to carry out the service. The surface must be adequately protected to avoid accidental staining from the permanent tint.
6. Collect metal tools from the UV cabinet, put them into a disinfectant solution on the trolley.
7. Prepare cotton wool: provide a selection of damp and dry cotton wool on the trolley, usually in small bowls which must be covered to keep clean and hygienic.
8. Display the materials and products required for the eye service on the trolley surface.
9. The beauty couch or chair should be protected with a long strip of disposable bed-roll placed over a freshly laundered sheet or usually a clean towelling couch cover.
10. For eye services the head of the couch should be slightly raised, not flat. This ensures client and beauty therapy comfort whilst the service is carried out. Incorrect working position can lead to postural aches and pains and possible long-term injury
11. Adjust the lighting – the lighting must not be too bright to avoid causing the client's eyes to water.
12. A small towel should be placed neatly at the head of the couch – this will be draped across the client's chest for hygiene and protection during the service. The bedroll or sheet will need to be changed, and freshly laundered towels replaced, before the next client.
13. Collect the client's record card and put it on the service trolley. A skin test record should be recorded if the client is receiving a permanent tinting or eyelash extension service.
14. Confirm that preparation of the work area meets with the senior beauty therapist's satisfaction.

BEST PRACTICE

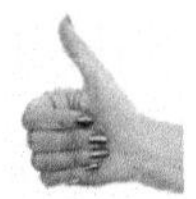

Protect the client's eyes with disposable eye shields when performing eyebrow shaping as the magnifying lamp if used may irritate the eyes.

Maintaining the work area

Clean, tidy and leave the work area in a suitable condition for further services.

- Dispose of the paper-tissue bedroll.
- Empty the bin that was used to collect waste in the work area. Replace the bin liner with a new one, if necessary. Handle carefully as permanent tinting materials will stain the skin or surfaces they come into contact with.

- Clean small bowls used to hold cotton wool in hot, soapy water; rinse the bowls and dry.
- It is a good idea to wear disposable protective gloves when cleaning up and disposing of waste products and materials after the service. Gloves help to avoid skin staining from permanent tint services and skin irritation from contact with chemicals used in the service.
- Clean small metal tools with surgical spirit and clean cotton wool before sterilizing them in the autoclave.
- Protective towels should be removed from the service area and laundered.
- Disinfect work surfaces.
- Return materials to the store area; ideally chemicals should be stored in a cool, dark, secure cupboard. Check that all bottle lids are tightly closed to prevent spillage and the product losing quality which will mean poor future results!
- If a product requires to be disposed of, i.e. the eyelash tint tube is empty, inform the relevant person for stock control before disposal and replacement. This will ensure adequate stock levels are maintained as replacement stock can be ordered.
- Return the client record card to the secure storage area for client data.

TOP TIP

Cleaning bowls

Care should be taken when cleaning bowls used for permanent tint, as the tint product will stain any materials it comes into contact with. Do not use your salon towels as they could be permanently stained.

TOP TIP

Eyelash extensions

Eyelash extensions may be required if applying an evening make-up or if extra definition is required for the eye area. Ask the beauty therapist if she will be requiring these. Place on the trolley, if required, when make-up service is being prepared for.

Preparing and maintaining the salon treatment work area for make-up service

Make-up is used to disguise and enhance the skin and facial features to help us achieve a particular look and also make a person feel more attractive and confident. Skilful application of different make-up products can reduce or draw attention to facial features and so create balance in the face. The final effect should always suit the client including her personality, lifestyle and the occasion for which the make-up is to be worn.

A large number of make-up products are available and a range should be available for the beauty therapist to select from to achieve the required effect.

Sterilization and disinfection

- Ensure tools and equipment are clean and sterile before use.
- Where possible, disposable applicators such as lip and mascara brushes are used during make-up application, and these should be costed into the service price. Make-up brushes should be cleaned after each use using a professional brush cleaner and then stored in the UV cabinet, ready for use.
- There should be at least three sets of make-up brushes available to allow for disinfection after each use. Brush cleaners care for and maintain brush hygiene and are a popular choice to maintain brush hygiene.
- Make-up sponges if made to do so, should be cleaned and disinfected after use, dried and stored in the UV cabinet, ready for use. Remember, many make-up sponges should be thrown away after use as they cannot be cleaned hygienically.
- The make-up palette should be placed in the UV cabinet after cleaning, ready for use. This is used to hold make-up products during application.

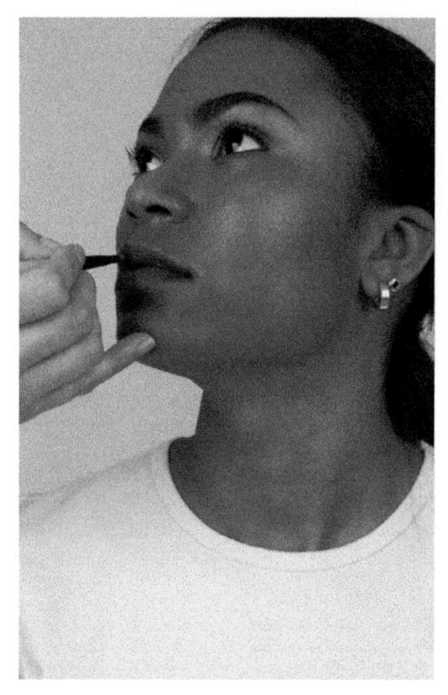

Make-up services

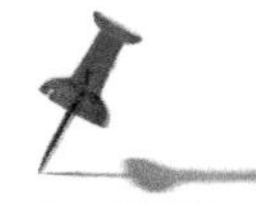

ALWAYS REMEMBER

Preparing make-up tools

Some salons have a professional make-up station with a shelf to place all the make-up products to be used.

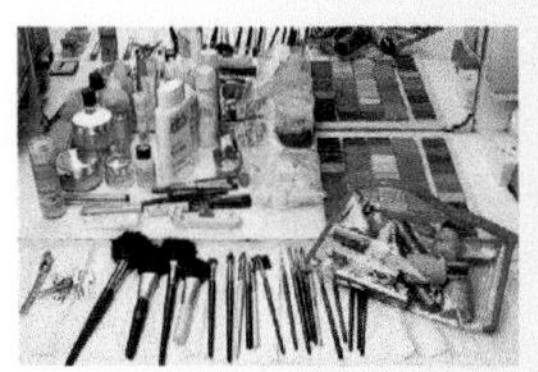

Make-up work station

- Cosmetic pencils, i.e. lip and eye pencils. should be sharpened before each use to make sure there is a fresh clean surface used for each client.
- Towels and headbands should be boil washed to destroy harmful microorganisms and prevent cross-infection. Often a headband is not used as it would spoil the hair if it has been styled. Large hair clips are ideal to keep scalp hair away from the client's face.
- Make-up capes used to protect the client's clothing, if made of fabric should be cleaned regularly.
- Wash your hands before handling clean equipment.

Refer to the equipment and materials checklist to make sure that you have all that is required for make-up service.

EQUIPMENT AND MATERIALS CHECKLIST FOR MAKE-UP SERVICE

SORISA	Couch, make-up station or beauty chair with sit-up and lie-down positions and an easy-to-clean surface	☐
SORISA	Trolley to hold all the necessary equipment and materials	☐
SORISA	A medium-sized towel or make-up cape to protect the client's clothing	☐
ELLISONS	Disposable tissue roll to cover the trolley surface	☐
ELLISONS	Headband to protect the client's hair and to keep hair away from the service area Hair clips to keep the client's hair away from the face area These can be used in preference to a headband Note: If the client has had her hair styled before make-up application, hair clips (in preference to a headband) will avoid spoiling the hair while offering protection from make-up products	☐

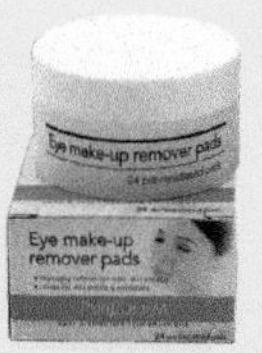

ELLISONS

Eye make-up remover – non-oily to cleanse the eye area to ensure effective make-up application and that the make-up will last ☐

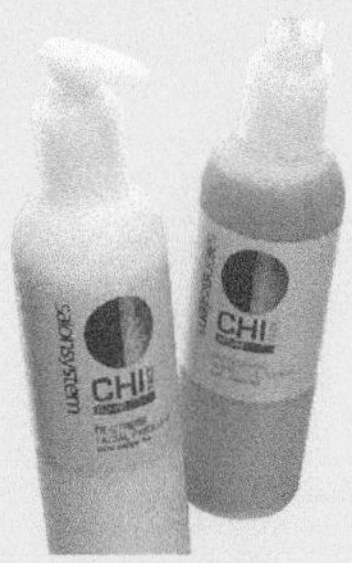

SALON SYSTEMS

Cleansing lotion – a range available to suit the different skin types: normal, dry, combination, oily, sensitive ☐

Toning lotion – a range available to suit the different skin types: normal, dry, combination, oily, sensitive ☐

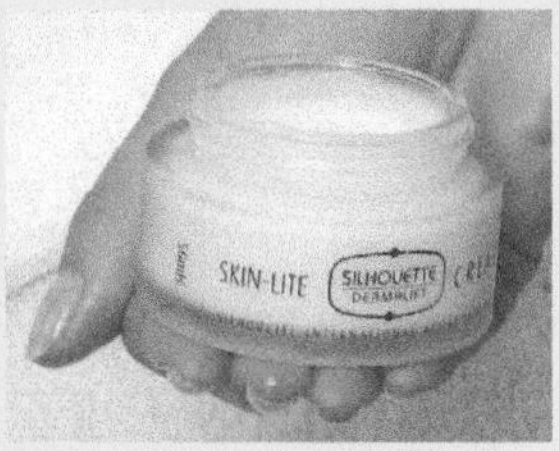

SILHOUETTE-DERMALIFT

Moisturiser – a range available to suit the different skin types: normal, dry, combination, oily, sensitive ☐

Note: Moisturiser should be a light formulation. If it is too oily the make-up will not last. Skin primers are popular to prepare the skin for make-up application

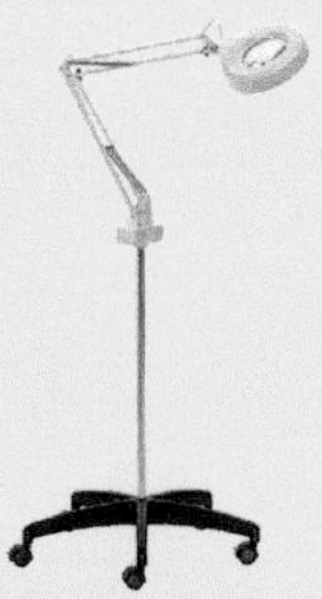

SORISA

Magnifying lamp to inspect the skin more closely following cleansing to identify any areas that require attention ☐

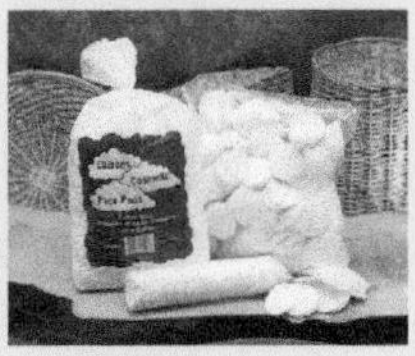

ELLISONS

Damp and dry cotton wool prepared for each client to apply and remove cleansing and make-up products ☐

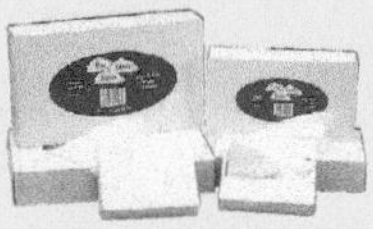

ELLISONS

Large white facial tissues to blot the skin after facial toning, and to protect the skin during make-up application ☐

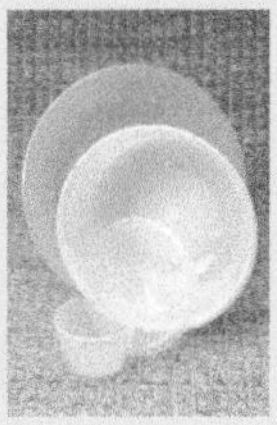

ELLISONS

Bowls to hold the prepared cotton wool ☐

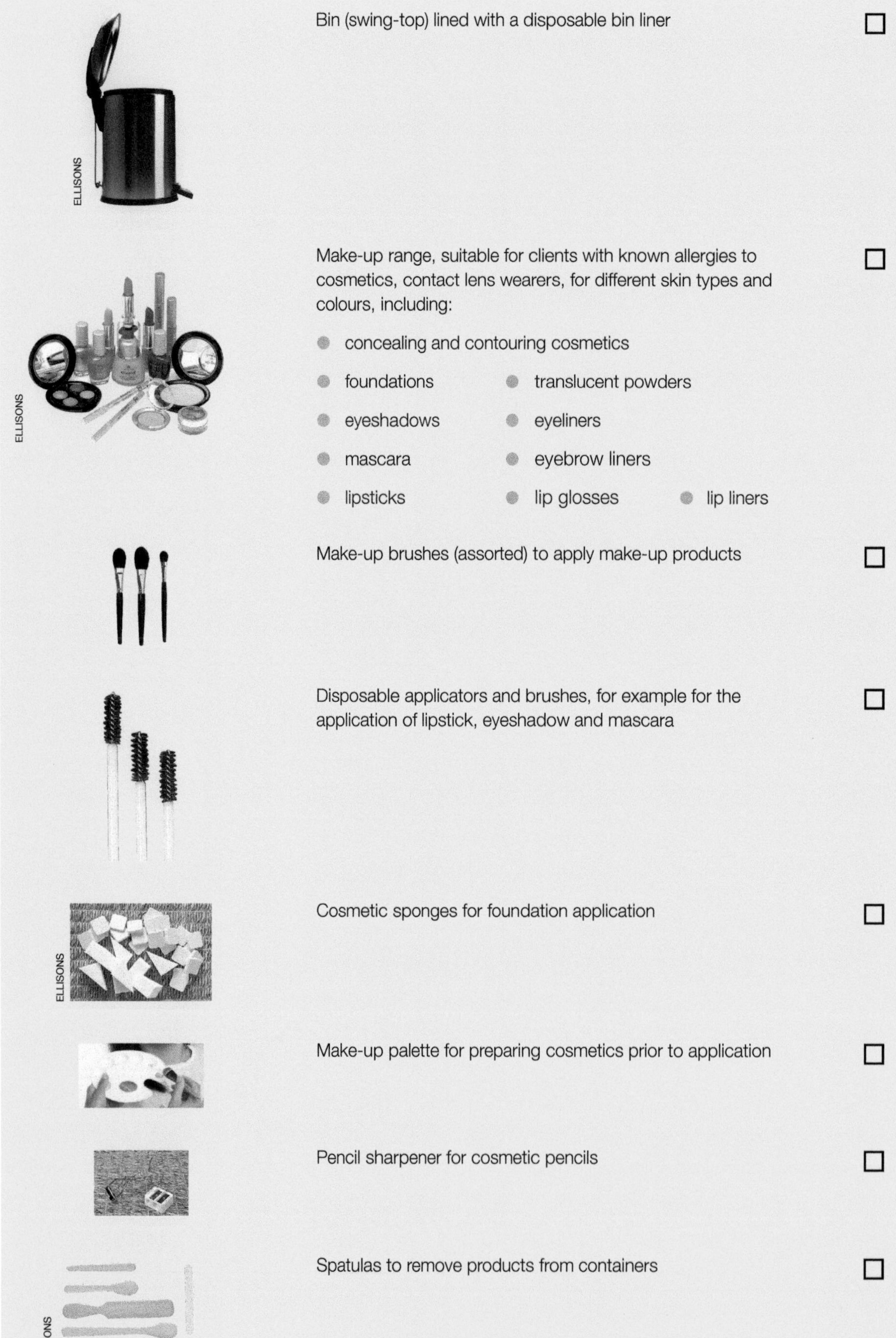

Bin (swing-top) lined with a disposable bin liner ☐

Make-up range, suitable for clients with known allergies to cosmetics, contact lens wearers, for different skin types and colours, including: ☐

- concealing and contouring cosmetics
- foundations
- translucent powders
- eyeshadows
- eyeliners
- mascara
- eyebrow liners
- lipsticks
- lip glosses
- lip liners

Make-up brushes (assorted) to apply make-up products ☐

Disposable applicators and brushes, for example for the application of lipstick, eyeshadow and mascara ☐

Cosmetic sponges for foundation application ☐

Make-up palette for preparing cosmetics prior to application ☐

Pencil sharpener for cosmetic pencils ☐

Spatulas to remove products from containers ☐

Orange sticks to remove products from small containers such as eyeshadows	☐
Mirror (clean) to discuss and show the client ongoing and at the end the effects achieved	☐
Client record card so that the client's details can be recorded before and after the service	☐
Aftercare leaflets – to provide guidance notes for the client to refer to on make-up products selected and their application to achieve the final result	☐

ELLISONS

Preparing the work area

1 The area should be clean and tidy.

2 There should be a clean covered, empty bin in the work area lined with a polythene bin liner.

3 Disinfect all work surfaces and cover with clean, disposable, paper tissue.

4 Check the trolley to make sure it has all that is needed to carry out the service.

5 Collect make-up tools from the UV cabinet, brushes, palette and sponges and place on the trolley.

6 Prepare cotton wool: provide a selection of damp and dry cotton wool placed on the trolley, usually held in small bowls which must be covered to keep clean and hygienic.

7 Adjust the lighting – the room should be well lit for make-up application.

8 Check the room temperature. Good ventilation is important – it should not be too warm or this will affect the application and durability of the make-up. Increase ventilation as necessary.

9 Place all equipment and materials on the trolley or work surface in front of a make-up mirror.

HEALTH & SAFETY

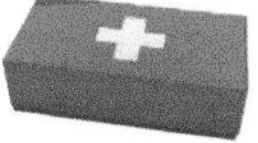

Disinfection in the UV cabinet
Allow 20 minutes for each side of an object to be disinfected in the UV cabinet. Thus 40 minutes is required for effective disinfection. Allow time for this process.

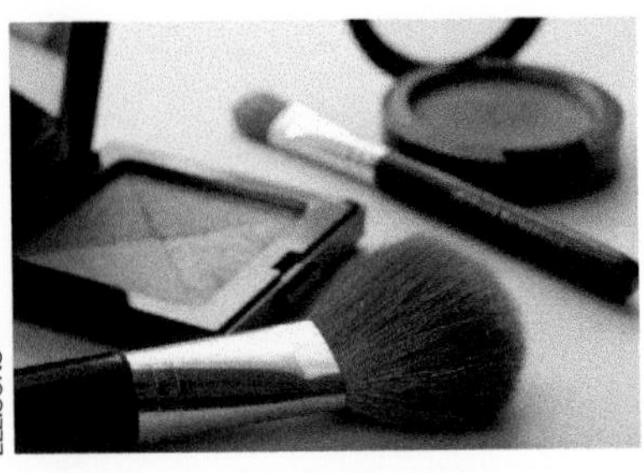
ELLISONS

Make-up products and brushes

10 Check the quality of the make-up sponges, replace with new ones if necessary. Make up sponges can only be used again if they are designed for this purpose and can be cleaned hygienically.

11 Sharpen make-up pencils to expose a non-contaminated clean surface.

12 Collect the client's record card and put it on the trolley.

13 Confirm that preparation of the work area meets with the senior beauty therapist's satisfaction.

Maintaining the work area

Clean, tidy and leave the work area in a suitable condition for further services.

- Dispose of the paper-tissue bedroll.
- Empty the bin that was used to collect waste in the work area. Replace the bin liner with a new one.
- Clean small bowls in hot, soapy water; rinse the bowls and dry.
- Clean the make-up brushes and make-up sponges in warm water and detergent; rinse thoroughly in clean water and allow them to dry naturally. Once dry, place in the UV cabinet. A professional alcohol-based brush cleaner can be used to clean brushes. The brushes are first cleaned as above. When dry they are briefly immersed in the alcohol solution and are then allowed to dry before placing in the UV cabinet.
- Clean the make-up palette in warm water and detergent, it might be necessary to remove stubborn marks with surgical spirit and clean cotton wool. Place in the UV cabinet.
- Ensure that the make-up products are clean, use a damp piece of cotton wool and surgical spirit to clean palettes and containers.
- Ensure the make-up mirror is clean; clean with a suitable cleaning product.
- Disinfect work surfaces.
- Protective towels and headband, if used, should be removed from the work area and laundered.
- If a product needs to be disposed of, e.g. mascara, inform the relevant person for stock control before disposal and replacement. This will ensure adequate stock levels are maintained as replacement stock can be ordered.
- Return the client record card to the secure storage area for client data.

HEALTH & SAFETY

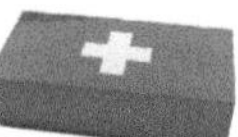

Laundry
Dirty laundry should be placed in a covered container until cleaned.

Preparing and maintaining the salon treatment work area for nail services

You are required to prepare and maintain the work area for the following nail services:

- manicure
- pedicure
- nail art
- nail enhancements.

Manicure is a service which aims to improve the appearance and condition of the hands, nails and skin.

Pedicure is a service which aims to improve the appearance and condition of the feet, nails and skin.

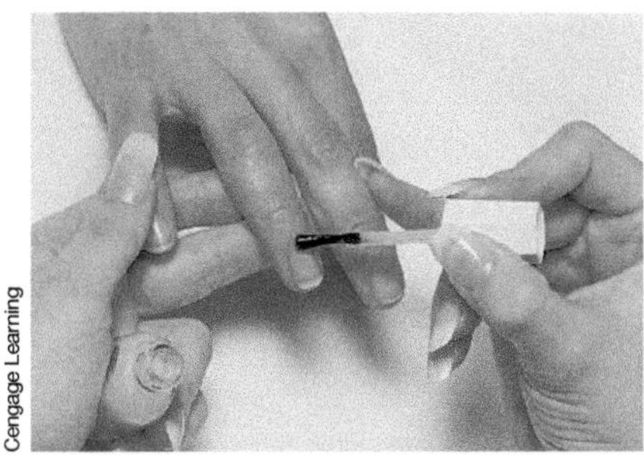

Cengage Learning

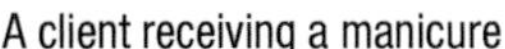

A client receiving a manicure

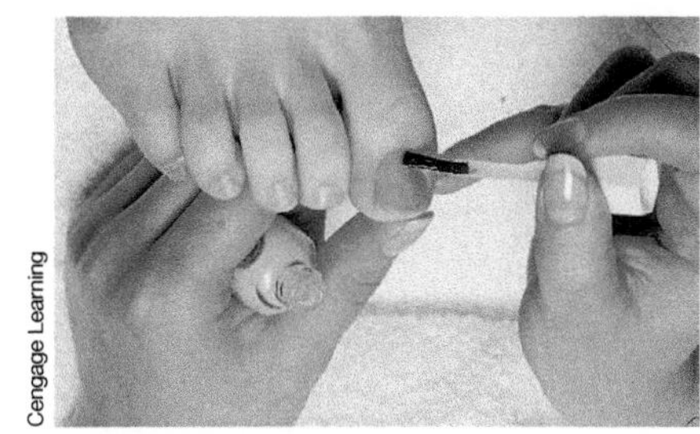

Cengage Learning

A client receiving a pedicure

In addition to the basic manicure and pedicure procedures, specialist therapeutic services may be applied.

These include:

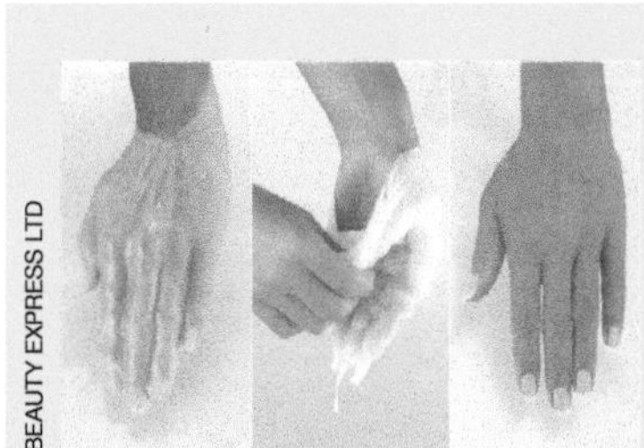

BEAUTY EXPRESS LTD

Paraffin wax service, a heat therapy service in which the hand or foot has heated liquid paraffin wax applied. This sets and creates a heat-maintaining barrier for the skin. It takes approximately 20 minutes for the wax to melt to the correct consistency for use, so this must be prepared well in advance of use.

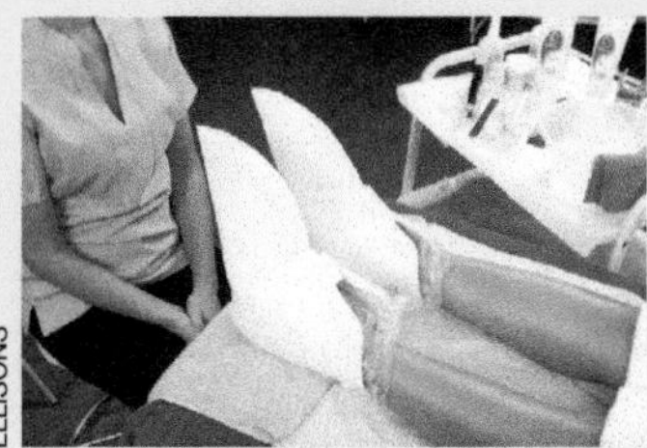

ELLISONS

Thermal booties, insulated boots for the feet are electrically heated to aid the absorption of service products to condition the skin of the feet.

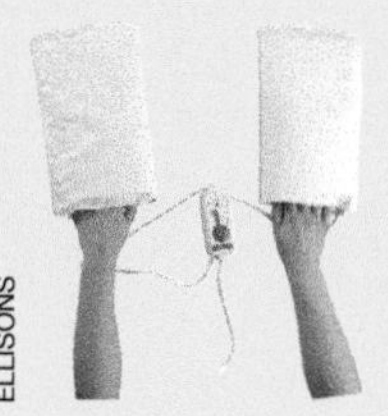

ELLISONS

Thermal mitts, insulated gloves for the hands are electrically heated to aid the absorption of skincare products to condition the skin of the hands and nails.

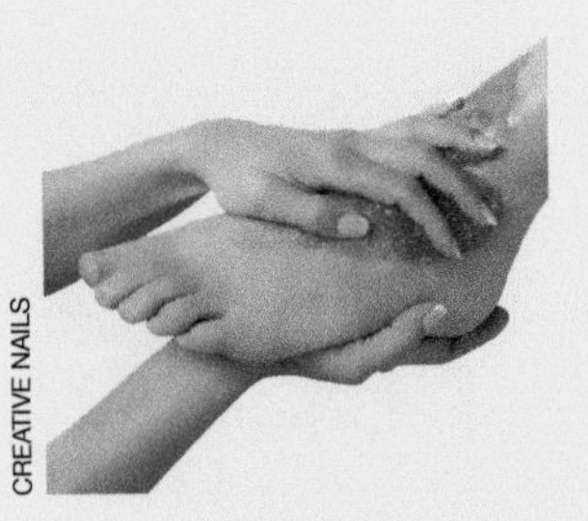
CREATIVE NAILS

Exfoliator cream can be applied to remove dead skin from the skin's surface which also softens the skin. The skin appears brighter after use as newer skin is shown.

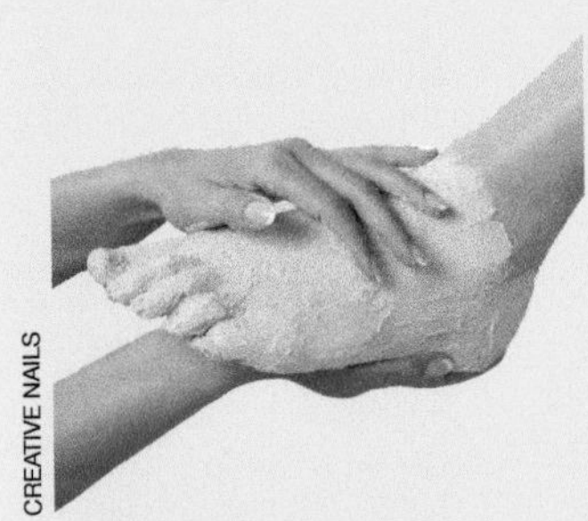
CREATIVE NAILS

Service masks, selected to stimulate, refresh or nourish the skin. The hands can be placed in thermal mitts to further improve the effects achieved.

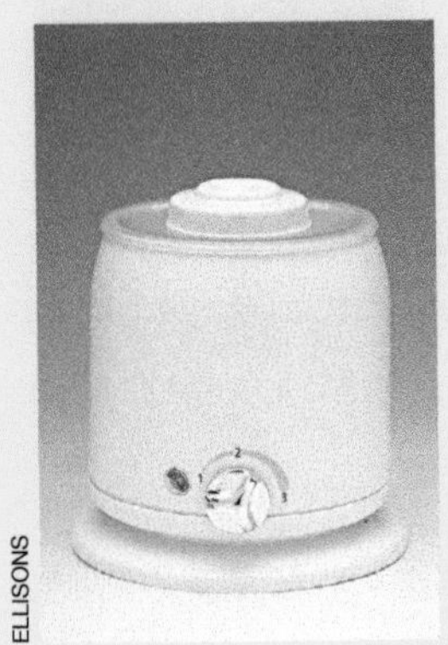
ELLISONS

Warm oil, oil is gently heated and applied to soften the skin and cuticles (the skin surrounding the nails). The hands can then be massaged using the oil as a hand massage medium.

TOP TIP

Exfoliator

The use of an exfoliator removes dead skin which naturally create a barrier to the absorption of other products. By removing the dead skin the effects of the product are improved. An exfoliator can be used on both the hands and the feet.

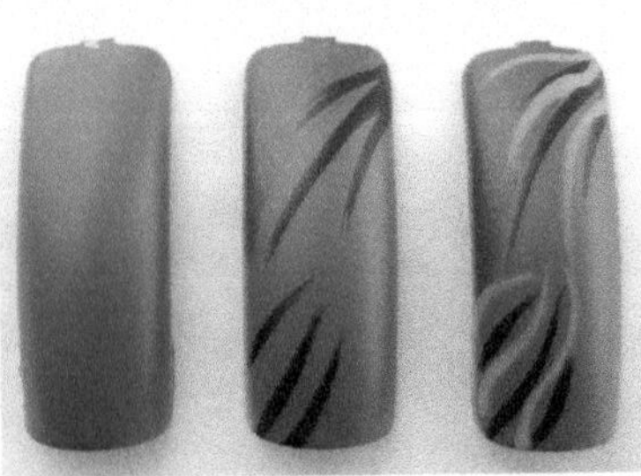
Basic nail art application technique called striping

Nail art

Nail art is decoration of the nails of the client's hands and feet applied to the natural or artificial nail, using nail art materials including nail polish, transfers, gemstones, glitters and foil to achieve different designs and effects.

Nail enhancement is where the nail is lengthened, strengthened or repaired using different nail enhancement systems. These include tips (plastic nail tips used to increase the length of the nail) and overlays (a thin coating applied to the natural nail or an application over the natural nail and tip) to create a natural finish.

The systems may be UV gel, liquid and powder or wrap.

Refer to the equipment and materials checklist to make sure that you have all that is required to perform each nail service.

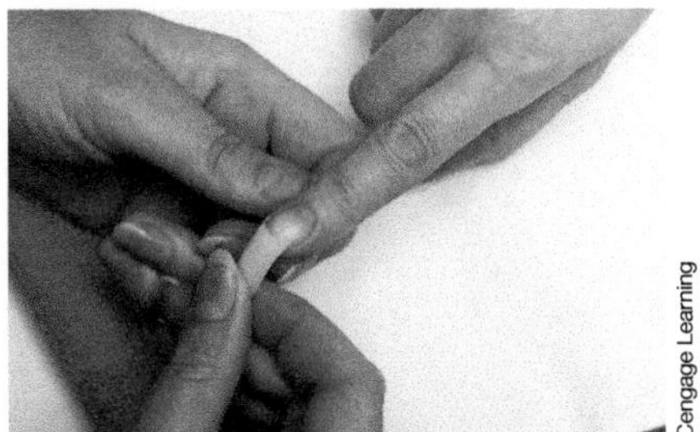

Cengage Learning

Nail tips

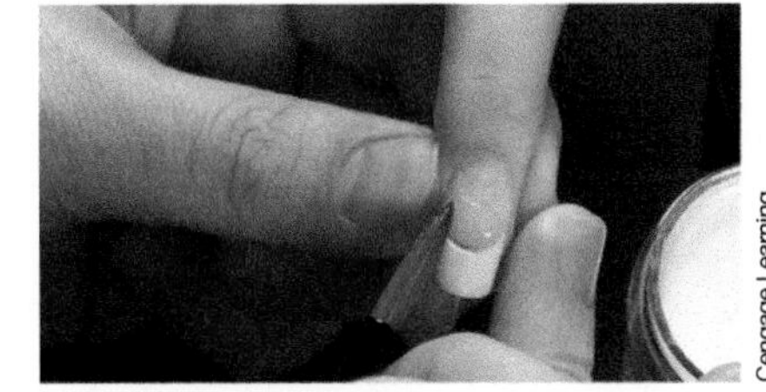

Cengage Learning

Nail tips and overlays

EQUIPMENT AND MATERIALS CHECKLIST FOR THE NAIL SERVICES: MANICURE, PEDICURE, NAIL ART AND NAIL ENHANCEMENTS

		MANICURE	*PEDICURE*	*NAIL ART*	*NAIL ENHANCEMENTS*
ELLISONS	Nail service table or trolley	☐	☐	☐	☐
THE DAYLIGHT COMPANY LTD	Lamp to improve lighting in the area for close work	☐	☐	☐	☐
BEAUTY EXPRESS LTD	Medium-sized towels: three for manicure, nail art, nail enhancements, five for pedicure	☐	☐	☐	☐
ELLISONS	Manicure pad or disposable tissue placed over the towels	☐	☐	☐	☐
ELLISONS	Small bowls lined with tissues (3) for clean cotton wool	☐	☐	☐	☐

		MANICURE	*PEDICURE*	*NAIL ART*	*NAIL ENHANCEMENTS*
ELLISONS	Dry cotton wool to apply and remove products	☐	☐	☐	☐
ELLISONS	Finger bowl for the client's fingers – to cleanse and soften the skin in warm water	☐		☐	
ELLISONS	Foot bowl or spa for the client's feet – to cleanse and soften the skin in warm water		☐		
ELLISONS	Emery board to file the nails to shape	☐	☐	☐	
ELLISONS	Files for nail enhancement service used for reducing and shaping the length of the nail tip and blending to create a smooth surface. The coarseness or 'grit' is graded dependent upon their purpose. A selection should be available				☐
ELLISONS	Blocks and buffers to provide a smooth, shiny surface to the nail surface during nail enhancement application				☐
ELLISONS	Orange sticks, tipped at either end with cotton wool, to apply products to the nails and to clean the nail	☐	☐	☐	☐
	Spatulas to remove products hygienically from their containers	☐	☐	☐	☐

	MANICURE	*PEDICURE*	*NAIL ART*	*NAIL ENHANCEMENTS*
Cuticle knife to remove skin from the nail	☐	☐	☐	☐
Hoof stick to push back the skin (the cuticle) around the bottom of the nail	☐	☐	☐	☐
Cuticle nippers to remove and neaten the appearance of overgrown cuticle	☐	☐	☐	☐
Nail scissors used to reduce the length of the nails, also to cut nail art and nail enhancement wrap material to size	☐		☐	☐
Tip cutters to cut the artificial nail structure to size				☐
Toenail clippers to shorten the length of the toenails		☐	☐	☐
Plastic glasses to protect the eyes when cutting the nails or reducing the length of nail tips	☐	☐	☐	☐
Safety mask to avoid the inhalation of nail dust when performing nail enhancement service				☐
Buffers to give the nail a sheen and to increase blood circulation to the nail	☐			
Tweezers to place and fix decorations to the nail			☐	

ELLISONS

ISTOCK/PROLL MEDIENDESIGN & FOTOGRAFIE

		MANICURE	PEDICURE	NAIL ART	NAIL ENHANCEMENTS
SALON SYSTEMS	Buffing paste, a coarse gritty nail product used to shine the nail plate when used with the buffer	☐			
ELLISONS	Detergent, to add to the warm water in the finger bowl or foot spa to cleanse and refresh the skin	☐	☐	☐	
ELLISONS	Callus file to remove excess skin from the feet		☐		
MAVALA	Hand cream, oil or lotion to soften and nourish the skin	☐			
CREATIVE NAILS	Foot cream, oil or lotion to soften and nourish the skin		☐		
SALON SYSTEMS	Skin/nail disinfectant to cleanse the skin/nail before service	☐	☐	☐	☐
	Base coat polish to provide a base to apply coloured polish and to prevent nail staining	☐	☐	☐	☐
JESSICA NAILS	Coloured polishes, a selection	☐	☐	☐	☐

		MANICURE	*PEDICURE*	*NAIL ART*	*NAIL ENHANCEMENTS*
MAVALA	Top coat to seal and protect nail polish colour providing durability	☐	☐	☐	☐
SALON SYSTEMS	Specialist nail service products such as nail strengthener	☐	☐	☐	
MAVALA	Non-acetone nail polish remover, to remove nail polish from the nail. Non-acetone formulation required for nail enhancements	☐	☐	☐	☐
SALON SYSTEMS	Nail polish drier to increase the speed of the polish hardening process	☐	☐	☐	☐
SALON SYSTEMS	Nail art materials Paints – specialist water-based paints Glitters Glitter dust and mixer – to add shimmer and create a design			☐	
MILLENIUM NAILS	Transfers – these may be either water-release (water will be required to apply them) or self-adhesive			☐	

		MANICURE	PEDICURE	NAIL ART	NAIL ENHANCEMENTS
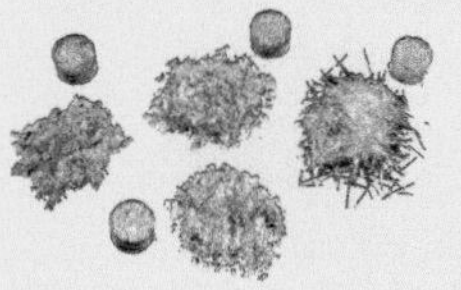 MILLENIUM NAILS	Foil strips, rolls or strips of metallic foil in various colours and designs, applied with a foil adhesive				
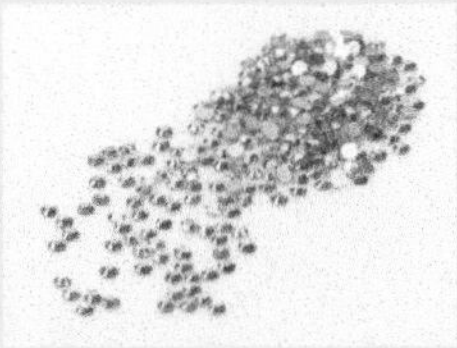 STAR NAILS	Polish secures – jewellery and tiny gems				
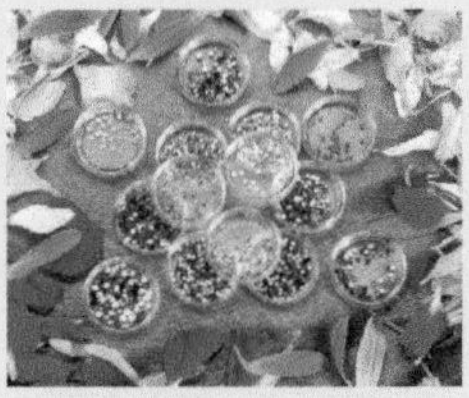	Gem stones such as rhinestones and flat stones				
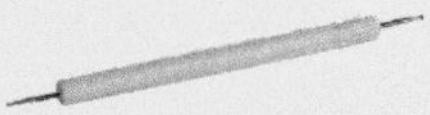 STAR NAILS	Dotting/marbling tool – used to apply dots of colour to the nail and to mix colours called 'marbling'				
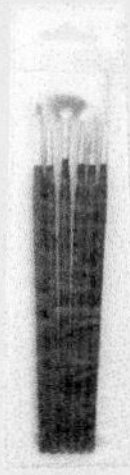	Nail art brushes to achieve different nail art application effects				
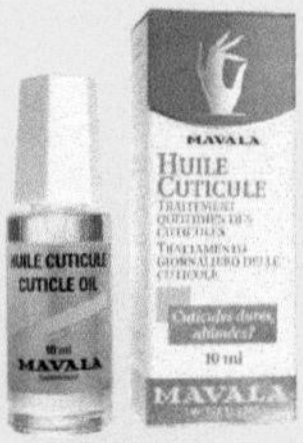 MAVALA	Cuticle remover to soften the skin of the cuticle and to aid its removal	☐	☐		
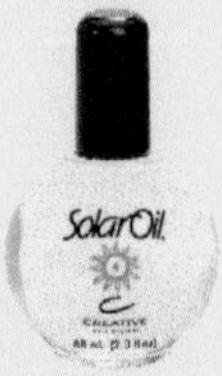 CREATIVE NAILS	Cuticle oil to soften and nourish the skin of the cuticle	☐	☐	☐	☐

		MANICURE	*PEDICURE*	*NAIL ART*	*NAIL ENHANCEMENTS*
	Cuticle massage cream to soften and nourish the skin of the cuticle	☐	☐		
SALON SYSTEMS	Jar of disinfecting solution to hold small metal and plastic nail service tools	☐	☐	☐	☐
SALON SYSTEMS	Paraffin wax service, specialist skin and nail service	☐	☐		
ELLISONS	Thermal booties, specialist skin and nail service		☐		
ELLISONS	Thermal mitts, specialist skin and nail service	☐	☐	☐	☐
SALON SYSTEMS	Exfoliator cream to remove dead skin cells from the service area	☐	☐		
CREATIVE NAILS	Service masks, specialist skin service	☐	☐		

		MANICURE	PEDICURE	NAIL ART	NAIL ENHANCEMENTS
BEAUTY EXPRESS LTD	Warm oil service, specialist skin and nail service	☐			
BEAUTY EXPRESS LTD	Plastic bags or plastic film to wrap the hands/feet after the application of a heat or service mask	☐	☐		
ELLISONS	Bin (swing-top) – lined with a disposable polythene bin liner	☐	☐	☐	☐
ELLISONS	Dappen dish – small glass dish to hold products during nail enhancement and nail art service application			☐	☐
SALON SYSTEMS	Nail tips: assorted styles and sizes				☐
SALON SYSTEMS	Adhesive to attach nail tips to the natural nails				☐
SALON SYSTEMS	Brushes to apply overlay product to the nails				☐

		MANICURE	PEDICURE	NAIL ART	NAIL ENHANCEMENTS
	Nail enhancement resources, these will differ dependent upon which nail system is used in your workplace (see images below)				☐
ELLISONS	Nail wrap nail enhancement resources				☐
ELLISONS	Acrylic nail enhancement resources				☐
ELLISONS	UV gel nail enhancement resources				☐
ELLISONS	Client's record card – to record the client's details before and after service	☐	☐	☐	☐
ELLISONS Nailcare Aftercare	Aftercare leaflets to provide guidance on how to care for the nails, hands/feet after the service	☐	☐	☐	☐

TOP TIP

Work area for nail services

Many salons have a nail service work station already prepared permanently for services.

Nail scissors

Your workplace may use specific scissors often termed 'stork scissors' for nail enhancement services.

Electric nail drills

Your salon may use electrical nail drills to blend nail enhancements, these should be placed safely away from water on the work station.

TOP TIP

Nail art designs

Have a range of prepared nail art designs, or photographic images for the beauty therapist to discuss with the client at consultation.

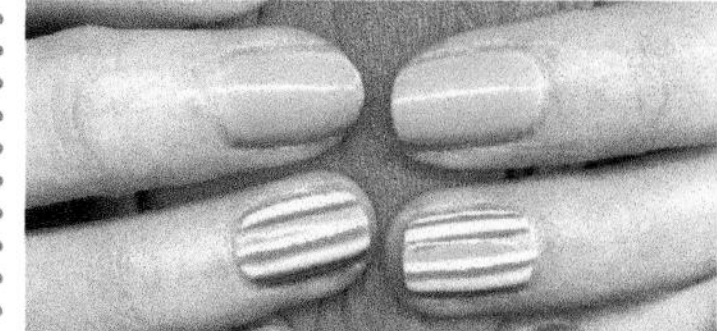

Nail art design

HEALTH & SAFETY

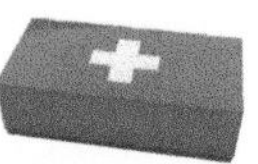

Poor ventilation will lead to eye and breathing problems for all in the work area.

HEALTH & SAFETY

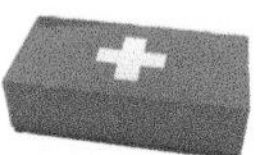

Use of electrical equipment
Place equipment on a stable trolley and make sure that the wires do not trail or are in such a position that they might cause an accident.

HEALTH & SAFETY

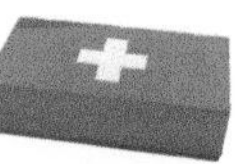

The client may also be offered protective plastic eyeshields when cutting the nails when performing nail enhancement service. If this is your workplace policy, two sets will be required.

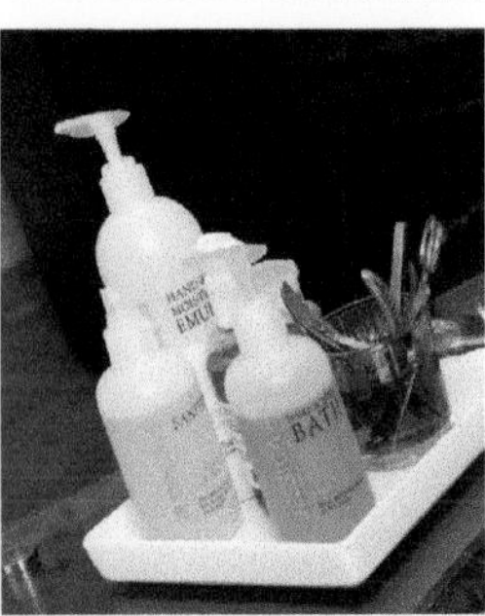

A prepared manicure station

HEALTH & SAFETY

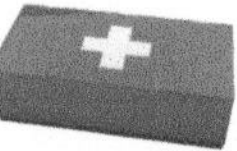

Positioning of the work station furniture and resources is important to prevent the beauty therapist stretching which could lead to long-term strain and injury called repetitive strain injury (RSI).

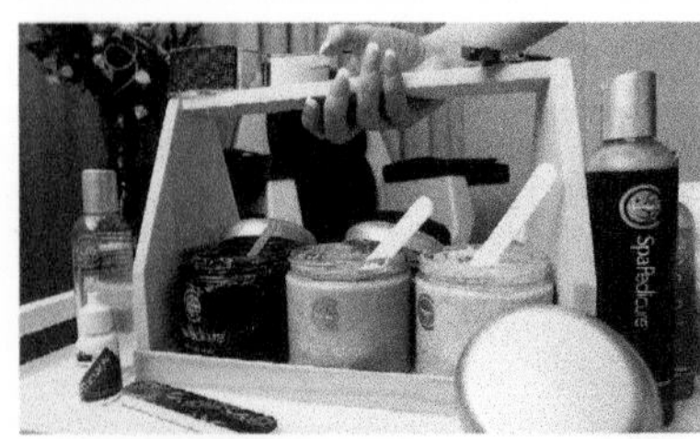

Pedicure products

Sterilization and disinfection

- Ensure tools and equipment are clean and sterile before use.
- Small metal tools should be sterilized after use. Clean them with surgical spirit and clean cotton wool and then sterilize them in the autoclave.
- Several sets of nail service tools are required to ensure that time is allowed for disinfection/sterilization after each service.
- Orange wood sticks, emery boards and nail files should be disposable and thrown away after use.
- Towels should be boil washed to destroy harmful microorganisms and prevent cross-infection.
- Wash your hands before handling clean equipment.

Preparing the treatment work area

1. The treatment area should be clean and tidy.
2. There should be a clean, covered empty bin in the treatment area lined with a polythene bin liner.
3. Disinfect all work surfaces and cover with clean disposable paper tissue.
4. Check the trolley to make sure it has everything necessary to carry out the service.
5. Check whether a heat therapy service is to be applied. If using warm paraffin wax, make sure there is sufficient wax in the heater. Adjust the temperature according to the manufacturer's instructions. Warm oil in the heater, following the manufacturer's instructions.
6. Check the ventilation is adequate. A ventilation system is required to remove fumes, chemicals and dust when performing nail enhancement service. The system must be suitable to take into consideration the number of nail technicians working in the area. Temperature must not be too warm as this can affect the application and setting properties of nail materials.
7. Collect the small metal/plastic tools from the UV cabinet and place them in the jar of disinfecting solution.
8. Put all materials neatly onto the trolley according to the nail service to be delivered.
9. A small table light might be needed for additional light when performing nail art and nail enhancement services.
10. For **manicure** or nail enhancement services to the hands, place a towel over the treatment work surface, then fold another towel into a pad and place it in the middle of the treatment work surface. The pad supports the client's forearm during service. Place a third towel over the pad. Position a chair on either side of the work station, one for the client and the other for the beauty therapist. For manicure, fill the finger bowl with warm water and detergent. Place a tissue or disposable manicure mat on top of the towels.
11. For **pedicure** and nail enhancement services to the feet, place a towel on the floor in between the beauty therapist and client. For pedicure, fill the foot bowl with warm water and detergent and put it on this towel. Five towels are required: one for the beauty therapist to place on her lap for protection, another should be provided to dry the client's feet, the other two are used to wrap the client's feet to keep them warm during pedicure service.

12 Collect the client's record card and put it on the service trolley.

13 Confirm the preparation of the work area meets with the senior beauty therapist's satisfaction.

Maintaining the treatment work area

Clean, tidy and prepare the treatment work area in a suitable condition for further services.

It is a good idea to wear gloves to protect your hands from chemicals used in the nail service, disinfectants when cleaning and contaminated waste.

- Dispose of the paper-tissue bedroll and other disposable items such as emery boards, spatulas and orange sticks.
- Empty the bin that was used to collect waste in the treatment area. Replace the bin liner with a new one. If any blood has been spilt, i.e. by accidentally cutting live skin, this waste is termed contaminated and should have been placed in a sealed, yellow bag. This should be disposed of correctly for waste classed as contaminated.
- Clean small bowls in hot, soapy water; rinse and dry.
- Clean all tools and metal equipment with surgical spirit and sterilize in the autoclave.
- Plastic equipment should be cleaned in hot soapy water, dried and placed in the UV cabinet.
- Dispose of the brushes used to apply paraffin wax; they cannot be cleaned.
- Clean brushes used to apply artificial nail systems in the appropriate brush cleaner solvent.
- The buffer, if used, should have the chamois leather cover cleaned in warm soapy water at 60°C. When dried, it should be placed in the UV cabinet to destroy the majority of microorganisms. The plastic handle should be wiped with surgical spirit.
- Clean mask brushes in hot, soapy water, dry and put in the UV cabinet.
- Electrical equipment should be cleaned to remove any dirt and debris following manufacturer's instructions. Switch off equipment before cleaning and use specialist equipment cleaner to clean. If the equipment is to be used again, switch on after cleaning.
- Replace and re-fill products as necessary.
- Clean the necks of bottles and jars to maintain hygiene and a high standard of presentation. Nail polish bottle necks should be cleaned regularly with clean cotton wool and nail polish remover to ensure that they close tightly or the polish will become thick in consistency and produce a poor finish if applied.
- Protective eye shields if worn should be cleaned to prevent cross-infection.
- Disinfect work surfaces. Remove any dust in the area as this may cause skin irritation and could affect the quality of the next service provided in the area, i.e. dust could spoil newly painted nails.
- Remove used towels from the service area and launder them.
- If a product needs to be disposed of, e.g. a nail polish, inform the relevant person for stock control before disposal and replacement. This will ensure adequate stock levels are maintained as replacement stock can be ordered.
- Return the client record card to the secure storage area for client data.

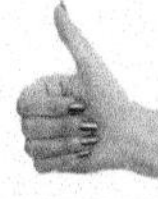

BEST PRACTICE

If a brush of poor quality is used for nail art or nail enhancement services – tell the relevant person that it needs replacing.

Poor quality brushes will affect the end result.

TOP TIP

Emery Board

The client is often offered the emery board used on them to take away following the service.

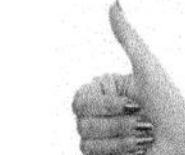

BEST PRACTICE

Code of Practice for nail services

Always follow the Habia nail service's Code of Practice and your workplace hygiene policy to maintain a safe, professional working environment.

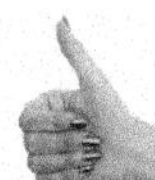

BEST PRACTICE

Client comfort

The client can become cold when not moving. Make an additional blanket available that can be provided to ensure client comfort if needed.

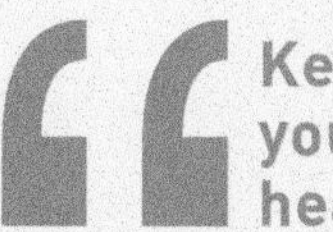

Keep a check on your client's health

Always check for contra-indications before commencing with any part of the service. Check with the senior beauty therapist if unsure.

Vicky Ann Kennedy

HEALTH & SAFETY

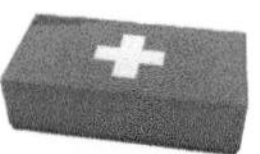

Disposable headbands
To avoid the laundering requirement of headbands, disposable paper headbands are an ideal hygienic alternative.

Preparing and maintaining the salon treatment work area for facial service

A facial is a service applied to the skin of the face that has a cleansing, toning, nourishing effect on the skin. The choice and application of products will depend upon the skin type of the client and their service needs.

Sterilization and disinfection

- Ensure tools and equipment are clean and sterile before use.
- Several sets of facial sponges and mask brushes will be required to ensure that time is allowed for disinfection/sterilization after each service.
- Towels and headbands should be boil washed to destroy harmful microorganisms and prevent cross-infection. It is a good idea to use disposable headbands as these can be thrown away after use.
- Wash your hands before handling clean equipment.

Refer to the equipment and material checklist to make sure that you have all that is required to perform facial services.

EQUIPMENT AND MATERIALS CHECKLIST FOR FACIAL SERVICE

SORISA

Couch or beauty chair with sit-up and lie-down positions and an easy-to-clean surface ☐

SORISA

Trolley to hold all the necessary equipment and materials ☐

SORISA

Large and medium-sized towels to protect the client's clothing and for the beauty therapist to dry their hands during service ☐

Note: The client could be offered a gown to wear: place a clean gown in the service area.

ELLISONS

Disposable tissue roll to cover the trolley surface and couch ☐

ELLISONS

Headband to protect the client's hair and to keep hair away from the service area ☐

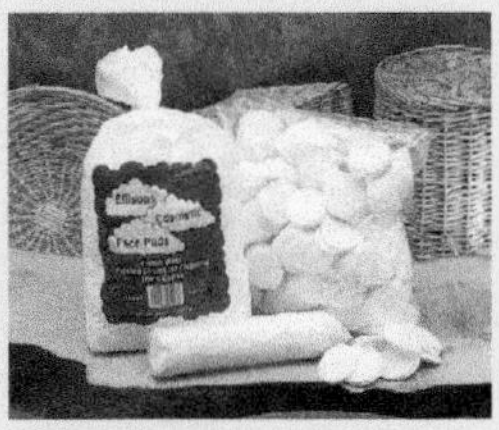

ELLISONS

Dampened, clean cotton wool, to remove skincare products ☐

Cotton wool eye pads pre-shaped round and dampened to place over the eyes during the mask service ☐

Note: Two further cotton wool eye pads will be required if facial steaming is being carried out to protect the delicate eye tissue

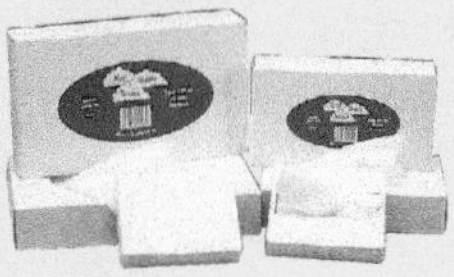

ELLISONS

Facial tissues to blot the skin dry after toner and following mask removal ☐

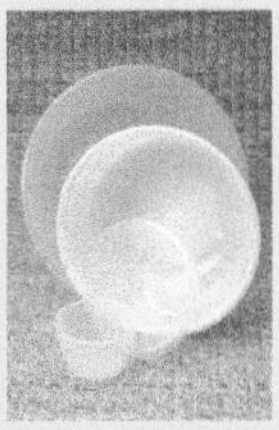

ELLISONS

Small bowls to store damp and dry cotton wool, mix service masks, hold cosmetic creams that have been dispensed ☐

Note: If a sink is not available for the beauty therapist, a large bowl will be required, filled with warm water to remove the mask

ELLISONS

Spatulas to remove products hygienically from containers and to tuck the client's hair underneath the headband to prevent soiling ☐

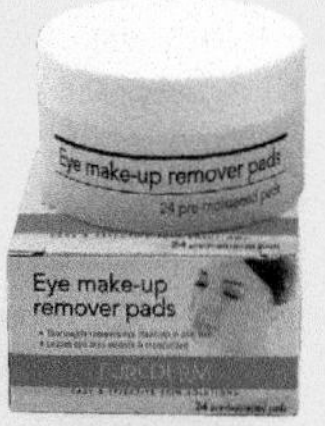

ELLISONS

*Non-oily or oily eye make-up remover to cleanse the eye area ☐

**Non-oily should be selected if the client is wearing eyelash extensions as oily eye make-up remover will loosen them

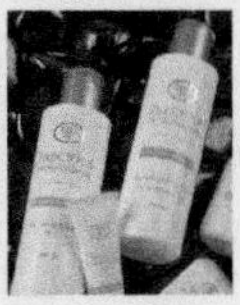

SALON SYSTEMS

Cleansing lotion – a range available to suit the different skin types: dry, combination, oily, and skin conditions: mature, sensitive, dehydrated ☐

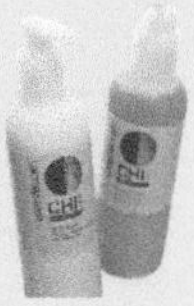

SALON SYSTEMS

Toning lotion – a range available to suit the different skin types: dry, combination, oily, and skin conditions: mature, sensitive, dehydrated ☐

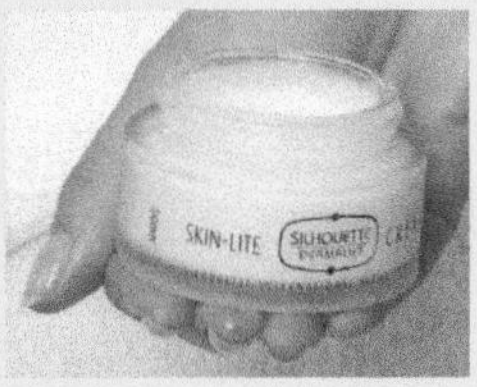

BEAUTY EXPRESS LTD

Moisturiser – a range available to suit the different skin types: dry, combination, oily, and skin conditions: mature, sensitive, dehydrated ☐

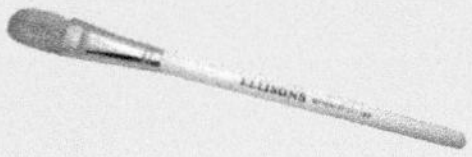

ELLISONS

Mask brush to apply facial masks ☐

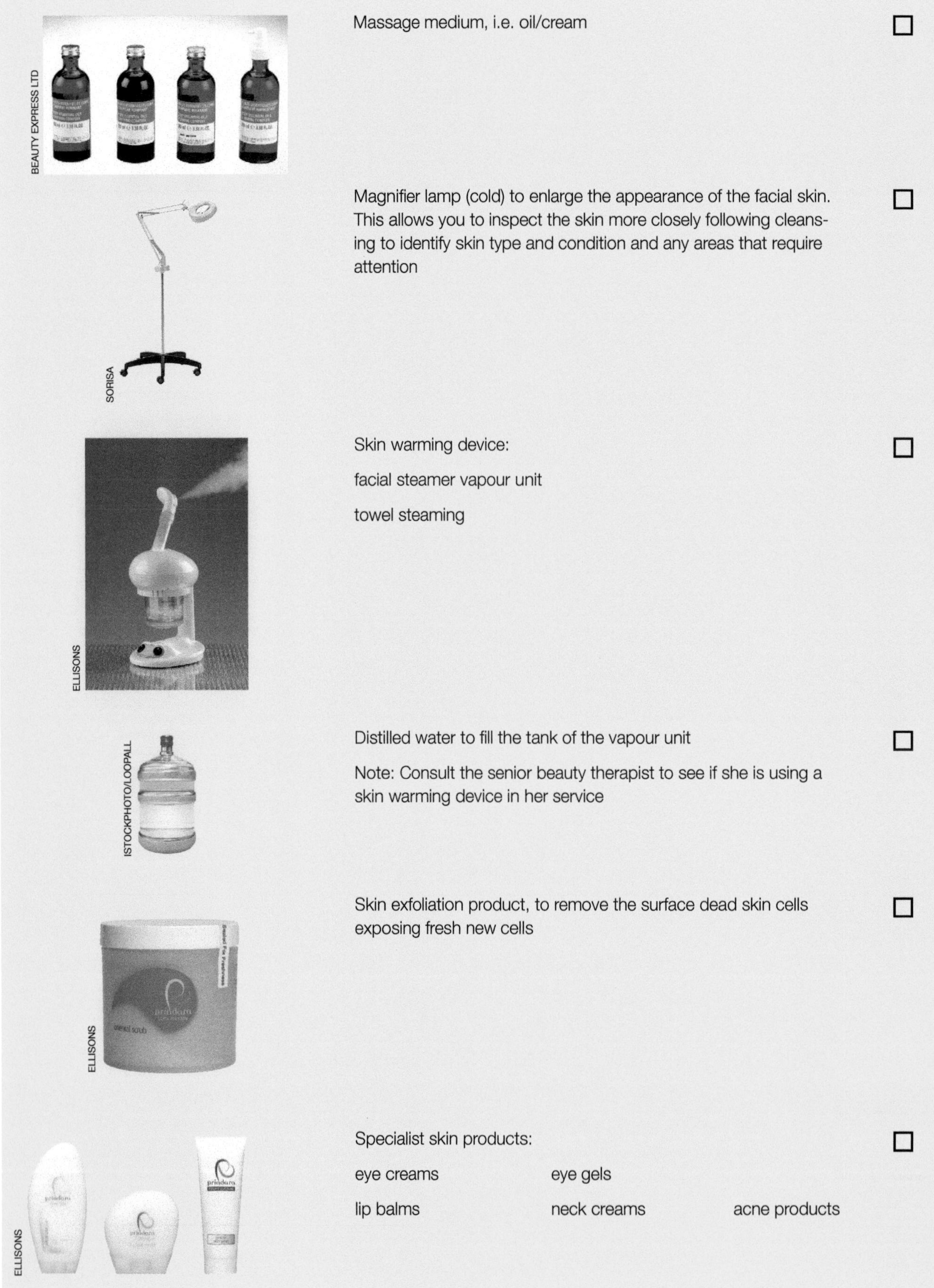

Massage medium, i.e. oil/cream ☐

Magnifier lamp (cold) to enlarge the appearance of the facial skin. This allows you to inspect the skin more closely following cleansing to identify skin type and condition and any areas that require attention ☐

Skin warming device: ☐

facial steamer vapour unit

towel steaming

Distilled water to fill the tank of the vapour unit ☐

Note: Consult the senior beauty therapist to see if she is using a skin warming device in her service

Skin exfoliation product, to remove the surface dead skin cells exposing fresh new cells ☐

Specialist skin products: ☐

eye creams — eye gels

lip balms — neck creams — acne products

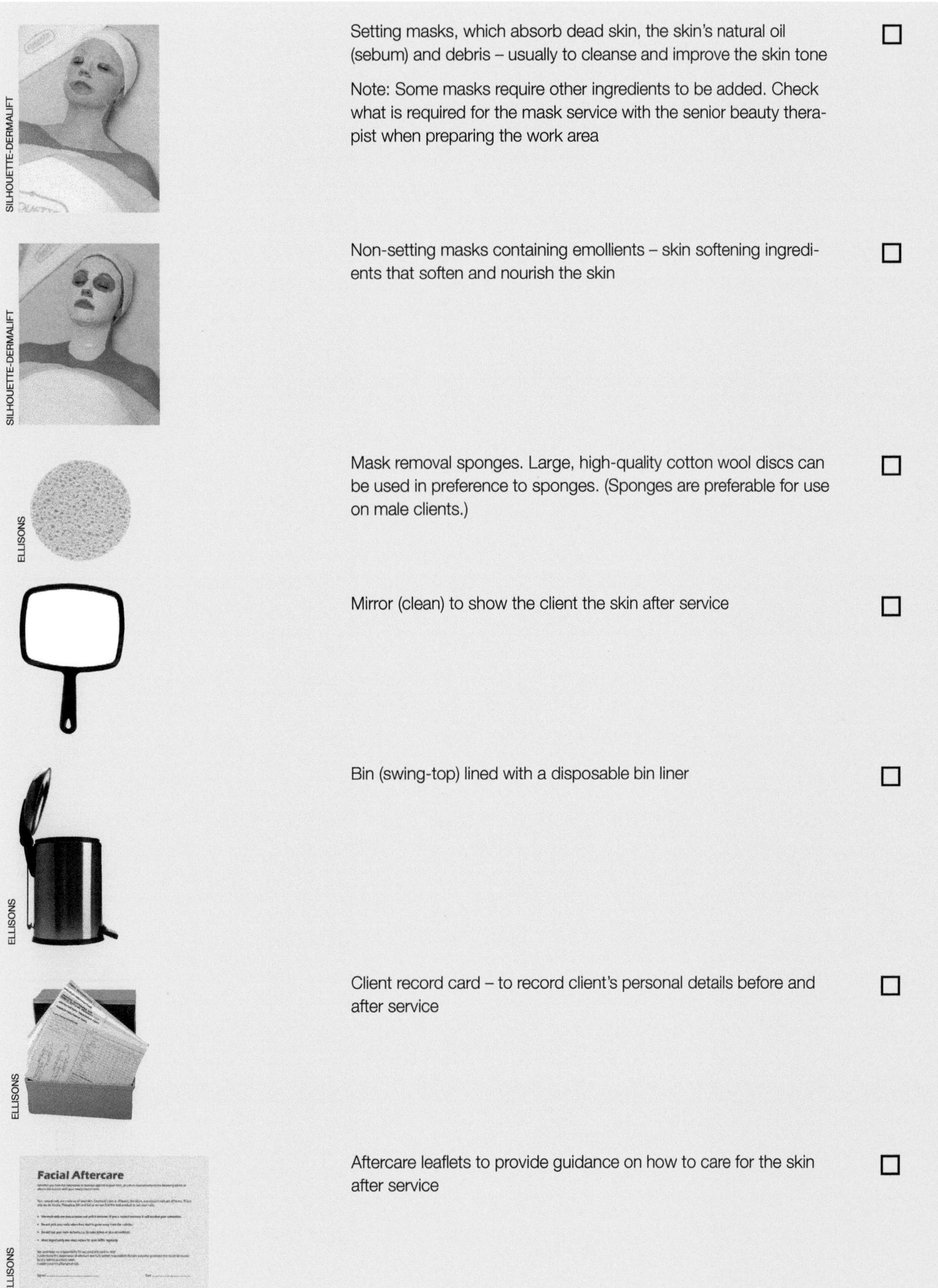

Setting masks, which absorb dead skin, the skin's natural oil (sebum) and debris – usually to cleanse and improve the skin tone ☐

Note: Some masks require other ingredients to be added. Check what is required for the mask service with the senior beauty therapist when preparing the work area

Non-setting masks containing emollients – skin softening ingredients that soften and nourish the skin ☐

Mask removal sponges. Large, high-quality cotton wool discs can be used in preference to sponges. (Sponges are preferable for use on male clients.) ☐

Mirror (clean) to show the client the skin after service ☐

Bin (swing-top) lined with a disposable bin liner ☐

Client record card – to record client's personal details before and after service ☐

Aftercare leaflets to provide guidance on how to care for the skin after service ☐

TOP TIP

Product labels

Position bottles so that labels can be easily read.

Packaging is often similar and can only be identified by the label name.

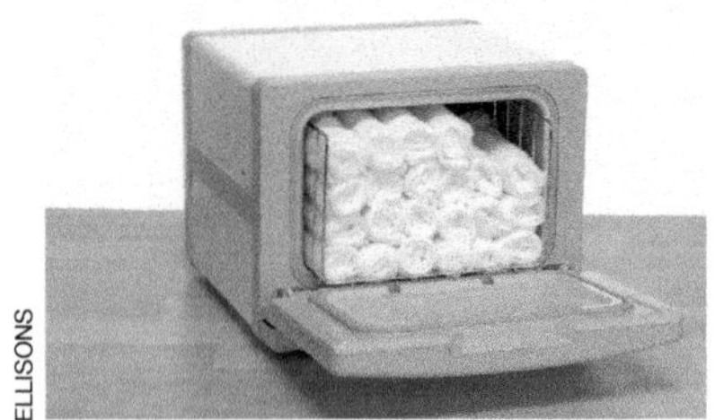
ELLISONS

A towel warmer

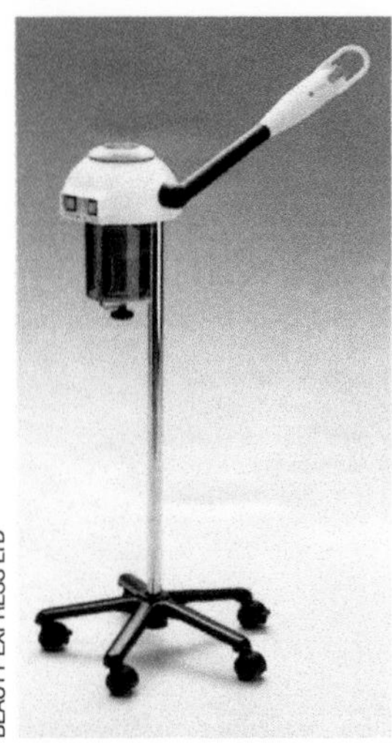
BEAUTY EXPRESS LTD

A facial steamer vapour unit

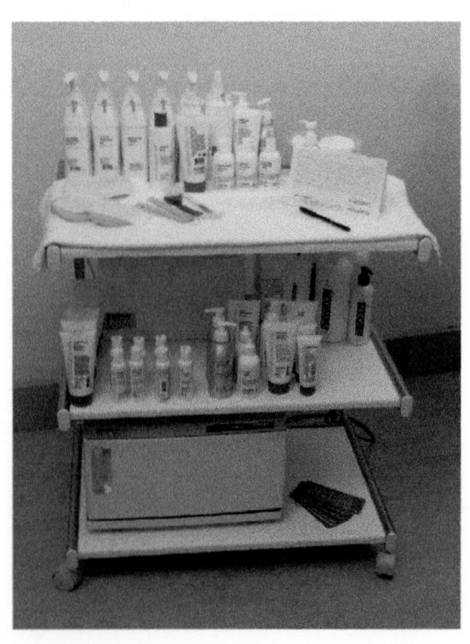

A prepared facial trolley

Preparing the treatment area

1. The area should be clean and tidy.
2. There should be a clean, covered empty bin lined with a polythene bin liner.
3. Disinfect all work surfaces and cover with clean disposable paper tissue.
4. Check the trolley to make sure it contains everything needed to carry out the service. All products should be clean and positioned in a logical order for use.
5. Collect facial equipment from the UV cabinet, mask brush and mask removal sponges and place on the trolley.
6. Prepare an adequate supply of cotton wool: provide a selection of damp and dry cotton wool placed on the trolley, usually in small bowls.
7. The beauty couch or chair should be protected with a long strip of disposable bed-roll placed over a freshly laundered sheet or usually a clean towelling couch cover.
8. Adjust the lighting – the room should be gently lit for facial service, to induce relaxation.
9. Check that the magnifying lamp is clean and in a good working area.
10. Check the room temperature, good ventilation is important – it should not be too warm.
11. A large towel, sheet or similar clean protective covering should be provided to cover the client's body and a small towel to drape across the client's chest and shoulders. Place these neatly on the service couch.
12. A clean gown can be provided, if the client prefers, to wear after removing outer clothing (a requirement if the client is receiving facial massage to the chest and shoulders).
13. If a skin-warming device is to be used, this should be prepared ready for use:
    a. Hot towels: clean, sterile towels should be placed in the towel warmer. Follow the manufacturer's guidelines for heating timings.
    b. Facial steamer vapour unit: fill the water tank with distilled water up to the maximum level. Switch on the machine at the mains, select the steam facility and heat the water until steam can be seen. Switch off the unit. This will save time as the water will now only need to be reheated.
14. Collect the client's record card and place on the trolley.
15. Confirm the preparation of the work area meets with the senior beauty therapist's satisfaction.

Maintaining the treatment area

Clean, tidy and prepare the work area in a suitable condition for further services.

- Dispose of the paper-tissue bedroll.
- Empty the bin that was used to collect waste in the treatment areas if necessary. Replace the bin liner with a new one. Clinical contaminated waste, usually from when extractions have occurred must be disposed of in accordance with the controlled Waste Regulations Act (1992). Always wear PPE when handling and disposing of clinical waste.
- Disinfect work surfaces.
- Clean bowls used in hot soapy water, rinse and dry.

- Clean the mask brushes in warm water and detergent, rinse thoroughly in clean water and allow them to dry naturally. Once dry, place them in the UV cabinet.
- Wash the mask-removal sponges in warm water and detergent and then sterilize in the autoclave. Place in the UV cabinet when dry, ready for use.
- Ensure the facial steamer, if used, is switched off and disconnected at the mains. Check the water level and refill with distilled water ready for future use.
- Used towels, including facial towels used to warm the skin, the headband and gown (if worn) should be removed from the service area and laundered.
- If a product needs to be disposed of, e.g. a facial mask, inform the relevant person for stock control before disposal and replacement. This will ensure adequate stock levels are maintained.
- Return the client record card to the secure storage area for client data.

GLOSSARY OF KEY WORDS

Cross-infection the transfer of contagious microorganisms by direct contact with another person or indirectly by contact with infected equipment.

Data Protection Act (1998) legislation designed to protect client privacy and confidentiality.

Disinfection the destruction of some, but not all microorganisms.

Environmental conditions the surroundings in which the service will be performed which should be correct at all times.

Eyebrow shaping service removal of eyebrow hair to maintain or create a new shape.

Eye services services applied to the eye area to enhance the appearance of the eye.

Eyelash and eyebrow tinting service the permanent colouring of the eyelash and/or eyebrow hair using a specialist dye to enhance their appearance.

Facial a service applied to the skin of the face; it has a skin cleansing, toning and nourishing effect.

Eyelash extensions threads of artificial hair attached to the natural eyelashes to make them appear thicker and longer.

Hygiene the recommended standard of cleanliness necessary in the salon to prevent cross-infection.

Legislation laws that affect the beauty therapy business and which relate to products and services, the business premises and environmental conditions, working practices and those employed.

Maintain to keep.

Make-up service the application of make-up cosmetics to enhance the skin and facial features.

Manicure service a service to improve the appearance of the hands, nails and skin.

Nail art nail decoration using nail art materials.

Nail enhancements lengthening, strengthening or repairing the nail using a nail enhancement system such as UV gel, liquid and powder or wrap.

Pedicure service a service to improve the appearance of the feet, nails and skin.

Preparation to get ready.

Record card personal information recorded for each client, also recording services received and retail product purchases.

Sterilization the destruction of all microorganisms.

Waxing the use of wax to remove hairs temporarily from the face and body.

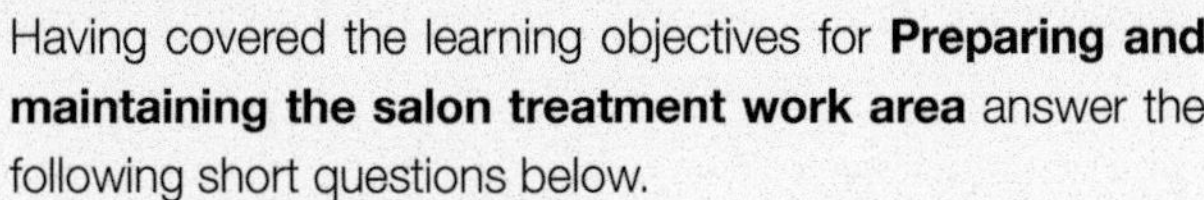

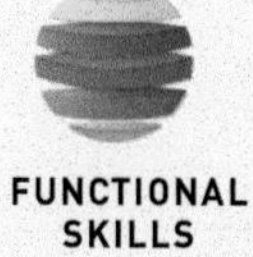

FUNCTIONAL SKILLS

Having covered the learning objectives for **Preparing and maintaining the salon treatment work area** answer the following short questions below.

The information covers:

- organizational and legal requirements
- preparing and maintaining treatment work areas.

Organizational and legal requirements

1 What are your responsibilities under the Health and Safety at Work Act?

2 Why is it important to keep accurate client records?

3 Why is it important that you wash your hands before preparing and maintaining the work area?

4 Why is it important to follow the senior beauty therapist's instructions for preparing the work area?

5 How can cross-infection be avoided when preparing the work area?

6 How can you ensure your own personal hygiene? Give three examples.

7 Name a piece of equipment used in sterilizing beauty therapy equipment.

8 Name a piece of equipment used to disinfect beauty therapy equipment.

9 Why should you know the storage requirements for different products?

10 Where should the client's records be stored after service?

Preparing and maintaining the treatment work areas

1 What must you consider when disposing of wax waste and nail service waste?

2 Why should the manufacturer's instructions always be followed when preparing materials and equipment?

3 Why should you regularly check the appointment book when planning your time to prepare and maintain the work areas for different services?

4 How should you aim to leave the work area after the service?

5 How would you clean the following:

a metal nail service tools

b make-up brushes

c wax heater

d eyelash tinting bowls

e facial mask brush and sponges.

6 Define the terms:

a sterilization

b disinfection.

7 Why must you check the environmental conditions for each service when preparing the work area for: heating, lighting, ventilation and general comfort?

5 Salon reception duties

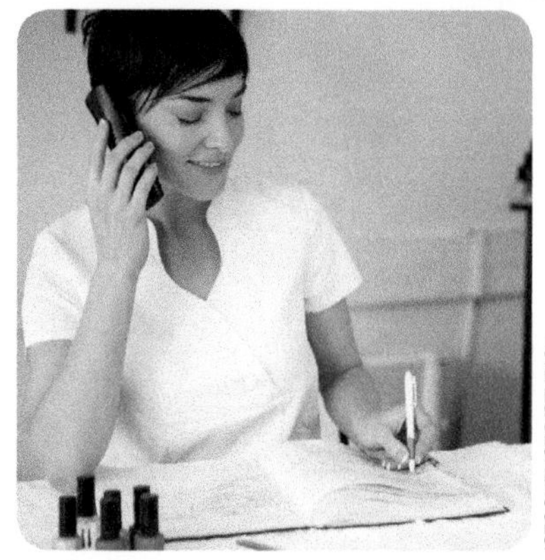
ISTOCKPHOTO/STUDIO9

Learning Objectives

This chapter covers the **Assist with salon reception duties** unit.

This unit is all about the skills and knowledge you will need to assist with reception procedures in the workplace. These include maintaining or keeping the reception area in a clean and organized manner; looking after clients when they arrive and leave; dealing with general enquiries (questions that the client may ask); making appointments face-to-face, by telephone and possibly handling on-line enquiries ensuring all necessary information linked to the booking is recorded following your workplace policy. It is important that the reception is managed well as it gives the client their first impression of the business. Often reception is a retail sales point, so you it is important to keep this area looking fresh and appealing with products that will invite interest in the way they are displayed and marketed. It is important to have an understanding of the workplace service and product range so that you can deal with enquiries within your responsibility. You have an important role to play when assisting with salon reception duties to create the best possible impression.

There are **three** learning outcomes which you must achieve competently:

1 **Maintain the reception area**

2 **Attend to clients and enquiries**

3 **Help to make appointments for salon reception services**

Your assessor will observe your performance on **at least three occasions, two of which will cover making appointments**.

From the **range** statement, you must show that you have:

- answered face to face and telephone **enquiries**
- made **appointments** over the telephone and face to face with clients
- recorded all the **appointment details** listed.

When assisting with reception duties it is important to use the skills and knowledge you have learnt in the following unit:

Health and Safety – Contribute to the development of effective working relationships

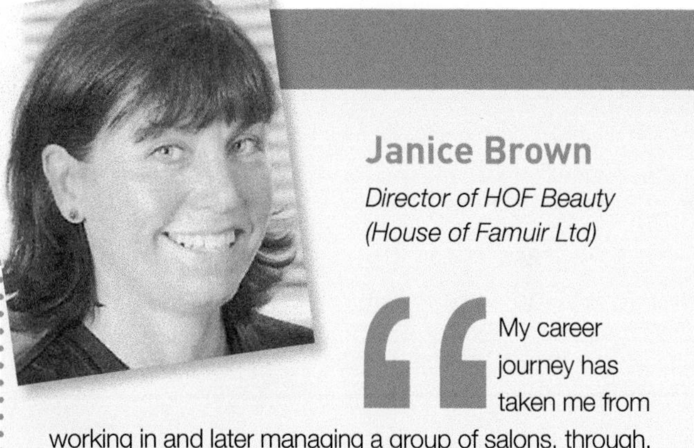

Janice Brown

Director of HOF Beauty (House of Famuir Ltd)

“My career journey has taken me from working in and later managing a group of salons, through, sales, teaching, training, research and development and I am currently director of HOF Beauty Ltd. Along the way I have specialized in electrolysis and other hair removal methods. I am the co-author of *The Encyclopedia of Hair Removal* along with Gill Morris. I am proud to say that I have been able to make a real difference to people’s lives by helping to correct skin, body and hair growth issues. I hope I have also been able to inspire and encourage fellow beauty therapists through the training I have provided. In the course of my career I have been fortunate enough to travel the world and work with wonderful people. Beauty therapy for me is not only a career but is a true passion.

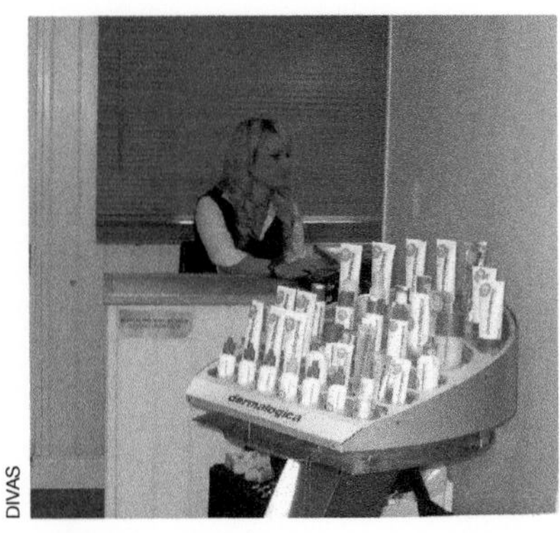

DIVAS

Beauty salon reception

Practical skills, knowledge and understanding

This table will help you to check your progress in gaining the necessary practical skills, knowledge and understanding for**: Assist with salon reception duties**.

Tick (), when you feel you have gained the practical skills, knowledge and understanding in each of the following areas:

	Practical skills, knowledge and understanding checklist	✓
1	Maintaining the reception area.	
2	Maintaining reception product displays including the removal of any faulty products.	
3	Knowing when and whom to report low levels of reception stationery and retail stock.	
4	Salon policy for reception client hospitality.	
5	Using good verbal and non-verbal communication and listening skills to suit the situation.	
6	Dealing with enquiries efficiently and competently.	
7	Knowing when to refer enquiries on and to whom.	
8	How to correctly record messages taken and know when to pass on information and to whom.	
9	Legal storage and access (right to use) client records in relation to the Data Protection Act (1998).	
10	How to capably deal with requests for appointments face to face or by telephone.	
11	Ensuring all appointment details are recorded so that they are easy to read, correct and confirmed for accuracy with the client as per salon policy. Remember this may be hand written in an appointment book or electronically on a computer.	
12	Knowing when to pass appointment requests on and to whom.	
13	To have a good understanding of salon services, products and pricings.	

When you have ticked all the areas you can, ask your assessor to assess you on **Assist with salon reception duties**. After practical assessment, your assessor might decide that you need to practise further to improve your skills. If so, your assessor will tell you how and where you need to improve to gain competence.

ALWAYS REMEMBER

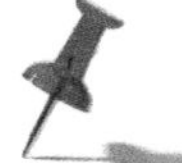

A positive welcome is important

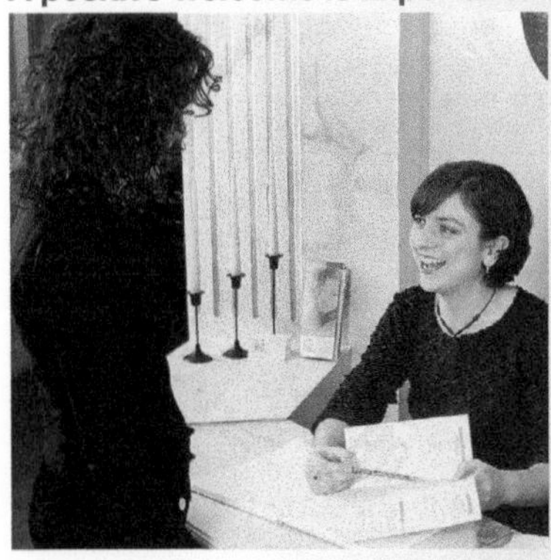

When working on reception, make sure clients get the right impression – a positive, confident welcome is important. Remember also, non-verbal communication is as important as verbal communication!

The reception area

The salon **reception** gives clients their first (and also their final) impression of the salon, whether this is on the telephone or in person on a visit to the salon. First impressions count, so make sure that clients get the right impression!

> By creating the right atmosphere on arrival at the salon, giving excellent service and paying attention to the client's needs you will encourage the client to return to you for their beauty therapy services.
>
> **Janice Brown**

Outcome 1: Maintain the reception area

Learn how to maintain the reception area by:
1 Keeping the reception area clean and tidy at all times.
2 Keeping product displays clean, neat and tidy at all times.
3 Promptly reporting low levels of reception stationery and retail products on display to the relevant person.
4 Promptly removing any faulty products from display and reporting them to the relevant person.
5 Offering clients hospitality following your salon's client care policies.

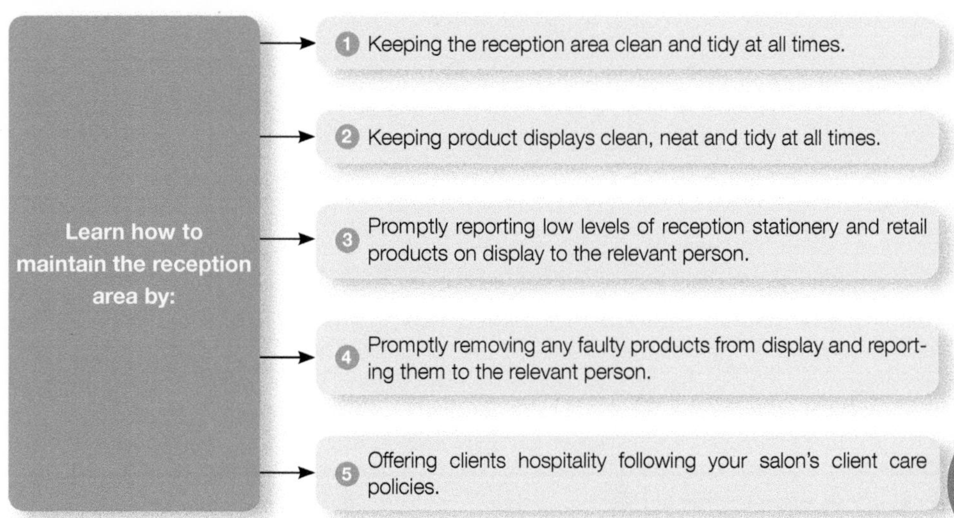

It is part of your responsibility to keep the reception area tidy and organized at all times, and to be quick to respond and pleasant when assisting with reception duties. The different duties you will be expected to perform in your reception role are listed below. Remember these must be within the limits of your own authority.

TOP TIP

Never miss opportunities to learn new things

If unsure about any request from a client or business visitor, explain that you will find somebody who will be able to answer their question. When you receive the answer, this will be something new you have now learnt.

The Assist with salon reception duties unit requires you to carry-out the following responsibilities:

Keep the reception area clean and tidy,
Ensure display areas look appealing, clean and are well stocked
Report any shortages of reception resources and retail products
Identify and inform the relevant person of faulty or damaged equipment and products
Show good client care and hospitality at all times
Refer any enquiries you are unable to deal with to the relevant person

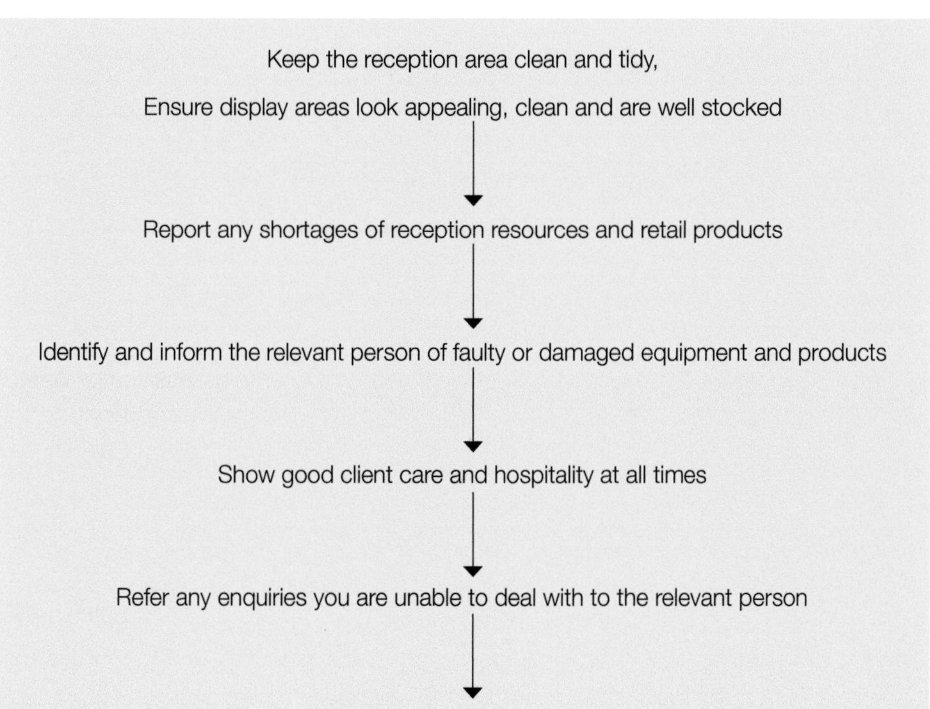

Accurately take messages and pass these on promptly

↓

Comply with the Data Protection Act (1998) regarding handling client records

↓

Handle appointments immediately, accurately identify client requirements

↓

Record all details accurately in the correct place and confirm appointment details with the client

↓

Refer any appointments you are unable to deal with to the relevant person

TOP TIP

Client attention

It is important to pay clients the right amount of attention – to ensure client satisfaction. This must always be considered in a situation when clients might be required to be kept waiting. Communicate with clients regularly to keep them updated if they are waiting for a service. Offer hospitality and alternative options if available.

Reception equipment and resources

The reception area should be uncluttered. The main equipment and furnishings required for an efficient reception include:

- A reception desk: the size of the desk will depend on the size of the workplace; some salons have several receptionists. The desk should include shelves and drawers, and some have an in-built lockable cash or security drawer. The desk should be at a convenient height for the client to communicate and for payment transactions. It should also be large enough to house the **appointment** book or **computer** (or both).
- A comfortable chair: the receptionist's chair should provide adequate back support.
- A computer: these are increasingly used in most salons because they can perform so many functions. They can be used to store data about clients, to book appointment schedules, to carry out automatic stock control, and to record business details such as accounts and marketing information. Space should be provided for a printer if required. Some computers can even be programmed to recommend specific services on the basis of personal data about the client.
- A calculator: this is used for simple financial calculations, especially if the salon does not have a computer.
- Stationery: examples include price lists, gift vouchers, appointment cards and a receipt pad.
- A notepad: for taking notes and recording messages.
- An address and contact book: this should hold all frequently used telephone numbers. These may also be stored electronically.
- A telephone and answering machine: this allows clients to contact you, even when the salon is closed, with appointment requests or even to let you know about an unavoidable change or cancellation: you can then reschedule appointments as quickly as possible. You can also programme your message to provide information when you are busy or the salon is closed.

- **Record cards**: these confidential cards record the personal details of each client registered at the salon. They should be kept in alphabetical order in a filing cabinet, a card-index box or electronically, and should be ready for collection by the beauty therapist when treating new or existing clients. Each card records:
  - the client's name, address and telephone number
  - any medical details
  - any contra-indications (such as allergies and contra-actions)
  - service aims and outcomes
  - services received, products used, and **retail** products purchased.
- Pens, pencils and an eraser: make sure these stay at the desk!
- A display cabinet: this can be used to store retail products, and any other merchandise sold by the salon; these items are referred to as retail products.
- Waste bin: a covered, lined waste bin may be provided at the reception area. Ensure this is emptied regularly following salon policy.

ALWAYS REMEMBER

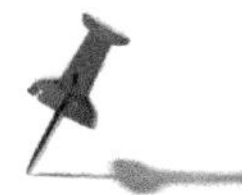

Price lists

Some salons put their price list in booklet form, detailing the services offered and explaining their benefits.

They may also publish them on their website if they have one. Accurate prices must be provided to the client to comply with the Prices Act (1974) requiring prices to be displayed.

ACTIVITY FUNCTIONAL SKILLS

Planning a reception area

Cost and design a reception area of your choice (to scale) appropriate to a small or large beauty salon. It may be specific to all beauty therapy services or specialised for nails and make-up or even eye treatments only. Discuss the choice of signage, the waiting area colour theme, wall and floor coverings, seating, and equipment, lighting and give the reasons for their selection. Consider client comfort, and health and safety.

To help you plan this you may refer to a specialist equipment supplier's brochure or online information for ideas.

Retail products and displays

Retail sales are very important to the beauty salon. They are a simple way of greatly increasing the income without too much extra time and effort. Clients need to be told about the retail products available. The retail display area should be kept well stocked and clear.

Maintain the appearance of the display area and retail stock by regularly:

- Dusting the display shelving and stock. If the salon is located on a busy main road it will quickly become dusty. Take care not to damage the packaging during cleaning.
- Rearrange the displays regularly to maintain client interest, for the promotion or advertising of new products and if products have been popular and the display needs to be restocked.

BEST PRACTICE

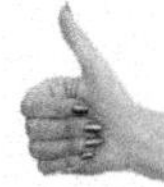

Eating and drinking at reception

The receptionist and other employees should not eat or drink at reception for reasons of hygiene and professorial appearance.

ALWAYS REMEMBER FUNCTIONAL SKILLS

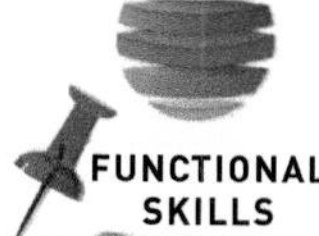

File contact details

Visitors to the salon might leave a business card, stating the name of their company, and the representative's name, address and telephone number. The receptionist should file these cards for future reference. Contact details are often stored electronically if the salon has a computer.

TOP TIP

Text communication

Some salons use texts to forward to clients directly to their mobile phones to remind them of future appointments, or if necessary to cancel/rearrange an appointment.

TOP TIP

Answering machines maintain communication with your clients

The answering machine is useful if for any reason all beauty receptionists are busy and the telephone cannot be answered. This avoids losing potential business.

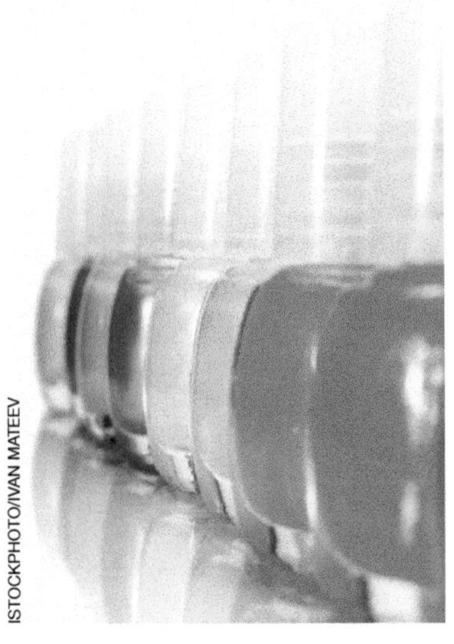

ISTOCKPHOTO/IVAN MATEEV

A nail product display showing colour range

TOP TIP

Reception Digital Marketing Media
Reception can be used to promote salon services. If your salon provides this facility, make sure the material is played and changed regularly to maintain client interest.

HEALTH & SAFETY

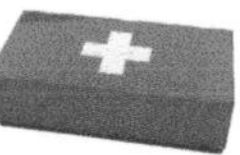

Cleaning
A large salon might employ a cleaner to maintain the hygiene of the reception area. In a smaller salon this might be the responsibility of the receptionist or the beauty therapists. Whoever is responsible, reception must be maintained to a high standard at all times. Only use cleaning products as recommended and store to prevent a health and safety hazard. Avoid general cleaning when there are clients in reception.

- Move the stock so that if new items arrive they will go to the back of the display shelf, and older ones are used first called stock rotation.
- Write down any damages to retail products. Damage can be recognized by spoilt packaging caused by leakage or damage to the container of the product. Report this to the relevant person if this occurs.
- Report any shortages of retail stock or reception **resources** and pass onto the relevant person. Keep accurate and up-to-date records.
- If there are testers for the client to try, make sure these are kept clean and in good condition.

Check that all the reception equipment and resources are always available, including retail products. Any shortages must be reported to the relevant person immediately. This ensures the smooth running of the reception area.

Client hospitality

Hospitality is friendliness and how you welcome your client to the salon.

Hospitality is important and shows the salon's commitment to client care. If a client arrives early for an appointment, or is likely to be delayed, offer a magazine or a refreshment such as coffee or water according to your salon's client care policy; magazines should be renewed regularly. It is also a pleasant gesture to have sweets on reception for clients.

Client records

Client record cards record personal details of each client registered at the salon. They should be kept in alphabetical order, if not stored electronically on a computer, and should be ready for collection by the beauty therapist on the client's arrival for an appointment.

The Data Protection Act (DPA) (1998)

The **Data Protection Act (1998)** was passed by Parliament to control the way information is handled and to give legal rights to people who have information stored about them. With more and more organizations using computers to store and process personal details, access to confidential information has become increasingly available.

This legislation is designed to protect the client's privacy and confidentiality. It is necessary to ask the client questions before the service can be finalized and the information obtained is recorded on the client record card. All information about a client is confidential and should be stored in a secure area following the client's service. This is usually at reception. When assisting with reception duties, you must only pass the client's confidential information to authorized people, and you must always store client records securely.

> “It is important that the client is given the right service and products in order to get the results they are after. You will need to have a basic knowledge of products and services when a client asks questions. If unsure you need to know who will be able to assist you.
>
> **Janice Brown**

The receptionist

Receptionists should have a smart appearance and be able to communicate effectively and professionally, creating the right impression.

As an assistant **receptionist**, your duties include:

- maintaining the reception area and retail displays
- looking after clients and visitors on arrival and departure
- assisting with scheduling appointments
- dealing with enquiries
- telling the appropriate beauty therapist that a client or visitor has arrived
- assisting with retail sales within your level of responsibility.

ALWAYS REMEMBER

Be careful not to interrupt when passing on information
If you need to pass information to another beauty therapist, never interrupt a client service. Wait until a suitable point in the service to communicate. If urgent information needs to be passed on, do so with minimum disruption. Make a note of what the message is and from whom to avoid forgetting!

BEST PRACTICE

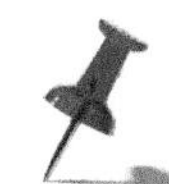

Impressions count
It is important that the attitude of the receptionist and their answer to any query is knowledgeable and extremely helpful. If insure always refer the question on to the relevant person explaining to the client at all times what you are doing.

The assistant receptionist should know:

- the name of each member of staff, their role and their area of responsibility, the salon's hours of opening, and the days and times when each beauty therapist is available
- the range of services or products offered by the salon, and their cost
- who to refer to if you receive different enquiries that you are unable to deal with or are not within your area of responsibility
- the person in your salon to whom you should refer reception problems
- any current discounts and special offers that the salon is promoting
- the benefits of each service and each retail product
- the approximate time taken to complete each service
- how to schedule follow-up services

You will also need to consider the last three points when **Preparing and maintaining the salon treatment area**

BEST PRACTICE

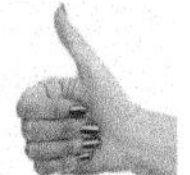

Wear a title badge
It is a good idea for receptionists to wear a badge indicating their name and position.

BEST PRACTICE

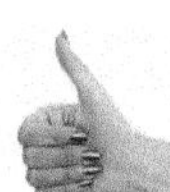

Non-verbal communication
If you are engaged on the telephone when a client arrives, look up and acknowledge the client's presence. This is an example of good interpersonal skills. The receptionist below demonstrates this perfectly.

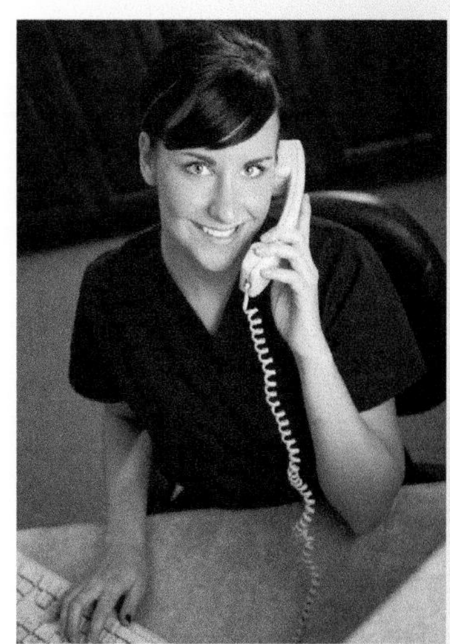

> Consultation is the key to a successful service. You may be asking yourself why you need to consult your client, you may feel you already know what they want, or see it as a card-filling task, so you should just get them on the couch and get started. However, you'd be wrong. Consultation is your opportunity to gain the information you need to enable you to give a safe service to meet your client's wants and needs. It is also your opportunity to impress the client with your knowledge and professionalism to ensure they build a trust in you and become a regular client. Always store client records securely.
>
> **Janice Brown**

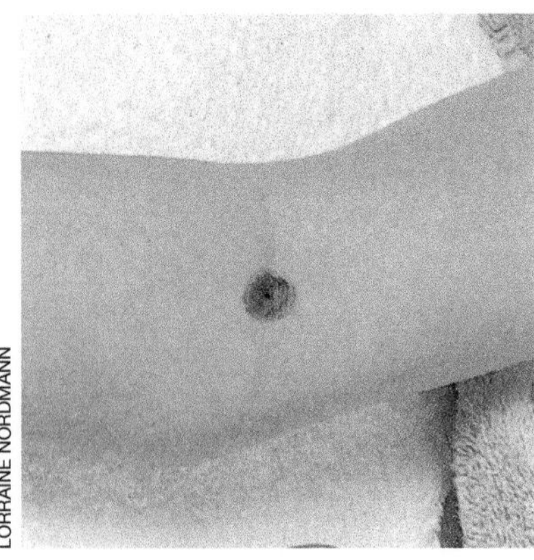

LORRAINE NORDMANN

A skin sensitivity test

You may also be required to perform **skin sensitivity tests**.

Skin sensitivity tests

Before clients receive certain services it might be necessary to carry out skin tests. The skin test is often carried out at reception, and the receptionist or assistant beauty therapist will be able to perform the test, after training. Every client should undergo a skin sensitivity test to check for ingredient intolerance which may lead to an allergic reaction, before a permanent tinting service to the eyelashes or eyebrows, or perming of the eyelashes. Further tests might be necessary, depending on the client's sensitivity, before services such as artificial eyelash service or wax depilation.

HEALTH & SAFETY

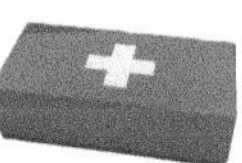

Keep the reception clear

As the receptionist, you should be familiar with the emergency procedure in case of an emergency. Make sure the reception area is free from any obstacles that could block the exit route in the event of an emergency. This will also remove potential hazards that may cause an accident. This is in compliance with the Workplace (Health, Safety and Welfare) Regulations (1992).

Outcome 2: Attend to clients and enquiries

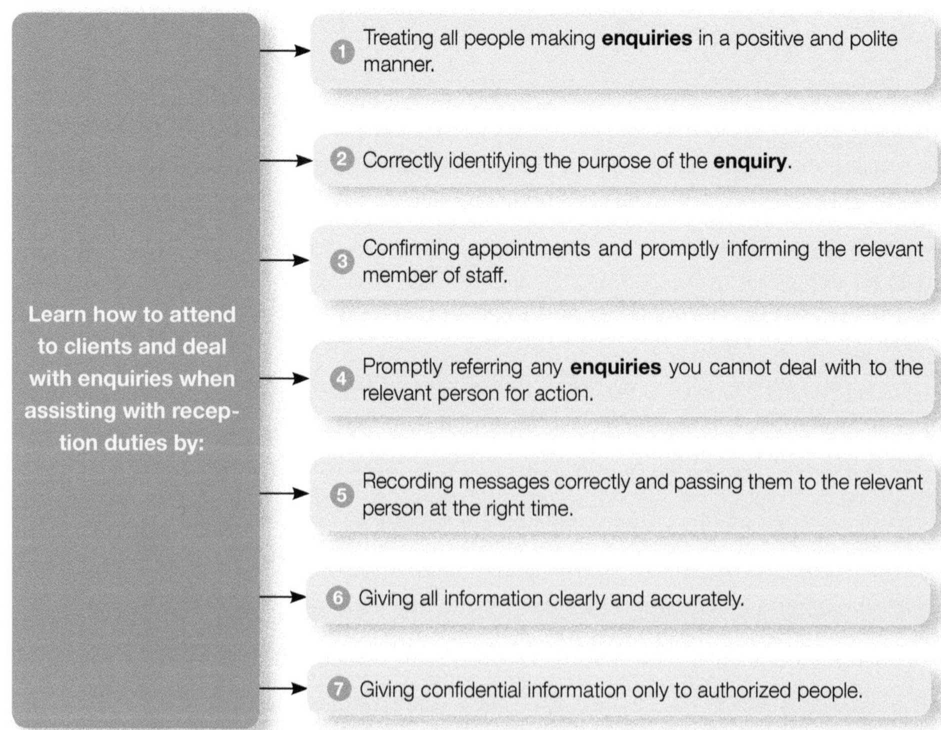

ALWAYS REMEMBER

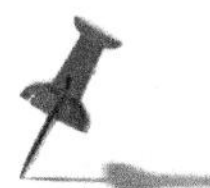

Visitors Book

Some businesses will request that visitors (non-clients, i.e. trade representatives) sign a visitors book. On arrival you should inform the member of staff they have arrived to see. You may then be required to direct them to the member of staff when available.

Attending to clients and dealing with enquiries

Act positively and confidently when attending to clients, visitors and their enquiries. Demonstrate good customer care skills at all times. Confirm their appointment and tell the beauty therapist of the client's arrival following your salon policy. If there is a delay inform the client immediately of this. If there is an **enquiry** answer this within the limits of your responsibility and refer any enquiry that you cannot deal with yourself to the relevant person as soon as possible, clearly and accurately.

All clients should feel valued. A client can be made to feel uncomfortable, ignored or important – and this can happen without you saying anything! Even without speaking you communicate by body language: with your eyes, your face and your body passing on some of your feelings. This is called **non-verbal communication**. How you look and how you behave in front of your clients is important. On meeting a client, always smile, make eye contact and greet them cheerfully – however bad your day is!

It is an important skill to be able to read and understand body language and the mood of clients. Looking at clients' body language will help you to be aware of their needs and what they expect and you can make sure that you respond accordingly. **Verbal communication** occurs when you talk directly to another person, either face to face or over the telephone. Always speak clearly and avoid slang. It is important to be a good listener: this will help you to know what the client wants and understand their personality.

Your tone of voice is important. You should always sound calm, cheerful, helpful, knowledgeable and professional. Your voice and manner should inspire confidence and trust.

Having a good posture will also positively affect your speech and professional appearance. You will sound and look more energized.

Always remember the **diversity** or range of people you will come into contact with. Diversity includes:

- personality
- beliefs and attitudes
- age
- religion, morality
- background and culture.

Diversity should be considered in all **communication**, respond to any enquiry and allow time for the client to respond. Consider if you feel you have dealt with their enquiry adequately. It is important that a client is listened to and responded to correctly.

Avoid all unsuitable topics such as sex, religion and politics. Never gossip with clients.

Interpersonal skills are behaviours – everything you say and do. Clients' opinions will be based upon your behaviour.

The following verbal and non-verbal **communication skills** are desirable in a receptionist:

- the ability to behave positively and confidently
- speak clearly
- have a friendly and smiling approach
- paying enough attention to the client and maintaining eye contact
- good listening skills
- showing interest in everything that is going on around the reception area
- giving each client individual attention and respect.

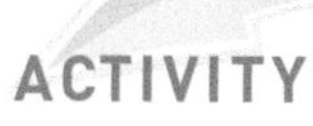

ACTIVITY

Telephone skills
What do you think is the most important use of the telephone in the workplace?

Telephone calls

Good telephone technique can win clients; poor technique can lose them. Here are some guidelines for good technique:

- Answer quickly: on average, callers are willing to wait up to 9 seconds: try to respond to the call within 6 seconds.
- Be prepared: have information and writing materials ready to hand. It should not normally be necessary to leave the caller waiting while you find something.
- Be welcoming and helpful: speak clearly, without mumbling, at the right speed. Speak clearly, and vary your tone. Sound interested, and never sharp.

Remember: the caller may be a new client ringing round several salons. The decision whether to visit your salon might depend on your attitude and the way you respond to the call.

ACTIVITY

Telephone calls
A telephone call is often the first contact the client has with the salon and is an important method of communication.

- How should the telephone be answered?
- What should you confirm if the client requires an eyelash tint?
- What action would you take if there was not enough time for the appointment at the time asked for?

TOP TIP

Your telephone manner

Don't consider the telephone ringing as an interruption. Always remember that clients matter – they ensure the success of your business!

A client who has received a poor response to a telephone call might tell friends or colleagues about it. If you receive an enquiry and are not sure of the answer, ask for help from a person with the relevant experience. Tell the client politely that you are unable to help but will get somebody who can.

TOP TIP

Cordless/mobile telephones

If the salon uses a cordless or mobile telephone, keep this in a central location where it can easily be found when it rings.

After each call, be sure to return the telephone to its normal location.

Here are some more ideas about good telephone technique:

- Smile – this will help you put across a warm, friendly reply to the caller.
- Speak clearly and alter the pitch of your voice as you speak, to create interest.
- As you answer, give the standard greeting for the salon, for example 'Good morning, Bodyworks Beauty Salon, Susan speaking. How can I help you?'
- Listen carefully to the caller's questions or requests. You will be speaking to a range of clients: you must respond suitably and helpfully to each.
- Consider the information the caller gives you and be sure to respond to what has been said or asked.
- Use the client's name, if you know it; this personalizes the call.
- Go over the main requests from the call to yourself; ask for further information if you need it.
- At the end, repeat the main points of the conversation clearly to check that you and the client have understood each other.
- Close the call pleasantly, for example 'Thank you for calling, Mrs Smith. Goodbye.'

ACTIVITY

Communicating with clients
Listen to experienced receptionists and notice how they communicate with clients.

If you receive a business call, or a call from a person seeking employment, always take the caller's name and telephone number. Your supervisor can then deal with the call as soon as they are free to do so.

Transferring calls

If you transfer a telephone call to another extension, explain what you are doing and thank the caller for waiting. If the extension to which you have transferred the call is not answered within nine rings, tell the caller that you will ask the person concerned to ring back as soon as possible. Take the caller's name and telephone number.

Taking messages

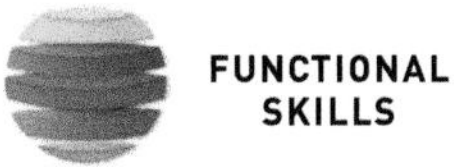

It is important that messages are recorded correctly and are passed on at the right time.

Messages should be recorded on a memorandum (memo) pad. Each message should record:

- who the message is for
- who the message was from
- the date and the time the message was received
- accurate details of the message
- the telephone number or address of the caller
- the signature of the person who took the message.

When taking a message, repeat the details you have recorded so that the caller can check that you've got it right. Pass the message to the correct person as soon as possible.

TELEPHONE MESSAGE RECEIVED			
To	Angela	Date	10.7.10
From	Jenny Heron	Time	9.30 am
Number	273451	Taken by	Sandra

Please ring Jenny Heron regarding her appointment on Saturday

A memo

Asking questions It is important to ask verbal questions to confirm and ensure that you are confident and understand what the client has asked you, or that the message has been taken correctly. Do not be embarrassed to do this, it will ensure you give an appropriate answer, make the correct decision and that client satisfaction will be achieved. You may ask 'open' or 'closed' questions. Always ask open questions if you need more information as these questions cannot be answered with 'yes' or 'no'. Open questions start with 'what', 'when', 'who' and 'why'. Closed questions are used when you need to check something quickly, these are answered with 'yes' or 'no'.

Dealing with a dissatisfied client at reception

Occasionally, a client might be dissatisfied. The receptionist is usually the first contact with the client and you might have to deal with dissatisfied, angry or awkward customers in a public place. Considerable skill is needed if you are to deal helpfully with a possibly damaging situation.

Never become angry or put yourself in an awkward position. Always remain polite and tactful, and communicate confidently and politely.

- Listen to the client as they describe their problems, without making judgement. Do not make excuses for yourself or for colleagues.

ACTIVITY

Listening to yourself

A pleasant speaking voice is a benefit. Do you think you could improve your speech or manner?

Record your voice as you answer a telephone enquiry, then play it back. How did you sound? This is how others hear you!

TOP TIP

Personal calls

Check the salon's policy on personal calls. Usually they are permitted only in emergencies. This is so staff are not distracted from clients and to keep the telephone free for clients to make appointments.

ACTIVITY

Finding the right approach

What telephone manner should you adopt when dealing with people who are:

- angry?
- talkative?
- nervous?
- confused?

ACTIVITY

Open and closed questions

Think of an 'open' and 'closed' question you may use when making an appointment for a leg waxing service. How did the way you asked the question differ to obtain the information needed?

ACTIVITY

Reception experiences

Pair with a colleague and share your experiences of a well managed and a badly managed reception.

ACTIVITY

Non-verbal communication

In discussion, you give signals that tell others whether you are listening or not.

What do you think the following signals indicate?

- a smile
- head tilted, and resting on one hand
- eyes looking around you
- eyes semi-closed
- head nodding
- fidgeting.

TOP TIP

Behaviour breeds behaviour

If you behave calmly, the client will become less angry. If you become angry, the client will become even angrier.

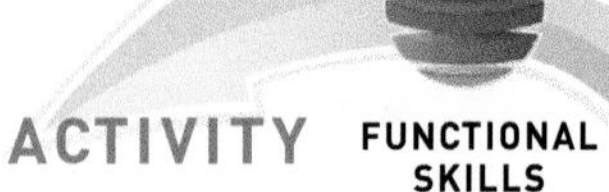

ACTIVITY FUNCTIONAL SKILLS

Do's and don'ts

List five important do's and five don'ts for the professional receptionist.

- Ask questions to check that you have all the details.
- If possible, agree on a course of action, offering an answer if you can. Check that the client has agreed to the planned course of action. It might be necessary to ask the salon manager before proposing a solution to the client: if you're not sure, always check first.
- Note the complaint by following salon policy recording: the date, the time, the client's name, the reason for the complaint and the agreed course of action.

Can you think of other body signals that indicate whether you are interested or not?

ACTIVITY

Reception scenarios

With colleagues, consider the following situations that might occur when working as a receptionist. What would you do in each situation?

- A client arrives very late for an appointment but insists that she is treated.
- A client questions the bill.
- A client comes in to complain about a previous service.

Remember you must protect client privacy and confidentiality by complying with the Data Protection Act (1984) at all times. Any information obtained from the client must only be available to those authorized to access the records.

Outcome 3: Help to make appointments for salon services

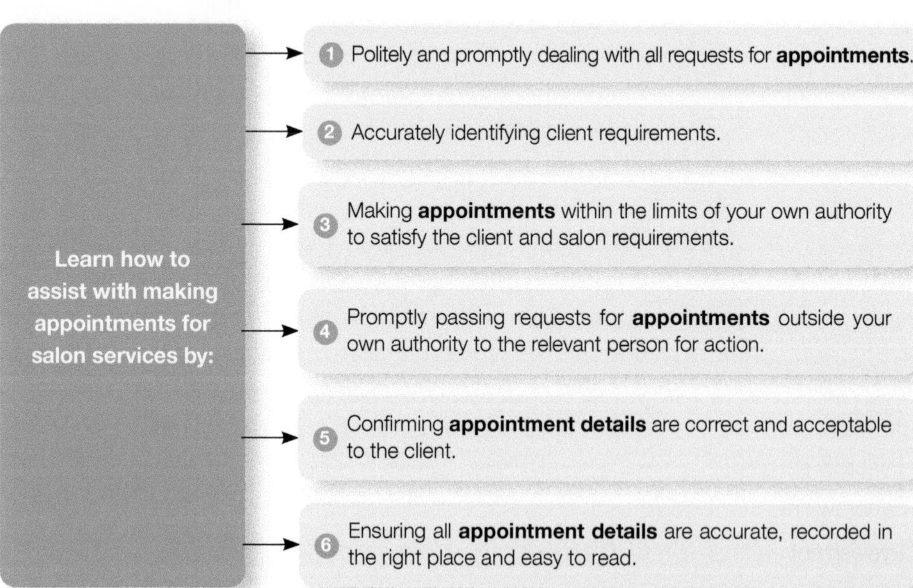

Making appointments

Making correct entries in the appointment book or salon computer is one of the most important duties of the receptionist. As assistant receptionist, you must understand the salon's appointment system, column headings, service times and any abbreviations used for the services.

Each beauty therapist will have their name at the head of a column. Entries in columns must not be changed without the agreement of the beauty therapist, unless they are absent, when a senior beauty therapist would reallocate the client bookings to ensure minimum disruption.

Information required

When clients call to make an appointment, their name and the service requested should be recorded. Allow enough time to carry out the required service. Take the client's telephone number in case the beauty therapist falls ill or is unable to keep the appointment for some other reason. If the client asks for a particular beauty therapist, be sure to enter the client's name in the correct column.

The hours of the day are recorded along the left-hand side of the appointment page, usually divided into 15-minute intervals. You need to know how long each service takes so that you can allow enough time for the beauty therapist to carry out the service in a safe, competent, professional manner. If you don't allow enough time, the beauty therapist will run late and this will affect all later appointments making them late too!. On the other hand, if you allow too much time, the beauty therapist's time will be wasted and the salon's earnings will be less than they could be. Suggested times to be allowed for each service are given in the service chapters. See the table below for a breakdown of services and their abbreviations (shortened form) and times allowed.

State the name of the beauty therapist who will be carrying out the service, the date and the time.

Finally, confirm or estimate the cost of the service to the client.

You could offer an **appointment card** to the client, to confirm the appointment. The card should record the service, the date, the day and the time. The beauty therapist's name might also be recorded.

Services are usually recorded in an abbreviated form. Everyone who uses the appointment page must be familiar with these abbreviations.

Service timings

If an appointment book is used, write each entry neatly and accurately. It is preferable to write in pencil: appointments can be amended by erasing and rewriting, keeping the book clean and clear.

Service	*Abbreviation*	*Service time allowed**
Cleanse and make-up (evening/special occasion)	C/M/up	45 mins
Cleanse and make-up (day)	C/M/up	45 mins
Eyebrow shaping	E/B reshape or trim	15 mins
Eyebrow tint	EBT	10 mins
Eyelash tint	ELT	20 mins
Manicure	Man	45 mins
Nail art	N/Art	5–10 mins (per nail)
Nail enhancements (this will vary dependant on the system used and service requirement)	N/En	120 mins

TOP TIP

Making service appointments

- Making appointments for **facials**, additional guidance is provided in chapter 6.
- Making appointments for **make-up**, additional guidance is provided in chapter 7.
- Making appointments for **nail services**, additional guidance is provided in chapter 6.

HEALTH & SAFETY

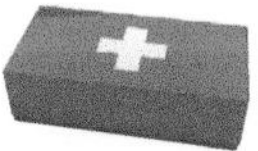

Health and Safety (Display Screen Equipment) Regulations (1992)
These regulations cover the use of visual display units (VDUs) and computer screens. They specify acceptable levels of radiation emissions from the screen and identify correct posture, seating position, permitted working heights and rest periods.

Service	*Abbreviation*	*Service time allowed**
Pedicure	Ped	50 mins
Leg wax: half	½ leg wax	30 mins
three-quarter	¾ leg wax	30–40 mins
full	Full-leg wax	45 mins
Bikini wax	B/wax	15 mins
Underarm wax	U/arm wax	15 mins
Arm wax	F/arm wax	30 mins
Facial wax	F/wax	10–20 mins
	Upper lip	10 mins
	chin	10 mins
Eyebrow wax	E/B wax	15 mins
Threading	EB/Thread	20 mins
	F/Thread	10–15 mins
	Upper lip	10 mins
	chin	10 mins
Ear pierce	E/P	15 mins
Facial	F	60 mins
Artificial eyelashes strip/ individual flare Full set 20 mins, partial 10 mins	F/Lash Full set 10 mins, partial 10 mins	10–20 mins

*Service time does not include preparation for service and consultation.

TOP TIP

Electronic bookings

Electronic appointment booking systems if used allow you to read the appointment schedule and add or edit appointments immediately.

Appointments can be made up to 6 weeks in advance. Often, clients will book their next appointment as they leave the current appointment. How far ahead the receptionist is able to book appointments will be different for each workplace.

When clients arrive for their service, draw a line (or tick) through their name to indicate that they have arrived. If using an electronic booking system use the appropriate entry.

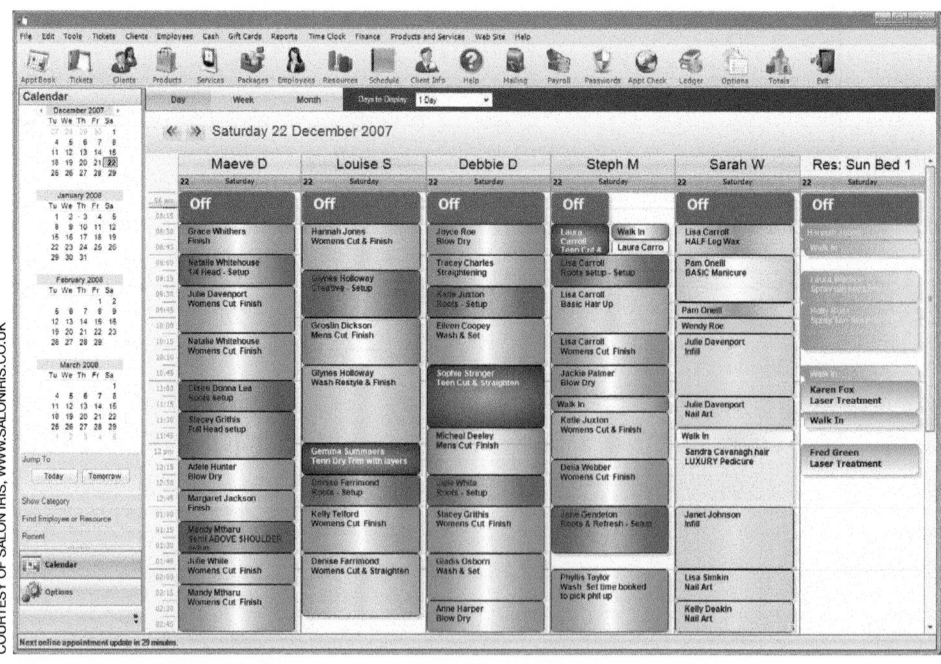

COURTESY OF SALON IRIS, WWW.SALONIRIS.CO.UK

Electronic client booking system

If a client cancels, indicate this on the appointment page immediately, usually with a large C written through the booking. This enables another client to take the appointment.

DAY SATURDAY DATE 15th JANUARY

THERAPIST	JAYNE	SUE	LIZ
9.00	Mrs Young	DNA	
9.15	1/2 leg wax	Jenny Newley	
9.30	Carol Kreen	ELT/EBT	
9.45	Full leg wax	EB trim	
10.00	B / Wax		
10.15		Sandra Smith	Fiona Smith
10.30	Ms Lord E/B wax	C / M / up	C / M / up
10.45			Strip / lash
11.00		Mrs Jones	
11.15		U/arm wax	
11.30		F/arm wax	Carol Brown
11.45			E/P
12.00			
12.15			
12.30	Nina Farrel		
12.45	Man		
1.00	Ped		
1.15		Sue Uip E/P	
1.30	1/2 leg wax	T Scott	
1.45		3/4 leg wax	
2.00	Karen Davies	U/arm wax	
2.15	Facial		
2.30			
2.45			Pat king
3.00			C / M / up
3.15	Anno Wood		Man
3.30	Man		
3.45	E/B Reshape		
4.00			

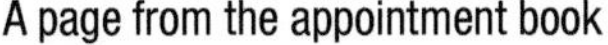

A page from the appointment book

If a client fails to arrive, the abbreviation DNA (did not arrive) is usually written over the booking. The client should then be telephoned to see if a re-booking is required.

Some salons have a policy of charging for a missed appointment.

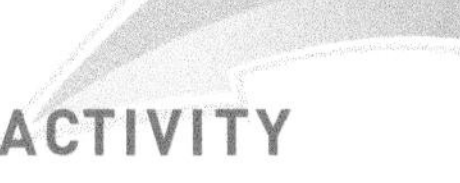

ACTIVITY

Careless booking

- What is careless booking?
- In what ways may careless booking affect the business?

The payment point

Every beauty therapy workplace will have a policy for handling cash and for operating the payment point. It is important that you are given training and are confident to take payment in the client's preferred method, which might be cash or a cash equivalent, e.g. gift voucher, cheque or payment card. You will be required to handle cash if you study salon reception duties at Level 2. Your responsibility is to be security conscious when working around the payment point . If you see anything unusual, pass this information on to the responsible person.

GLOSSARY OF KEY WORDS

Appointment arrangement made for a client to receive a service on a particular date and time

Communication exchange of information and the development of understanding between people

Computer electronic machine that holds data on the business

Confidential Information this may include conversation that you have had with a client or colleague, details recorded on client record cards and client and staff personal details, e.g. addresses and telephone numbers

Confidentiality keeping information or data private. In order to gain trust between your self and the client it is important to keep client information confidential.

Data Protection Act (1998) legislation designed to protect client privacy and confidentiality

Enquiry question presented by clients or business contacts to find out more information

Health and Safety (Display Screen Equipment) Regulations (1992) these regulations cover the use of visual display units (VDUs) and computer screens. They specify acceptable levels of radiation emissions from the screen and correct working posture, permitted working heights and rest periods

Hospitality friendliness and care for clients at reception, being helpful, i.e. offering refreshments and magazines while waiting for a service

Messages communication of information to another person in written or verbal form

Non-verbal communication communicating by using body language, i.e. using your eyes, face and body for transmitting your feelings

Reception an area in the salon where clients are received and their enquiries dealt with, either in person or by telephone

Receptionist person responsible for maintaining the reception area, scheduling appointments, dealing with enquiries and taking messages

Record cards personal information recorded for each client, recording services received and retail product purchases

Resources needs of various kinds, people, stock, facilities

Retail selling of goods, i.e. products that clients use at home

Skin sensitivity tests assessment of a client's tolerance/sensitivity to a particular substance to check suitability before a service is provided

Verbal communication occurs when you talk directly to another person, either face to face or over the telephone

ASSESSMENT OF KNOWLEDGE AND UNDERSTANDING

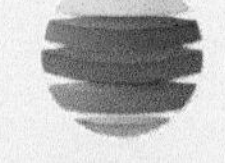

FUNCTIONAL SKILLS

Having covered the learning objectives for **asssist with salon reception duties** – test what you need to know and understand by answering the following short questions below. The information covers:

- salon and legal requirements
- communication
- salon services, products and pricing
- making appointments.

Salon and legal requirements

1 You have a duty to handle client records when assisting with reception. What legislation must you comply with when handling this confidential information?

2 State **three** duties of the salon receptionist.

3 What is your role in maintaining the standard of reception area?

4 If, as assistant receptionist, you were unable to give appropriate information to a client, what action would you take?

5 If a client is likely to be delayed for an appointment, who will you need to communicate with and with what regularity?

6 What are your workplace procedures for making and recording appointments?

Communication

1 How can you make a client feel welcomed at reception? Give **three** examples of good client hospitality.

2 When taking a message, what **five** things should be recorded?

3 What do you understand by the following methods of communication:
- verbal communication
- non-verbal communication.

4 Give **three** examples of positive body language.

5 If a client was dissatisfied with a service they had received, how would you deal with this client?

6 Give **three** examples of good telephone technique.

7 When is it necessary to ask questions when communicating with clients? Give **three examples**.

8 When is it necessary to use 'open' questions?

Salon services, products and pricing

1 Name **five** pieces of equipment or resources required for use in the reception area, and state the purpose of each.

2 Why is it important that you know the salon services that are available and their cost and timing?

3 How can you help in increasing the sales of retail products?

4 What action would you take if you found stock to be spoilt when restocking the display area?

5 Why is it important to tell the relevant person if you notice low stock levels of reception resources, e.g. price lists?

6 Why is it important to know about the retail products available in your workplace and their cost?

Making appointments

1 When making an appointment for a client, what information should be requested from the client?

2 When making an appointment for a client requesting a specific day/time:

- What do you need to check initially in the appointment book?
- What information do you need to obtain from the client?

3 What do you need to check first of all in the appointment book?

4 What information do you need to find out from the client?

5 Why is it important that appointments are made correctly?

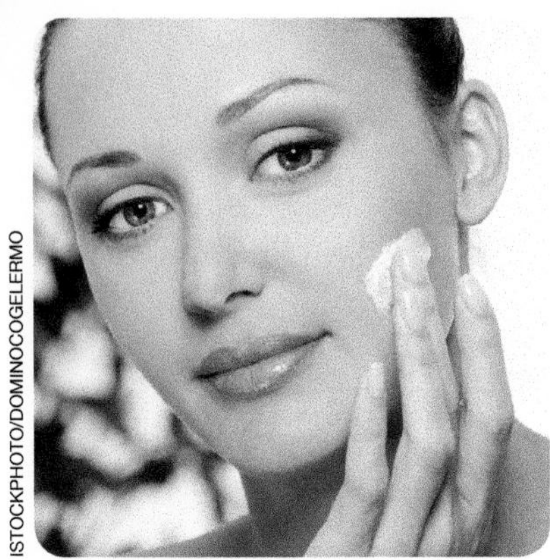

6 Facial skincare

Learning Objectives

This chapter covers the **Assist with facial skincare services** unit.

This unit is all about the skills needed to assist you with facial services in the workplace.

There are **four** learning outcomes which you must achieve competently:

1. **Maintain safe and effective working methods when assisting with facial services**
2. **Consult, plan and prepare for facial services with clients**
3. **Carry out facial services**
4. **Provide aftercare advice**

Your assessor will observe your performance on **at least three separate occasions which will be recorded**.

From the **range** statement, you must show that you have:

- used all **consultation techniques**
- identified all **skin types**
- carried out all types of **preparation of the client**
- used all types of **facial products**
- given all types of **advice**.

When providing facial skincare services it is important to use the skills you have learnt in the following chapters:

- **Health and Safety**
- **Developing positive working relationships**
- **Preparing and maintaining the salon treatment work area**

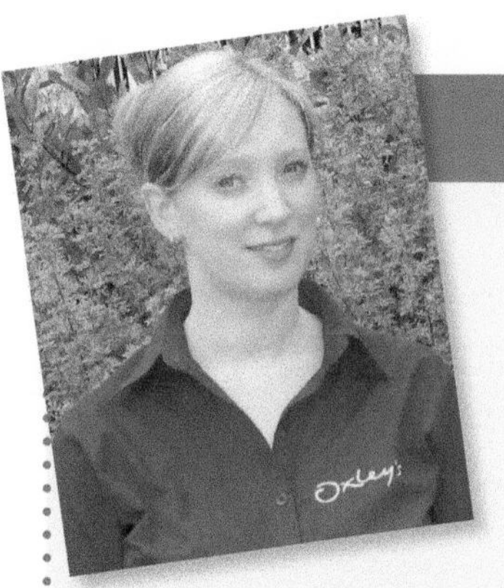

ROLE MODEL

Sally-Anne Braithwaite

Front of House Manager, Oxley's at Ambleside Blue Fish Spa

"My current job role as Front of House Manager includes all sorts of responsibilities such as running reception, meeting and greeting customers, product sales and helping with marketing and accounts.

When I first started the job in October 2006 I was new to the beauty industry and had to learn all aspects of the job as I went along. I was trained up to have a good knowledge of all the services we have to offer, which I feel is a very important part of my role. Now I am part of a great team and have a very rewarding and enjoyable job.

Practical skills, knowledge and understanding

The table shown here will help you to check your progress in gaining the necessary practical skills, knowledge and understanding for **assisting with facial skincare services**.

Tick (✓), when you feel you have gained the practical skills, knowledge and understanding in each of the following areas:

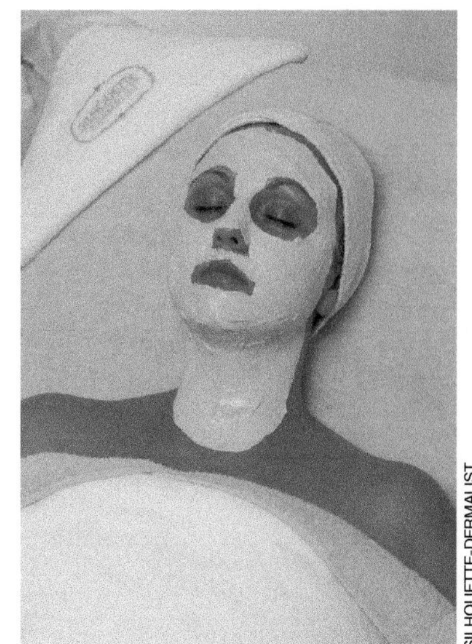

SILHOUETTE-DERMALIST

Client with face mask applied

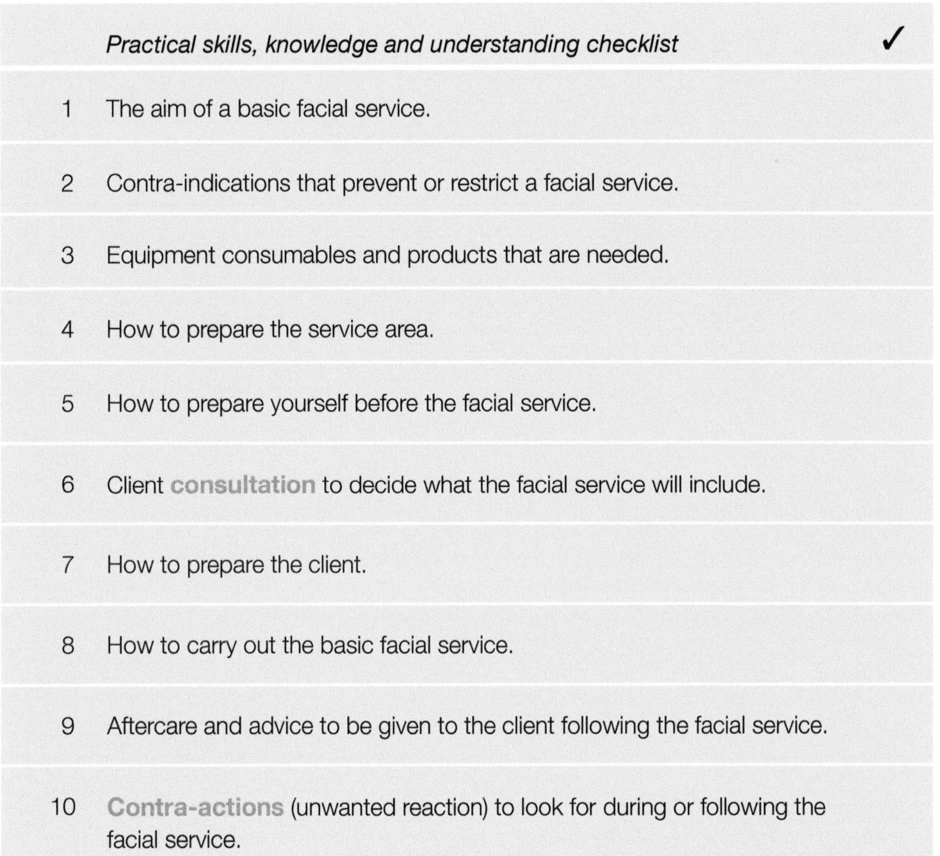

	Practical skills, knowledge and understanding checklist	✓
1	The aim of a basic facial service.	
2	Contra-indications that prevent or restrict a facial service.	
3	Equipment consumables and products that are needed.	
4	How to prepare the service area.	
5	How to prepare yourself before the facial service.	
6	Client consultation to decide what the facial service will include.	
7	How to prepare the client.	
8	How to carry out the basic facial service.	
9	Aftercare and advice to be given to the client following the facial service.	
10	Contra-actions (unwanted reaction) to look for during or following the facial service.	

When you have ticked all the areas you can, ask your assessor to assess you on **Assisting with facial skincare services**. After practical assessment, your assessor might decide that you need to practise further to improve your skills. If so, your assessor will tell you how and where you need to improve to gain competence.

After assessment of your knowledge and understanding there may be 'gaps' that need to be studied further. Your assessor will tell you what you need to study to achieve the required level of knowledge and understanding.

Facial services

As well as looking after the skin from the inside, by maintaining a healthy diet, it needs care from the outside – it must be kept clean and it must be nourished.

When it is functioning normally, the skin becomes oily and sweat appears on its surface. The natural oil in the skin (called sebum) can easily build up on the skin's surface and block the skin's natural openings – the pores – on the surface of the skin; This is called skin congestion and can lead to infection seen as 'spots'. Facial cosmetics, including self-tanning products can cause blockages. Skincare facial services help keep the skin healthy and improve how it functions.

The basic facial service you will provide aims to improve the overall external appearance and condition of the skin by the application of suitable skincare services and products for the client's skin. Internally the skins functions will also be benefited. The facial service includes:

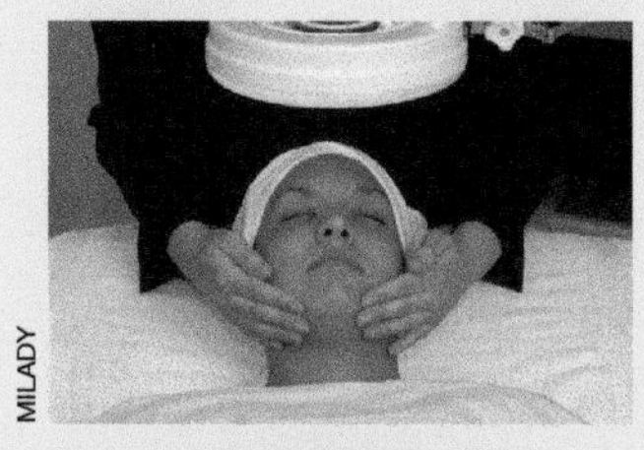

Consultation and skin analysis

Consultation and **skin analysis** to decide the client's skin type and service needs

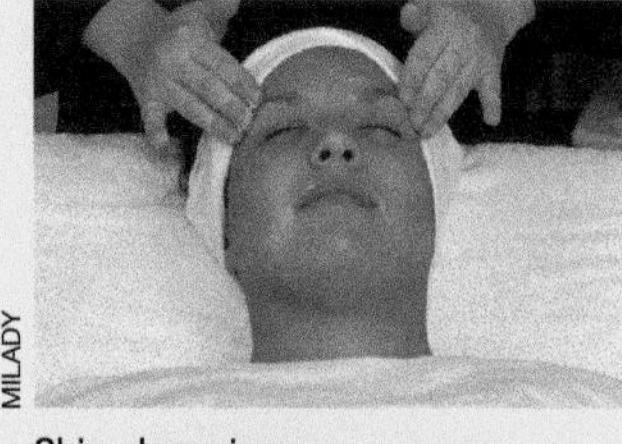

Skin cleansing

Skin cleansing to remove surface dirt, make-up and skin debris, such as dead skin, oil and sweat

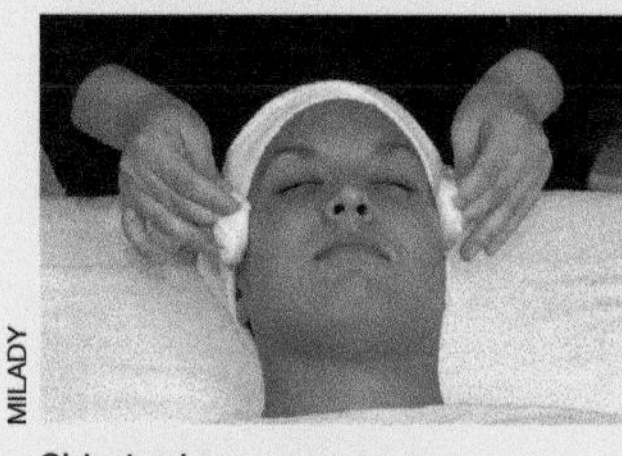

Skin toning

Skin toning to remove cleansing products and refresh and tighten the skin's surface

> A good knowledge of the products and the benefits of the service is essential when carrying out each service.
> **Sally-Anne Braithwaite**

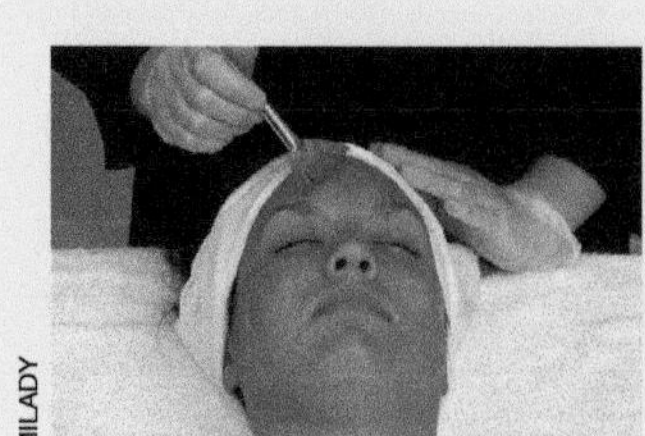

The application of a face mask

The application of a face mask to cleanse, calm or nourish the skin – whatever the skin needs

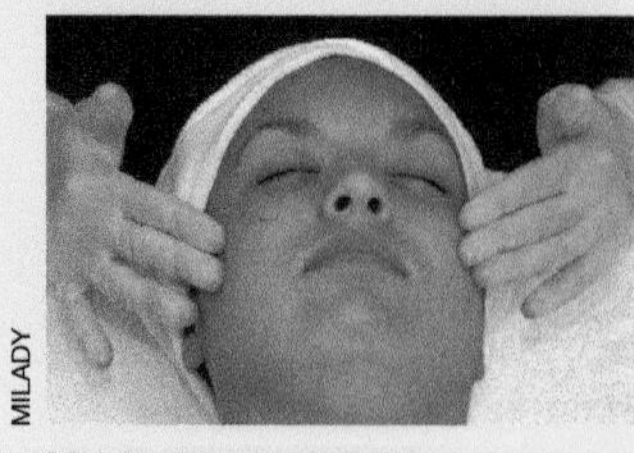

Moisturiser application

Moisturiser application to protect and add moisture to the skin

The skin is different in appearance, according to our race, sex and age. It changes from season-to-season, year-to-year and can be a mirror of our general health, lifestyle and diet. The way the different parts of the skin works gives us our skin type, e.g. dry, oily or combination.

Anatomy and physiology of the skin

You need to know about the skin, its structure and function (how it works) so that you can improve its appearance and understand how it should be cared for properly.

Basic functions of the skin

The skin has many functions; the main functions are listed below.

Protection The skin helps to protect the body from harmful substances and conditions, and cushions the other parts of the body underneath it from physical injury. The outer surface of the skin is bactericidal, which means it helps to prevent the growth of harmful microorganisms (minute organisms - invisible to the human eye). The skin is tough and waterproof which forms a barrier that prevents the absorption of many substances into the skin, and also prevents the skin losing water, which would cause it to dry out. Cells in the skin contain a pigment called **melanin**, which gives us our skin colour and helps protect the body from the harmful rays of UV light. The amount of melanin in the skin can differ between individuals and between races. In darker skin, melanin is present in larger amounts throughout all the layers of the part of the skin, known as the 'epidermis'.

Heat regulation The normal body temperature is maintained at 36.8–37°C.

Body temperature is controlled generally by heat loss through the skin and by sweating.

If the body temperature is increased by 0.25–0.5°C, the **sweat glands** secrete sweat to cool the skin's surface. The body is cooled by the loss of heat used to evaporate (turning the liquid into a vapour) the sweat from the skin's surface.

If the body becomes too warm there is an increase in **blood** flow into the blood capillaries (tiny vessels carrying blood) in the skin. The blood capillaries widen and heat is lost from the skin's surface.

Absorption The skin can absorb substances, i.e. moisturiser ingredients. This means on occasions it must be protected to avoid damage, i.e. from harmful chemicals.

Excretion Small amounts of waste products are removed from the body in sweat by a process called excretion.

Secretion The skin secretes a natural oil called sebum which provides the skin's surface with a waterproof anti-bactericidal coating, preventing harm from microorganisms the skin losing water from its tissues.

Sensations The skin allows the feelings of **touch**, **pressure**, **heat** and **cold**, and allows us to recognize objects by their feel and shape and can cause the body to react to prevent harm i.e. touching a hot object will cause you to move your hand away quickly. These are recognized by **nerve** endings in the skin called *sensory nerve endings*.

Basic structure of the skin

The skin is the largest organ in the body, making up one-eighth of the body's total weight. It is made up of microscopic cells, which provide a tough, flexible covering, with many important functions. Each **cell** contains structures surrounded by a chemical substance called protoplasm. The actions of these cells are necessary for our general health. If the cells cannot function properly, a disorder results.

Each cell is surrounded by a coating called the cell membrane. This membrane is porous, allowing food to enter and waste materials to leave, keeping it healthy.

HEALTH & SAFETY

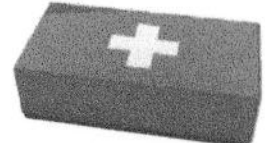

Allergic reactions

If the skin is allergic or sensitive to something this shows as an allergic reaction. The skin becomes red, itchy and swollen. At the consultation you must check whether a client is allergic to anything so that you don't cause an allergic reaction. Remember to carry out a skin sensitivity test, checking client suitability if at all unsure.

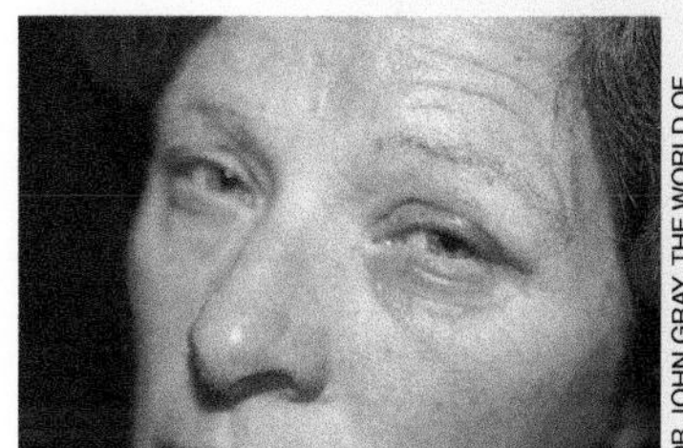

DR JOHN GRAY, THE WORLD OF SKINCARE

Client with an allergic reaction

TOP TIP

Remember the skin's functions by remembering SHAPES
S ensation
H eat regulation
A bsorption
P rotection
E xcretion
S ecretion

ACTIVITY

What ingredients in facial skincare products may a client be allergic to?

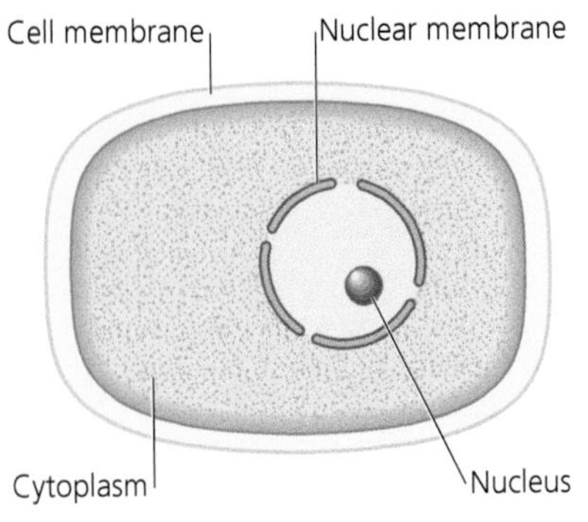

A cell

In the centre of the cell is the **nucleus**, which contains the **chromosomes**, long pieces of DNA that carry the genes we have inherited from our parents, making us who we are. Genes are responsible for cell reproduction and functioning.

The liquid that surrounds the nucleus is called the cell **cytoplasm**.

If we used a microscope to look inside the skin we would be able to see two distinct layers: the **epidermis** (the top layer of the skin) and the **dermis**. Found below the epidermis and the dermis is a further layer, the **subcutaneous tissue layer** or **fat layer**.

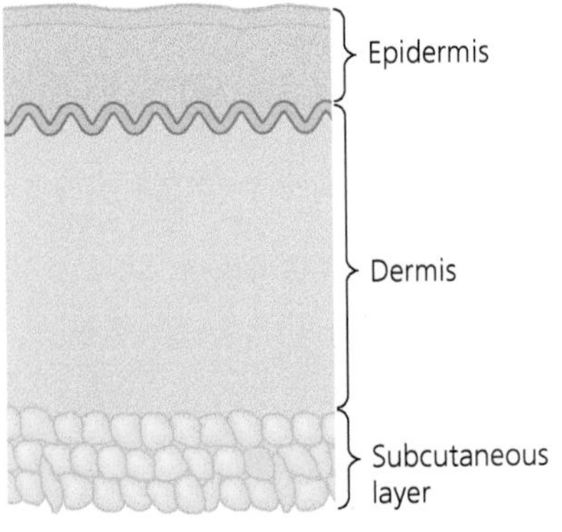

The skin

The epidermis

The main function of the epidermis is to protect the deeper living structures in the body from harm by the outside or external environment.

The epidermis is found above the dermis layer. It is composed of **five** layers, with the outer layer being the skin we can see and touch. This is the most important layer of the skin with regard to the application of skincare products. Each layer of the epidermis can be recognized by the shape of its cells.

Over a period of about 4 weeks, cells move from the bottom layer of the epidermis to the top layer – the skin's surface – changing in shape and structure as they move through the different layers.

ALWAYS REMEMBER

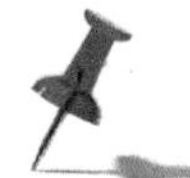

Keratin
The main type of cell in the epidermis is the keratinocyte, which produces a substance called keratin. Keratin makes the skin tough and reduces the entry of materials into the skin. Keratin is the main substance that forms hair and nails.

ALWAYS REMEMBER

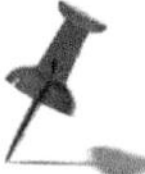

DNA
Found in the nucleus, DNA makes up our unique genes, which create who we are. If a chromosome is missing or there are additional chromosomes this can affect a person's health and their physical development.

The process of cellular change

The cell is formed

↓

The cell becomes fully developed

It changes in structure and moves upwards and outwards

↓

It moves upwards towards the skin's surface and becomes an empty shell which is shed from the skin's surface

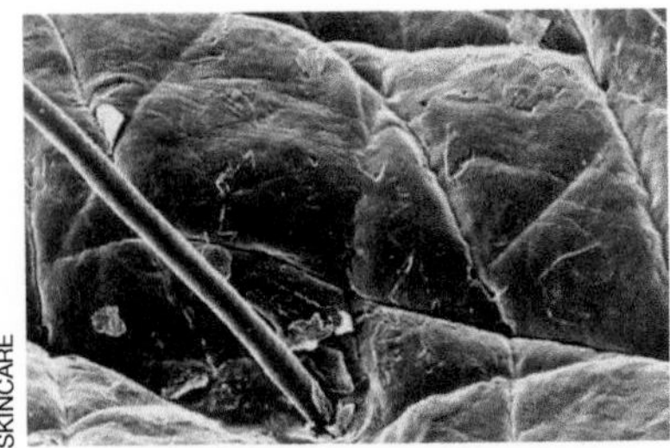

DR JOHN GRAY, THE WORLD OF SKINCARE

The outer layer of the skin's epidermis with hair shaft shown viewed with a microscope

The five layers of the epidermis are listed below. Sometimes they are referred to by other names, so these have been listed also.

1 *stratum corneum* or cornified layer

2 *stratum lucidum* or clear layer or lucid layer

3 *stratum granulosum* or granular layer

4 *stratum mucosum* or *spinosum* or prickle-cell layer

5 *stratum germinativum* or basal layer.

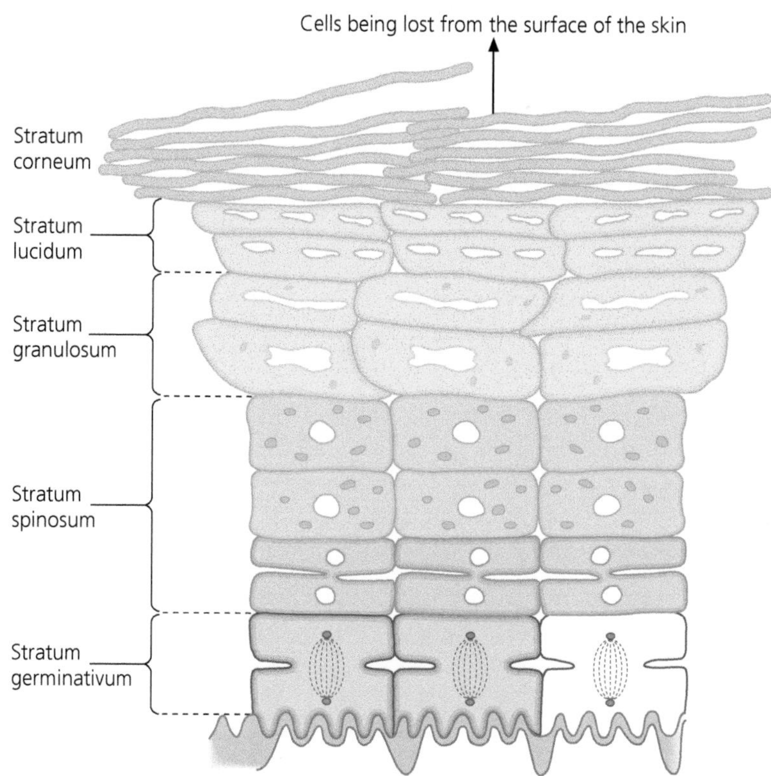

Five layers of the epidermis

Stratum corneum or cornified or horny layer This outer layer is formed from several layers of flattened, scale-like overlapping cells, made up mainly of keratin. These help to reflect and protect the skin's surface from UV light; darker skin can tolerate stronger UV light and also have a thicker stratum corneum than less pigmented, lighter skin.

It takes about 4 weeks for the epidermal cells to reach the stratum corneum from the stratum germinativum. The cells are then lost in a process called **desquamation**. The epidermis grows more slowly as we age and the skin appears thinner in some areas such as around the eyes, where small veins and capillaries can be seen through the skin.

Stratum lucidum or clear layer or lucid layer This layer is seen only in non-hairy areas of the skin such as the palms of the hands and soles of the feet. The cells here lack a nucleus and are filled with clear substances called *eledin*.

Stratum granulosum or granular layer This is composed of two or three layers of flattish cells. The nucleus of the cell has begun to break up, creating granules within the cell cytoplasm. These granules later form keratin.

Stratum mucosum or spinosum or prickle-cell layer The stratum spinosum or prickle-cell layer is formed from between two and six rows of cells that have a surface of spiky spines, which connect to surrounding cells. Each cell has a large nucleus filled with fluid.

ALWAYS REMEMBER

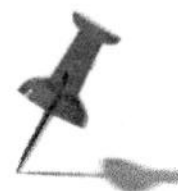

Stratum is simply the Latin word for layer. Therefore this word appears before the name of each epidermal layer.

ALWAYS REMEMBER

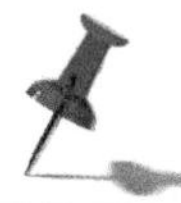

Removing dead cells

When we cleanse the skin and apply specialist skin products, such as a service mask, we remove dead cells from the surface of the epidermis. Every 5 days on average we shed a complete surface layer.

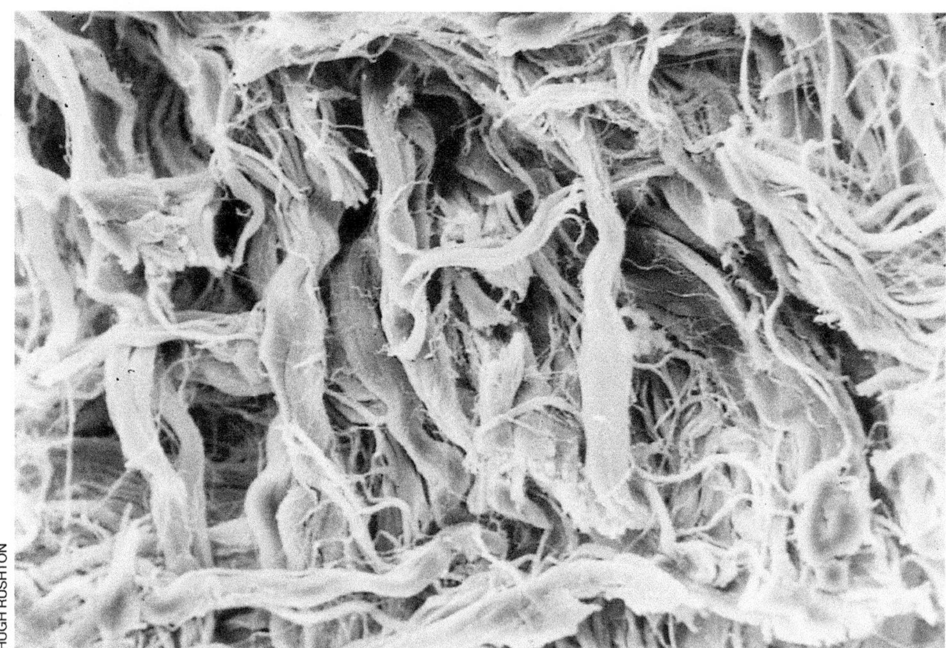

HUGH RUSHTON

Collagen and elastin fibre

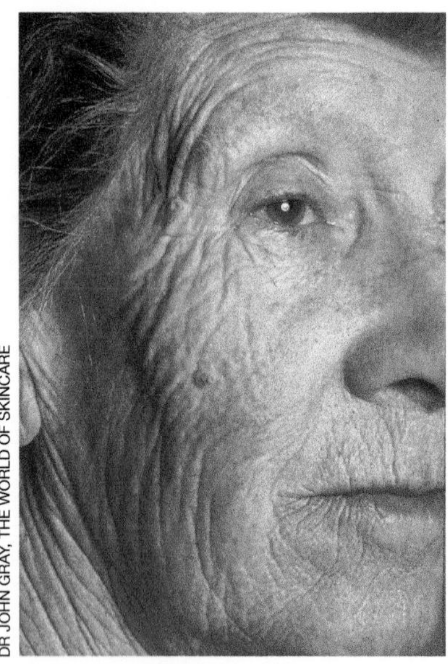

DR JOHN GRAY, THE WORLD OF SKINCARE

Aged skin – the skin has visibly lost its elasticity and strength

Stratum germinativum or basal layer This is the deepest layer of the epidermis. It is formed from a single layer of column-shaped cells. These cells divide constantly and produce new cells. **Melanocytes** are found in this layer; these are the cells that produce the skin pigment melanin and give the skin its colour. The amount and distribution of melanocytes varies according to race. In a white skinned person the melanin tends to be destroyed when it reaches the granular layer of the epidermis. With stimulation from artificial or natural UV light, however, melanin is also in the upper layers of epidermis.

In black skin melanin is in larger amounts throughout all the layers of the epidermis, giving a high level of protection. This increased protection allows less UV into the dermis layer below, reducing the UV light ageing effect. The amount and supply of melanin through the epidermis also means that people with dark skins are at less risk of skin cancer.

The dermis

The dermis is the inner part of the skin found underneath the epidermis. It is much thicker than the epidermis and contains a network of **fibres** that give skin its strength and elasticity. There are two types of fibres:

- yellow elastin gives the skin its elasticity
- white collagen gives the skin its strength.

As the skin begins to age, this network loses strength and elasticity, seen as facial lines and slack skin.

The dermis also contains other structures such as **blood vessels**, **lymph** vessels and nerves.

There are different types of nerves, which can sense touch, pressure and temperature. They inform us about the outside world and what is happening on the skin's surface. They are more numerous in sensitive parts of the skin such as the lips and the fingertips.

Near the surface of the dermis are tiny structures called dermal **papillae** in the papillary dermis layer. These contain nerve endings and blood capillaries which supply the upper epidermis with nutrition.

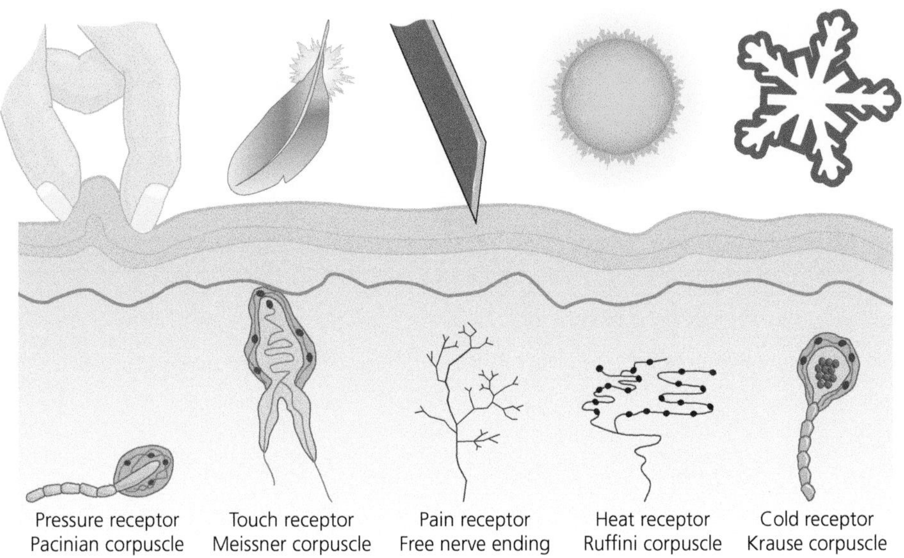

Sensory nerves to receive sensations

> **TOP TIP**
>
> **Blood supply**
>
> When you massage the skin's surface when applying cleansing products, you increase the blood supply to the skin and so help the removal of waste products from the skin. This improves the health and functioning of the skin. You will know this has happened as the skin will feel warm and may appear redder or darker in colour dependent upon the skin's natural pigmentation.

The blood supply to the skin Food and oxygen, which are necessary for the skin's health and growth, are carried to the dermis in the blood. The blood vessels that bring blood to the dermis also take away some waste products. Other waste products (e.g. used blood cells) are carried away by the lymph vessels that carry waste.

Skin appendages Within the dermis are additional structures called **skin appendages**. These include:

- sweat glands
- hair follicles, which produce hair
- **sebaceous glands**
- nails.

Sweat glands Sweat glands are small tubes in the skin, found in the epidermis and dermis. They are found all over the body, especially on the soles of the feet and palms of the hands. The main function of the sweat glands is to control the body temperature. Sweat, a fluid, flows onto the skin's surface through a sweat pore, where it is lost by the heating action of the skin creating a cooling effect. We each have 2–5 million sweat glands. Fluid loss and control of body temperature are important to prevent the body overheating, especially in hot, humid countries.

For this reason, perhaps, sweat glands are larger and more abundant in black skin than white skin.

Pores allow the absorption of some facial products into the skin. The facial service is aimed at cleansing the pores with facial cleansers and masks.

The pores may become enlarged because of blockages caused by dirt, dead skin cells and cosmetics. The application of **toning lotion** creates a skin tightening effect upon the skin's surface, slightly reducing the size of the pores.

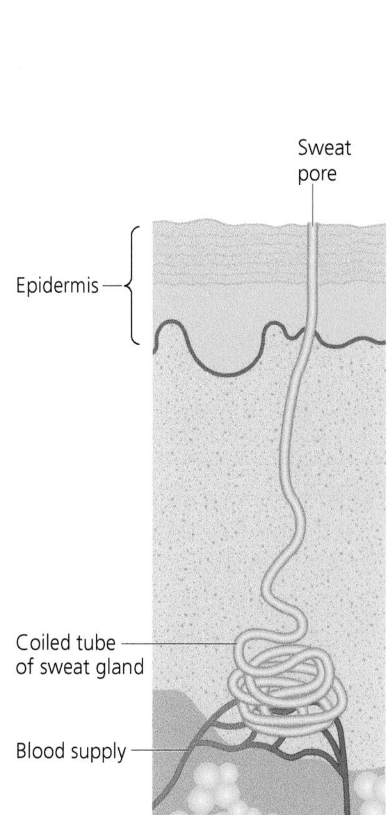

A sweat gland

Hair follicles **Hair follicles** are small tubes in the epidermis and dermis of the skin. They are found all over the body except on the palms of the hands and soles of the feet. At the bottom of each follicle is a cluster of cells, this is called the matrix, that divide here and move up the hair follicle, changing in structure forming a hair.

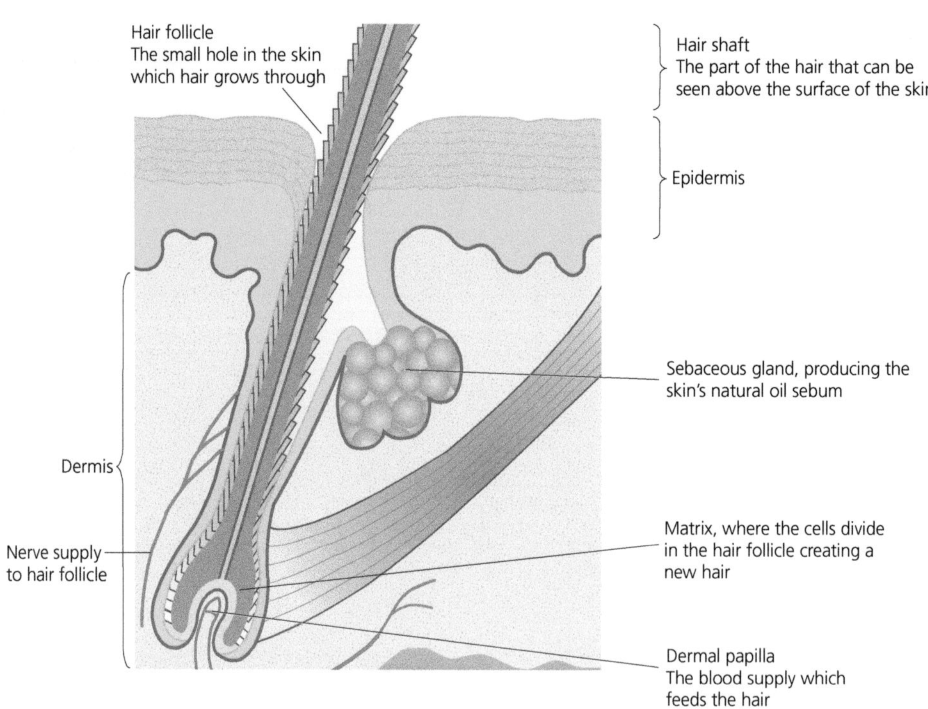

Cross-section of the skin, hair and hair follicle

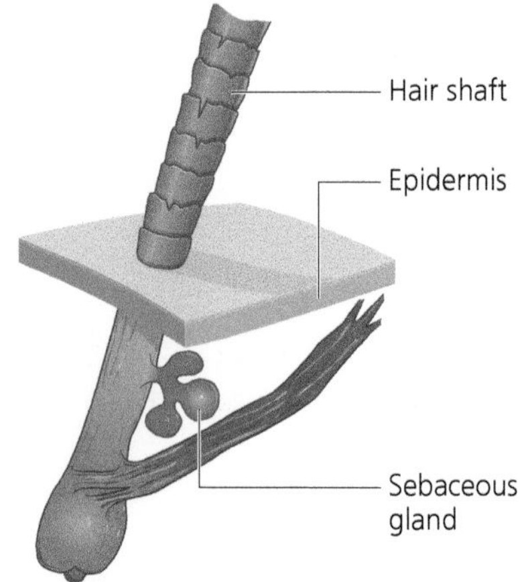

Sebaceous gland

Sebaceous glands Sebaceous glands produce the skins natural oil sebum. They are found all over the body, except the palms of the hands and soles of the feet. The cells of the sebaceous gland break down to form **sebum**. The activity of the sebaceous gland increases at puberty, when stimulated by a chemical messenger carried in the blood called a hormone. In adults, the activity slows down again. Men secrete slightly more sebum than women. With ageing we therefore produce less oil and the skin becomes drier. The sebaceous glands on black skin are larger and more numerous than on white skin.

Sebum has bactericidal and fungicidal properties, which help slow the growth of harmful microorganisms on the skin surface, which could lead to skin disease. Sebum also prevents loss of moisture from the surface of the skin. Cosmetic moisturisers copy sebum in providing an oily covering for the skin's surface to reduce moisture loss.

The acid mantle Sweat and sebum combine on the skin's surface to create an acid film, this is called the **acid mantle**. This has a protective function and slows the growth of bacteria and fungi.

TOP TIP

Sebum and skin types

An overactive sebaceous gland produces a large amount of sebum (too much) and results in an 'oily' skin type.

If the sebaceous gland is underactive, it produces less sebum (too little) and the skin is termed 'dry'.

ALWAYS REMEMBER

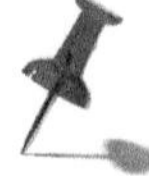

Protecting the skin's acid mantle

Some products that come into contact with the skin (such as some soaps) disturb the skin's acid mantle. If these products are used on the skin, the acid mantle will take several hours to return to its normal state and the skin might become irritated, reddened and sensitive during this time.

Black skin

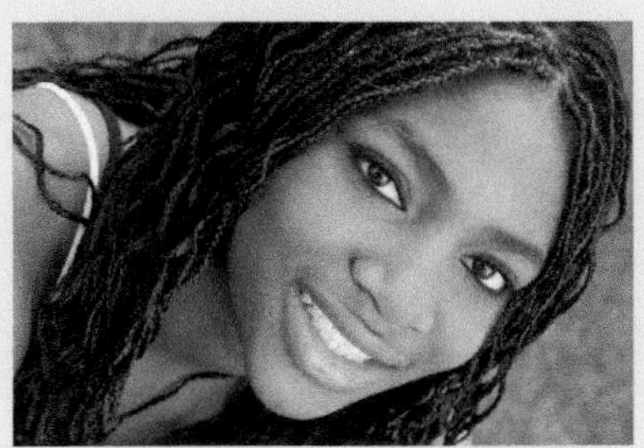

Skin colour is dark and ranges in tone to black

Care must be taken when treating a blemished skin as scars may occur appearing as darker patches as the skin heals Areas of skin that is darker than the surrounding area is known as hyper-pigmentation

Loss of pigment can also occur where the skin appears lighter called vitiligo

Male black skin may have a tendency towards pseudo folliculitis, an inflammatory skin disorder where the facial hairs becomes trapped in the skin becoming ingrown

Dermatosis papulosis nigra, also called flesh moles can occur. These are hyper-pigmented marks usually seen on the cheeks

Asian skin

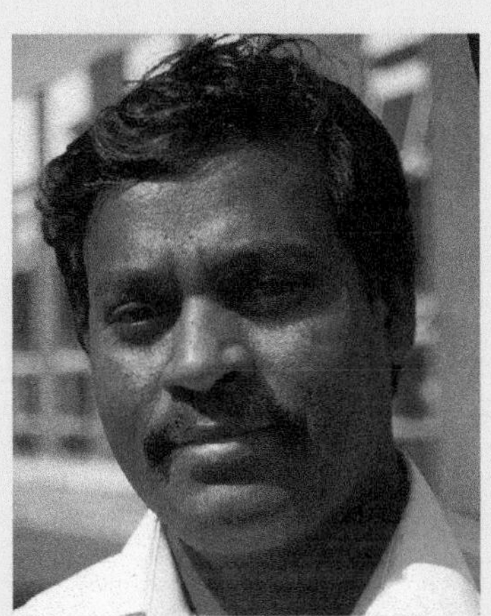

Skin colour is light to dark in tone due to increased melanin with yellow undertones
Hyper-pigmentation can easily occur as darker patches of skin and scarring can occur as skin blemishes heal. This also increases in appearance with age

White skin

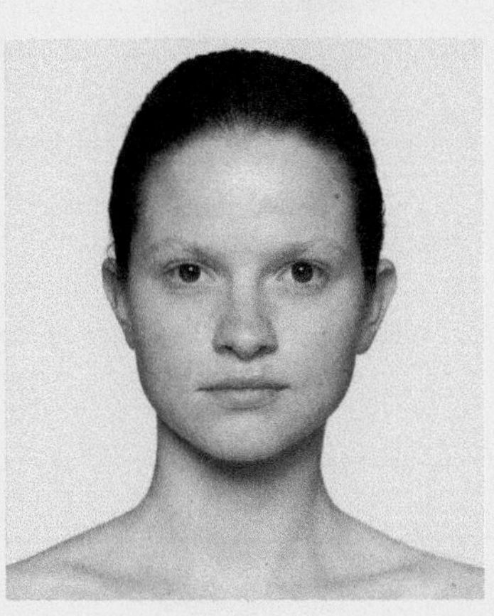

The skin colour is pink with less uneven supply of melanin in the skin. This can result in pigmentation patches called 'freckles' or ephelides

Oriental Asian skin

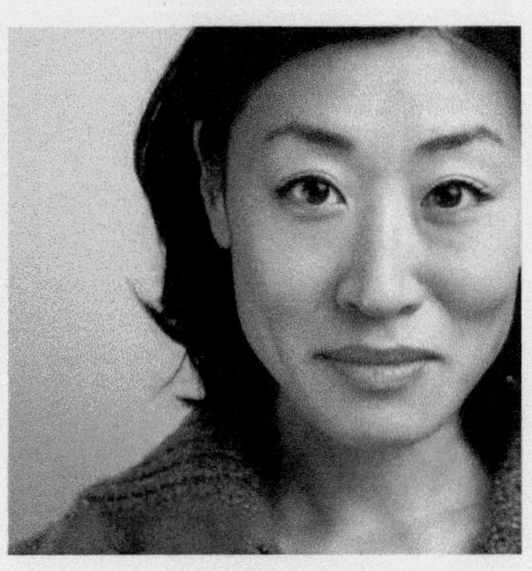

Contains more melanin with a yellowish tone. This skin is usually oily with larger pores in the oily areas. Hyper-pigmentation can easily occur. Scarring can occur as skin blemishes heal

Skin types

How the skin functions and how we care for it give us our skin type. The basic skin types that you need to be able to recognize and treat are:

- oily (also known as greasy)
- dry
- combination.

A skin analysis – an inspection of the client's skin usually by using a piece of equipment called a magnifying lamp. This helps us to decide skin type by what we can see.

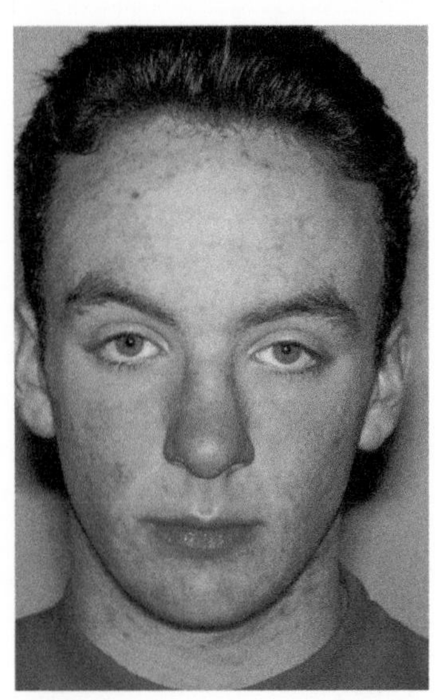

Oily skin

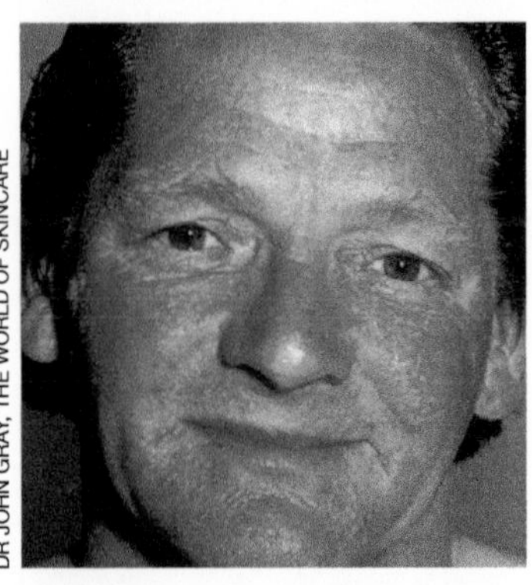

DR JOHN GRAY, THE WORLD OF SKINCARE

Dry skin

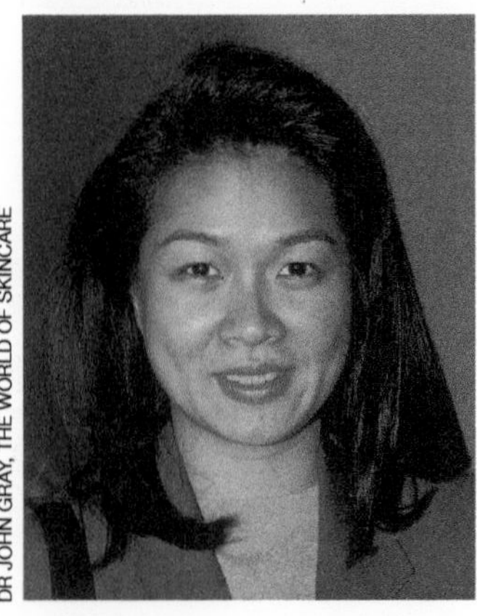

DR JOHN GRAY, THE WORLD OF SKINCARE

Combination skin

How to recognize different skin types

Oily skin The sebaceous glands that produce the skin's natural oil, sebum, are very active, especially at puberty (sexual maturity). An increase in sebum production can often lead to the appearance of skin blemishes, spots, known as pustules, and blackheads, known as comedones. Sebaceous gland activity begins to slow down in a person's twenties.

Oily skin:

- has large pores
- has a coarse skin texture (not smooth)
- appears thick
- appears shiny due to too much sebum production
- has good skin strength (tone) because of the protective effect of sebum
- might show certain skin disorders, e.g. comedones (blackheads), pustules and papules (blemishes caused by bacterial infection of the skin).

Dry skin Dry skin is lacking in sebum, moisture (water) or both. Because sebum limits the loss of moisture from the skin's surface, skin with insufficient sebum loses moisture more quickly becoming **dehydrated**. A dehydrated skin is one that has lost water from its tissues. A dry skin:

- has small tight pores
- has poor moisture content
- has a thin, coarse texture
- often shows patches of flaking skin
- often has sensitive areas, showing broken capillaries as a result of reduced sebum protection
- might contain milia (sebaceous blockages, accumulated in the hair follicle) – these appear as small, hard, pearly white lumps that are often seen around the eye area.

Combination skin This skin is partly dry and partly oily. The oily parts are generally the chin, nose and forehead known as the **T-zone**. The upper cheeks might also show signs of oiliness but the rest of the face and neck is dry. In a combination skin:

- there are enlarged pores in the T-zone and small-to-medium-sized pores in the cheek area

- the moisture content is high in the oily areas but poor in the dry areas
- the skin is coarse and thick in the oily areas but thinner in the dry areas
- the skin may show sensitivity in the dry areas
- the **skin tone** is good in the oily areas but poor in the dry areas
- there may be blemishes such as pustules and comedones at the T-zone
- milia and broken capillaries might appear in the dry areas, commonly on the cheeks and near the eyes.

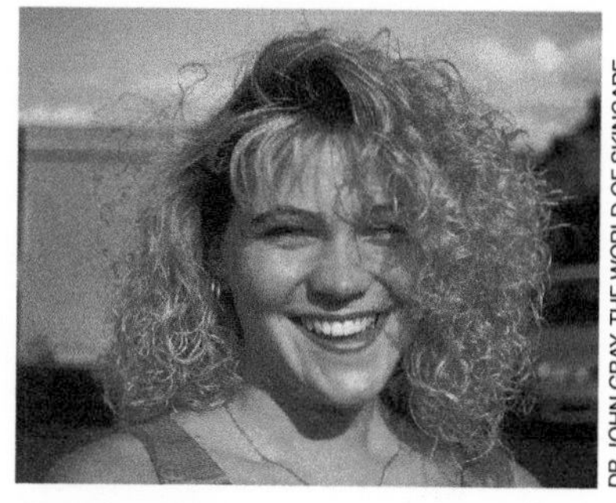

DR JOHN GRAY, THE WORLD OF SKINCARE

Sensitive skin

Sensitive skin Sensitive skin usually accompanies a dry skin type, but not always. The characteristics of sensitive skin are these:

- the skin may show high colouring as it is easily irritated
- there are usually broken capillaries in the cheek area
- the skin feels warm to the touch
- there is superficial flaking of the skin
- the skin may show high colouring and tightness after skin cleansing, if it is sensitive to pressure.

In black skin, instead of the redness shown by Caucasian skin, irritation shows up as a darker patch.

Allergic skin **Allergic skin** is irritated by external allergens or irritants – substances that cause sensitivity. The allergens inflame the skin and might damage its protective function. At the consultation, always check with the client if she has any allergies, and if so what?

Contact with an **allergen**, especially if repeated, can cause skin disorders such as eczema and dermatitis (see Chapter 2 for more information). If a skin is sensitive, use hypoallergenic products – these products do not contain any of the known allergens such as perfume.

ALWAYS REMEMBER

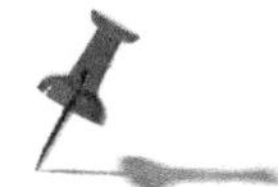

Pustules are red blemishes with pus present showing bacterial infection.

Papules are red blemishes without pus. A papule may become infected and become a pustule.

Comedones are a plug of sebum which turns black in contact with the air and is often termed as a 'blackhead'.

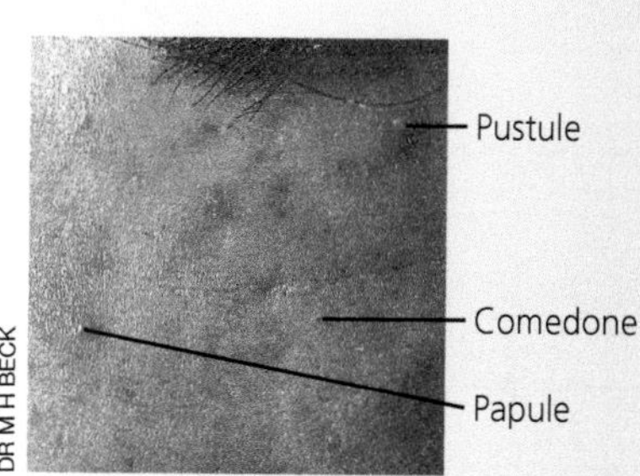

DR M H BECK

Pustules, papules and comedones

Step-by-step: Basic facial service

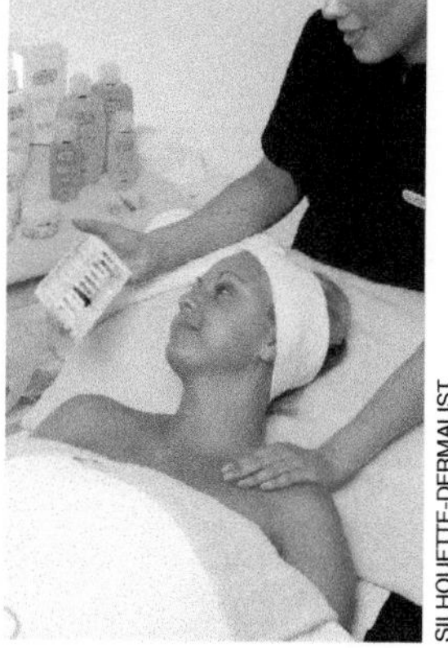

SILHOUETTE-DERMALIST

1 Consultation

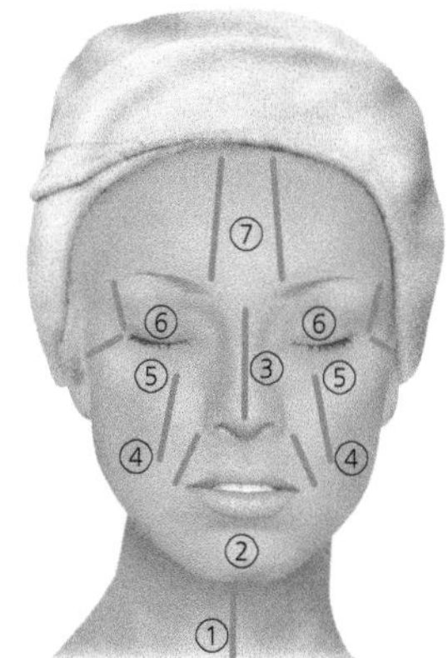

2 Skin analysis

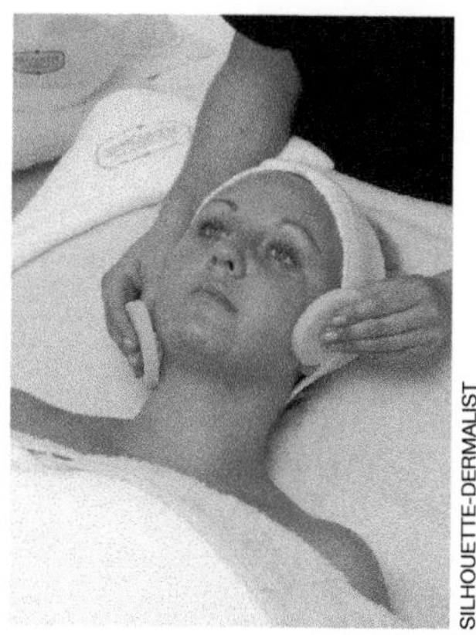

SILHOUETTE-DERMALIST

3 **Superficial cleanse**

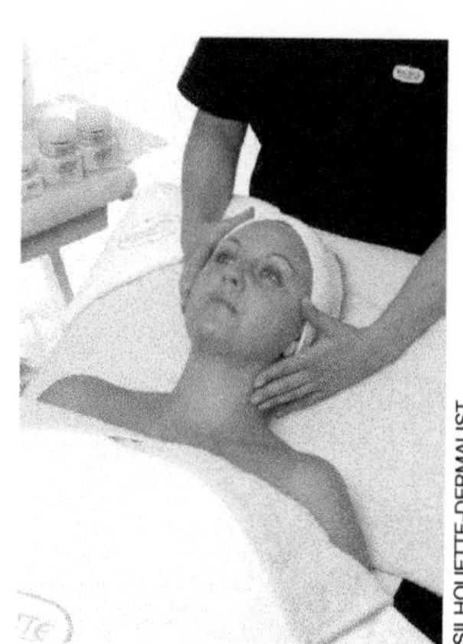

SILHOUETTE-DERMALIST

4 Deep cleanse

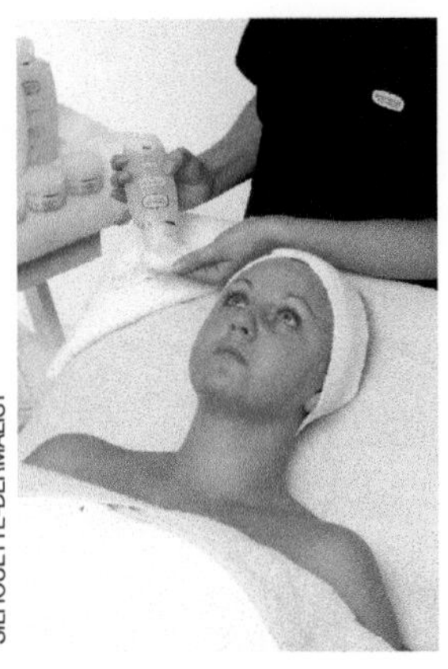
SILHOUETTE-DERMALIST

5 Skin toning

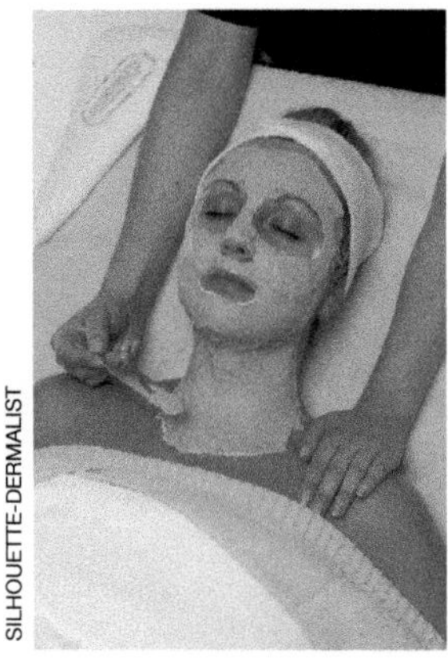
SILHOUETTE-DERMALIST

6 Mask application

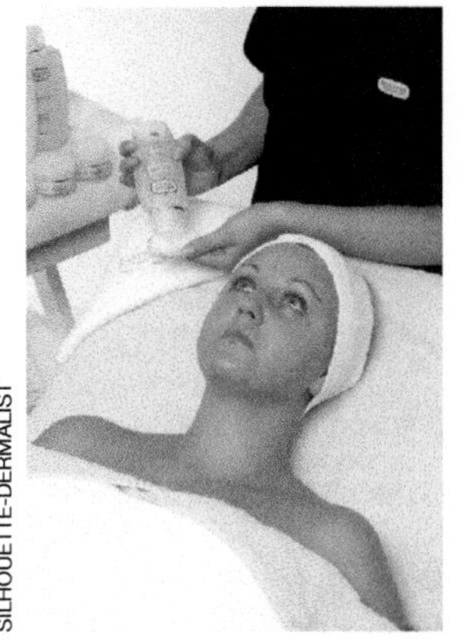
SILHOUETTE-DERMALIST

7 Skin toning following mask removal

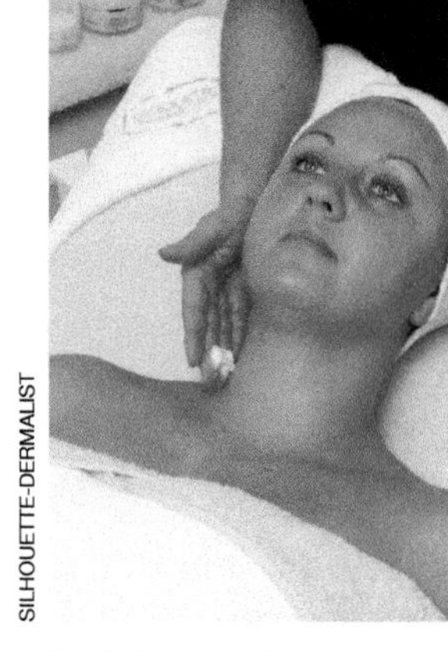
SILHOUETTE-DERMALIST

8 Skin moisturising

ACTIVITY FUNCTIONAL SKILLS

Deciding skin type

Refer to the illustration below. What skin characteristics would you expect to see in each of the numbered areas? Answer this for each of the **skin types** discussed.

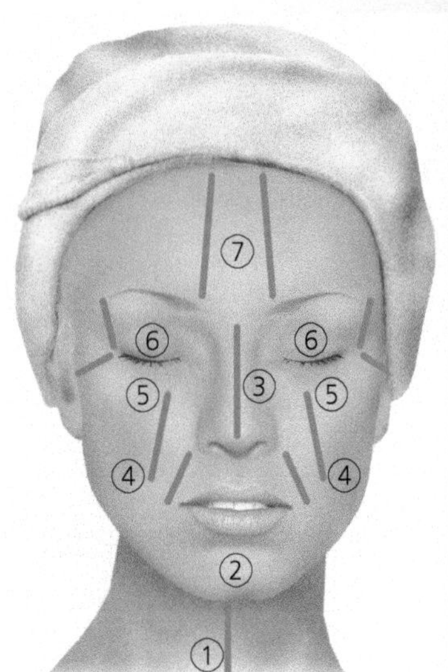

ACTIVITY FUNCTIONAL SKILLS

Timing

What is the time allowed for a basic facial service?

Why is it important to complete the service in this time?

Think of three reasons for each question above.

Outcome 1: Maintain safe and effective working methods when assisting with facial services

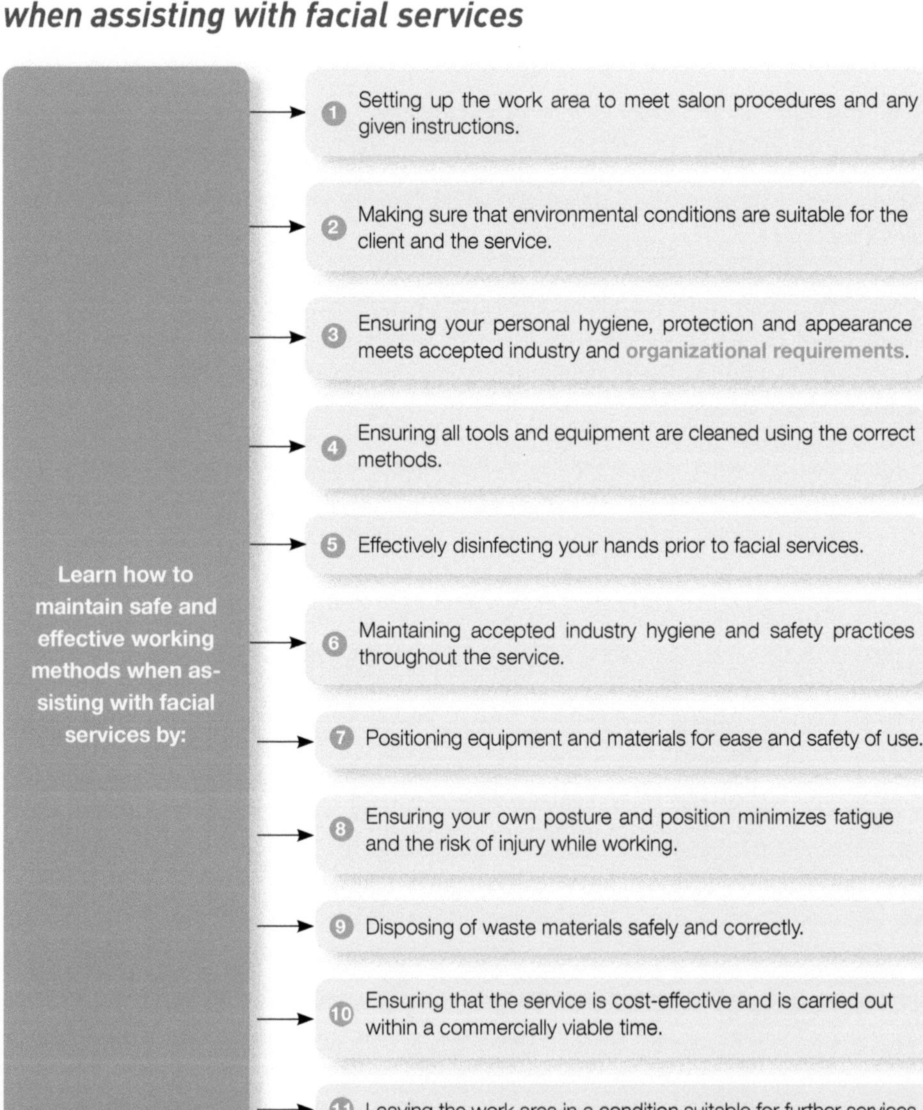

> Someone who is well presented, willing to learn, works well with others and a confident communicator makes a good impression.
>
> **Sally-Anne Braithwaite**

Making the appointment

When assisting with reception duties you may be required to make a facial service appointment. The following will help you in your job role.

When a client makes an appointment for a basic facial service, the receptionist should ask a few basic questions:

- What is the client's name and telephone number? This will help you to get the client's **record card** ready before they arrive for the service. The telephone number is important in case you need to cancel the service for any reason, e.g. the beauty therapist is ill.
- Which beauty therapist does the client want to book with? If a particular beauty therapist is needed you will have to check on availability.
- When does the client want the service, i.e. day/date and time? If any of these are not available, suggest another time or day as near to this as possible.
- Has the client had the facial before? If they have not, ask if they have any questions they would like to ask in relation to the service.
- Does the client want to book any other services as well as the basic facial service? Always look at opportunities to increase service bookings: the salon needs to keep busy!

Remember, when making an appointment it is important to allow enough time to complete the service properly. It is also important for the beauty therapist to be able to complete the service in a commercially acceptable time. Allow 30 minutes for a basic facial service. This does not include the consultation and preparation time.

> Recognize the needs of each individual client and work to build a positive relationship with them. Show a genuine interest in them and their lifestyle, family and hobbies, etc. and your client will come to trust you and listen to your recommendations.
>
> **Sally-Anne Braithwaite**

The Data Protection Act 1998 Since the introduction of the **Data Protection Act 1998** these details are confidential, or private. All information relating to a client should be stored securely. Only those staff with permission to access it can do so. Therefore, as soon as all service details have been recorded on the record card, the client's details should be stored securely. It is important that all details are accurate and up-to-date.

Equipment, materials and products used in a basic facial service It is important that you understand the purpose of the different equipment, materials and products and any related health and safety practice related to their use.

Product	*Use*	*Health and safety practice*
ELLISONS Bowls – various sizes	Can be used to hold client jewellery; skincare preparations; cotton wool; warm water to remove face mask	Clean after use with a detergent, disinfect, rinse and dry If using for water, keep on a stable surface to avoid spillage

Product	*Use*	*Health and safety practice*
Skin cleanser	This is usually a mixture of oil and water that is able to dissolve grease, make-up and other substances from the skin's surface Various cleansing preparations are available to the beauty therapist whose formulations are designed to treat the different skin types and conditions	If a client has sensitive skin, use a hypo-allergenic product. These will help to prevent skin irritation Use the correct cleansing product for the skin type to avoid skin irritation or sensitivity Avoid the use of too much **cleanser** around the eye area to avoid cleanser entering the eye and causing eye irritation
Skin toner	Applied after the skin has been cleansed Toning lotions remove any remaining cleanser and skincare preparations from the skin's surface They also create a skin-tightening effect, making the pores smaller Various toning preparations are available, in formulations for the different skin types	If a client has sensitive skin, use a hypo-allergenic product. Use the correct toning product for the skin type to avoid skin irritation or sensitivity Replace lids immediately following use to avoid spillage Gently blot the skin dry following toning lotion application with a soft facial tissue to avoid stimulating the skin too much as the toner evaporates or disappears from the skin's surface
Make-up remover	Eye make-up remover cleanses the eyelids and eyelashes, gently dissolving make-up if worn. It also conditions the delicate skin Formulated as a lotion or gel, it is designed to remove either water-based or oil-based products (or both)	If a client has sensitive skin, use a hypo-allergenic product Support the delicate eye tissue with the hand when cleansing the eye to avoid stretching the skin Avoid using too much eye make-up remover as it may enter the eye causing irritation Never apply pressure over the eyeball when cleansing the eye area
Moisturiser	The skin needs water to keep it soft and supple. Moisture level is constantly being lost. The application of a cosmetic moisturiser helps to maintain the natural oil and moisture balance by locking moisture into the skin, providing protection and hydration. The basic formulation of a moisturiser is oil and water	If a client has sensitive skin, use a hypo-allergenic product Always use a spatula to remove moisturiser if in an open container to prevent contamination Return lids immediately for **hygiene** and to prevent the quality of the product spoiling
Face mask	A cleansing preparation using different ingredients to absorb, cleanse, tighten (astringents), soften (emollients) and calm and soothe (desensitizers)	Clean the container following use Ensure that the product is taken from an open container using a clean spatula. Never place the mask brush on the client's skin and return to the product otherwise contamination will occur

Product	*Use*	*Health and safety practice*
ELLISONS Mask brush	Used to apply face mask to the skin of the face and neck. Usually consists of a plastic handle with synthetic (not natural hair) bristles	Clean in hot soapy water, allow to dry. It may be stored in the UV cabinet or alternatively in a lined, covered container

Before the service

Before the service is carried out you will need to prepare the work area, yourself and the client for the service.

Equipment and materials Before carrying out the basic facial, check that you have all the necessary equipment and materials at hand. Refer to the equipment and materials checklist to make sure that you have all that is required to perform a basic facial service. Tick next to each item on the checklist to help you as you prepare the work area.

EQUIPMENT AND MATERIALS CHECKLIST FOR FACIAL SERVICE

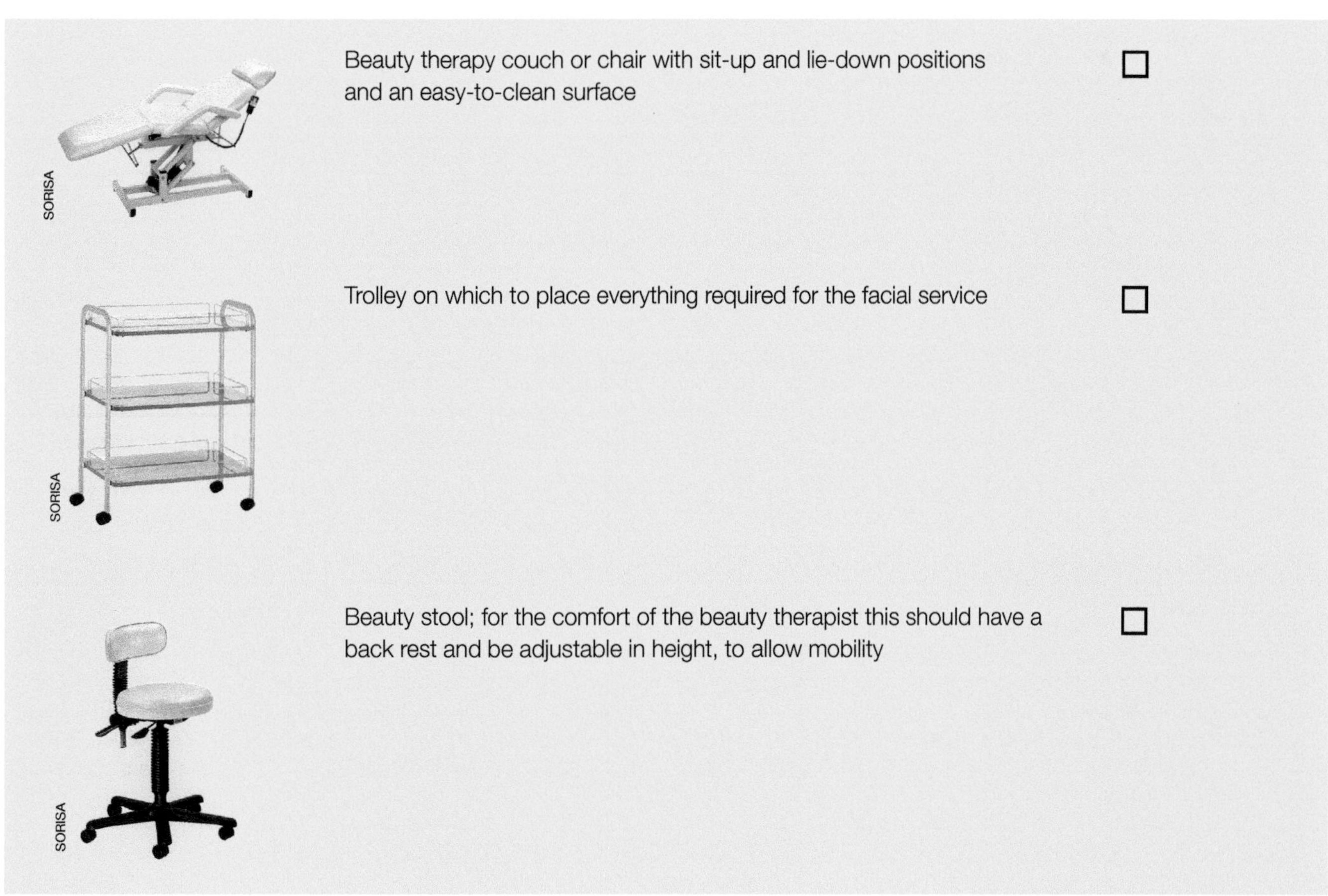

SORISA	Beauty therapy couch or chair with sit-up and lie-down positions and an easy-to-clean surface	☐
SORISA	Trolley on which to place everything required for the facial service	☐
SORISA	Beauty stool; for the comfort of the beauty therapist this should have a back rest and be adjustable in height, to allow mobility	☐

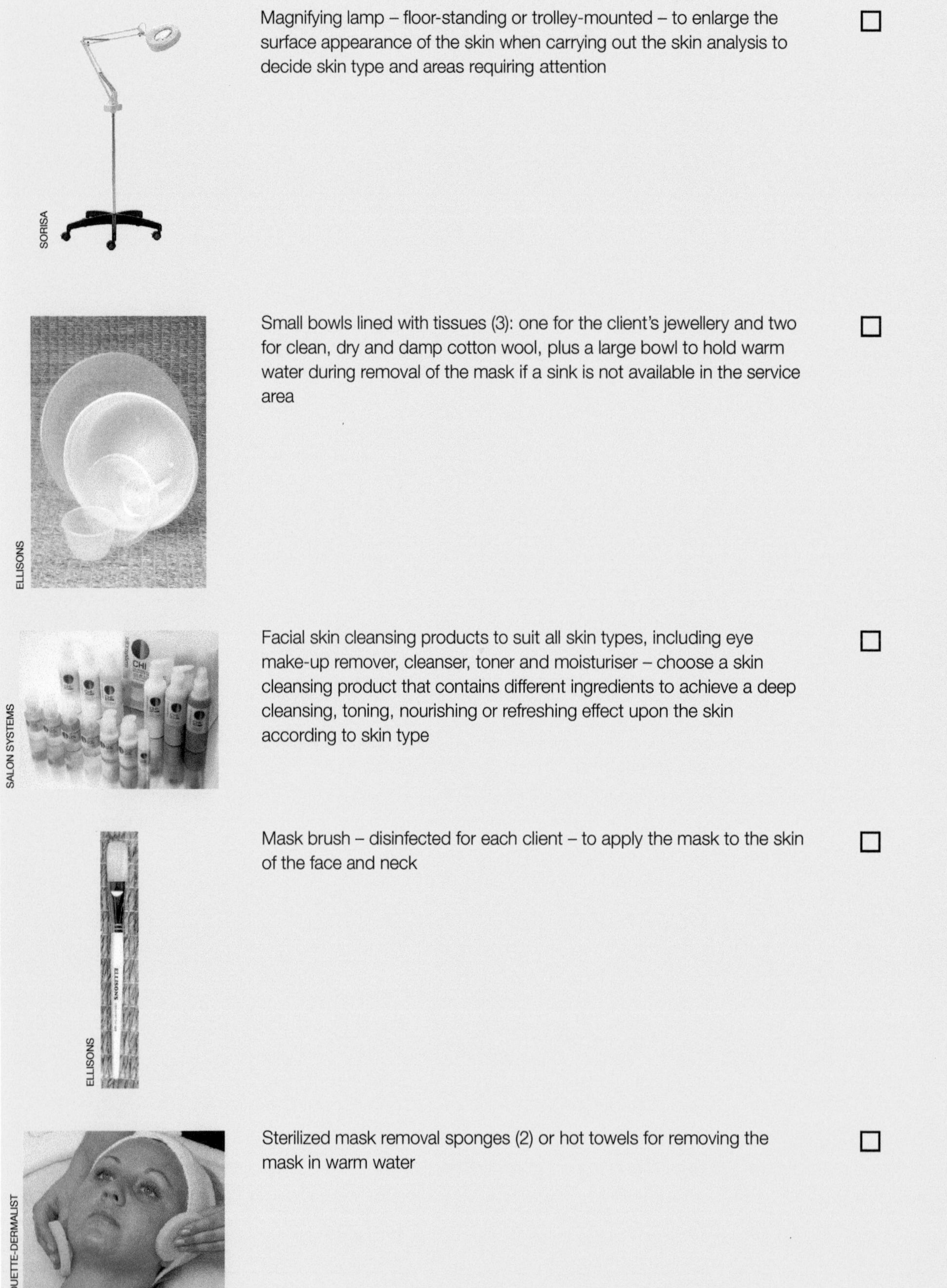

Magnifying lamp – floor-standing or trolley-mounted – to enlarge the surface appearance of the skin when carrying out the skin analysis to decide skin type and areas requiring attention ☐

Small bowls lined with tissues (3): one for the client's jewellery and two for clean, dry and damp cotton wool, plus a large bowl to hold warm water during removal of the mask if a sink is not available in the service area ☐

Facial skin cleansing products to suit all skin types, including eye make-up remover, cleanser, toner and moisturiser – choose a skin cleansing product that contains different ingredients to achieve a deep cleansing, toning, nourishing or refreshing effect upon the skin according to skin type ☐

Mask brush – disinfected for each client – to apply the mask to the skin of the face and neck ☐

Sterilized mask removal sponges (2) or hot towels for removing the mask in warm water ☐

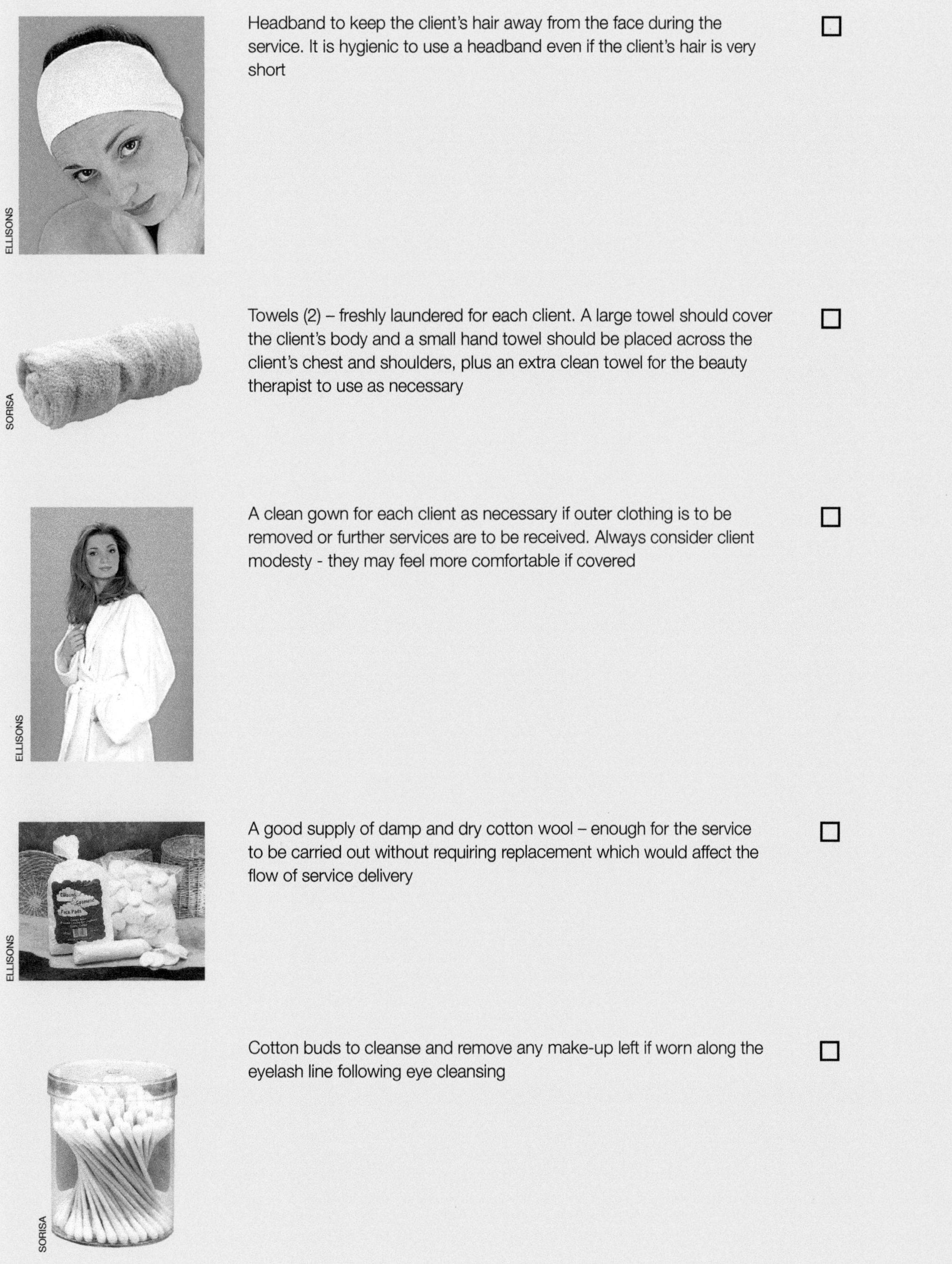

Headband to keep the client's hair away from the face during the service. It is hygienic to use a headband even if the client's hair is very short ☐

Towels (2) – freshly laundered for each client. A large towel should cover the client's body and a small hand towel should be placed across the client's chest and shoulders, plus an extra clean towel for the beauty therapist to use as necessary ☐

A clean gown for each client as necessary if outer clothing is to be removed or further services are to be received. Always consider client modesty - they may feel more comfortable if covered ☐

A good supply of damp and dry cotton wool – enough for the service to be carried out without requiring replacement which would affect the flow of service delivery ☐

Cotton buds to cleanse and remove any make-up left if worn along the eyelash line following eye cleansing ☐

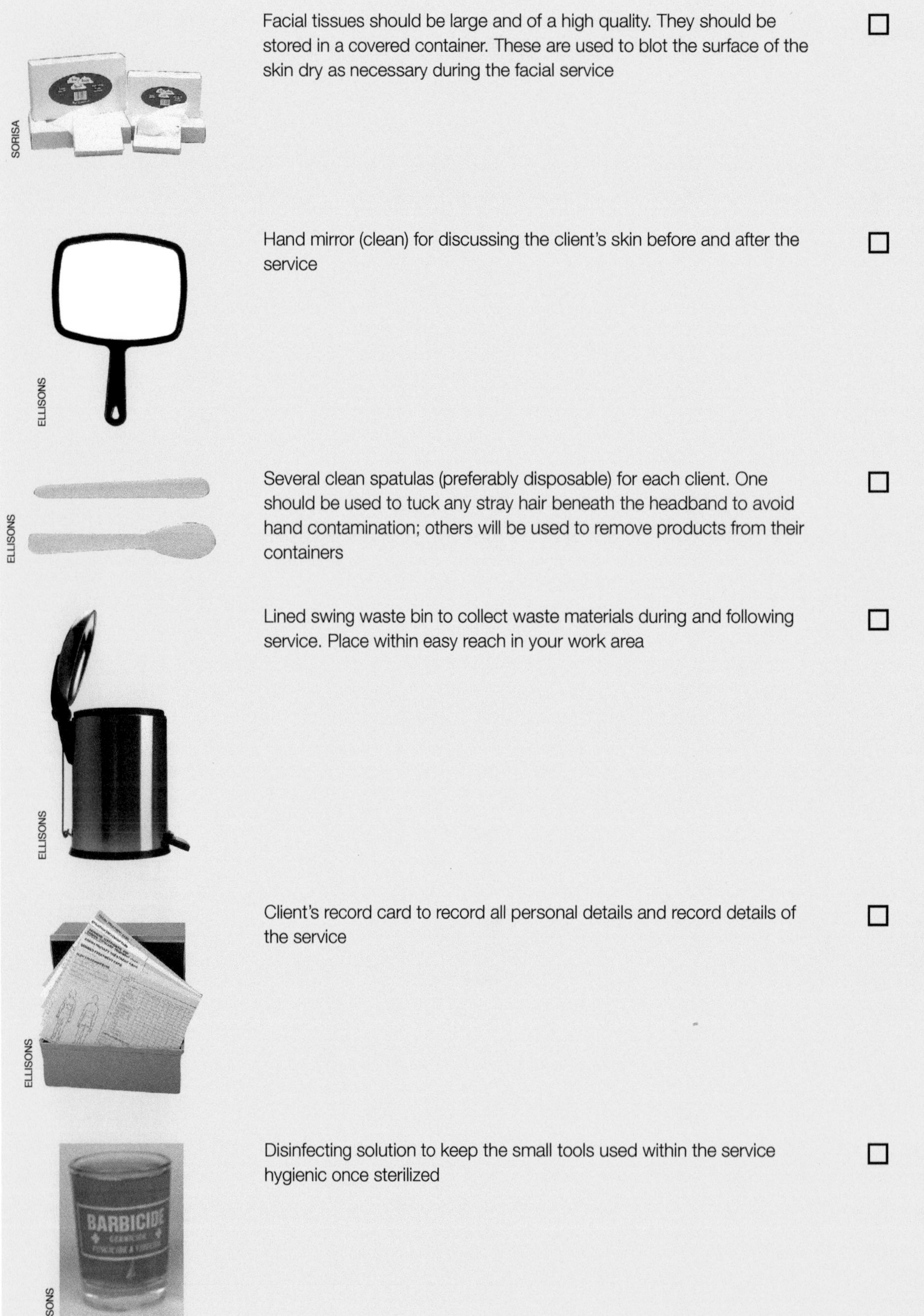

Facial tissues should be large and of a high quality. They should be stored in a covered container. These are used to blot the surface of the skin dry as necessary during the facial service ☐

Hand mirror (clean) for discussing the client's skin before and after the service ☐

Several clean spatulas (preferably disposable) for each client. One should be used to tuck any stray hair beneath the headband to avoid hand contamination; others will be used to remove products from their containers ☐

Lined swing waste bin to collect waste materials during and following service. Place within easy reach in your work area ☐

Client's record card to record all personal details and record details of the service ☐

Disinfecting solution to keep the small tools used within the service hygienic once sterilized ☐

Sterilization and disinfection It is important that good hygienic practice is considered before, throughout and after the client service. This will help prevent **cross-infection** – the transfer of harmful bacteria/microorganisms from one person to another. All equipment should be sterilized or **disinfected** using the most suitable method before use on each client.

Hygiene checks

- Ensure that all tools and equipment are clean and sterile before use.
- Disinfect work surfaces regularly.
- Use disposable items whenever possible. Throw away immediately after use in a covered, lined waste container.
- Follow hygienic **working practices** at all times.
- Maintain a high standard of personal hygiene at all times.
- Always check that you are helping to keep the work area in an **aseptic** condition, a situation described as trying to destroy bacteria.

Hygiene equipment

Equipment	*Hygiene practice*
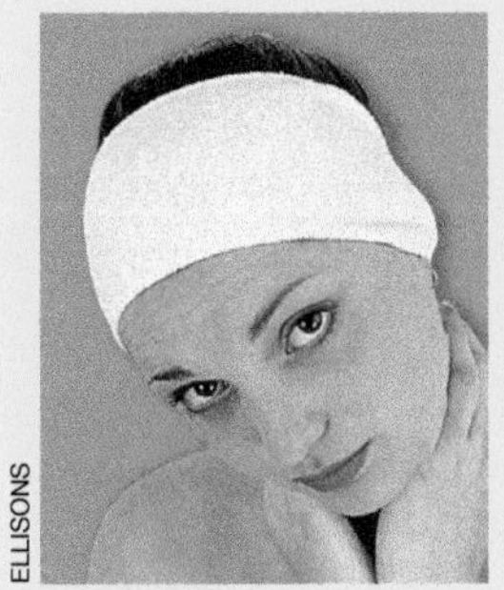 ELLISONS Headband	A clean, freshly laundered headband should be provided for each client to prevent cross-infection. Several should be available to allow for drying time. Alternatively use a disposable headband which can be thrown away after use
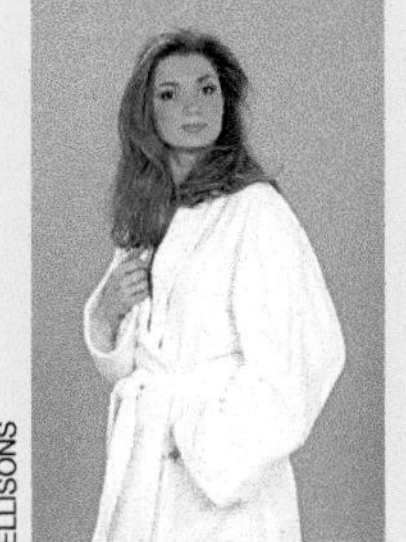 ELLISONS Gowns and towels	All towels should be boil washed at 60°C to kill harmful microorganisms following use. Clean towels and gowns should be provided for each client to prevent cross-infection
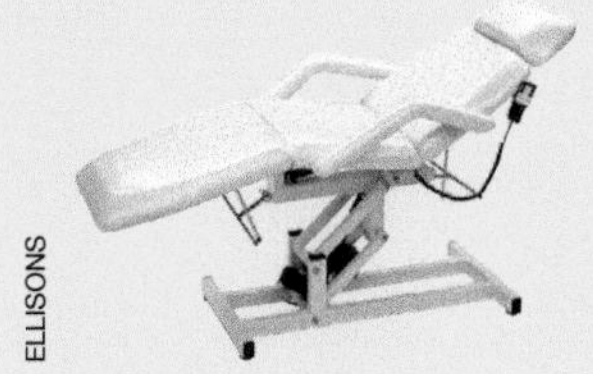 ELLISONS Beauty couch or chair	The beauty couch should have an easy-to-clean surface. It should be cleaned daily with warm water and detergent. The surface of the couch should be protected with clean towels and clean disposable paper roll for each client. Ideally it should be adjustable in height to meet all client's needs

HEALTH & SAFETY

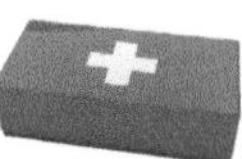

The autoclave

The autoclave – a sterilizing unit similar to a pressure cooker – makes steam as the water inside it boils. A temperature of 121–134°C is reached and sterilizes anything inside the autoclave. However, this system is only suitable for beauty therapy equipment that can withstand high temperatures – check first.

HEALTH & SAFETY

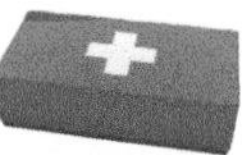

Eye make-up remover

If the client is wearing waterproof mascara, use an eye make-up remover designed to remove oil-based make-up.

Non-oily make-up remover should be selected for a client wearing false eyelashes to prevent them being removed.

Always check with the senior beauty therapist that you are selecting the correct product.

TOP TIP

Disposable headbands are ideal as a clean headband is immediately available without the need for laundering.

TOP TIP

Magnifying lamps

The magnifying lamp will provide the extra light required to magnify the surface of the skin during skin analysis to allow correct naming of skin type.

Protect the client's eyes with a suitable shield to avoid irritation of the eyes with the bright light.

TOP TIP

Work area

The work area should be left ready for the next client on service completion.

Waste products should be disposed of correctly following local council waste regulations.

If you are free, assist other colleagues to tidy the area after service to maintain the work area in readiness for the next client.

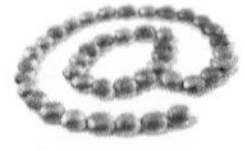

COURSEMATE

For a video on preparation of the treatment room, please see this book's accompanying CourseMate.

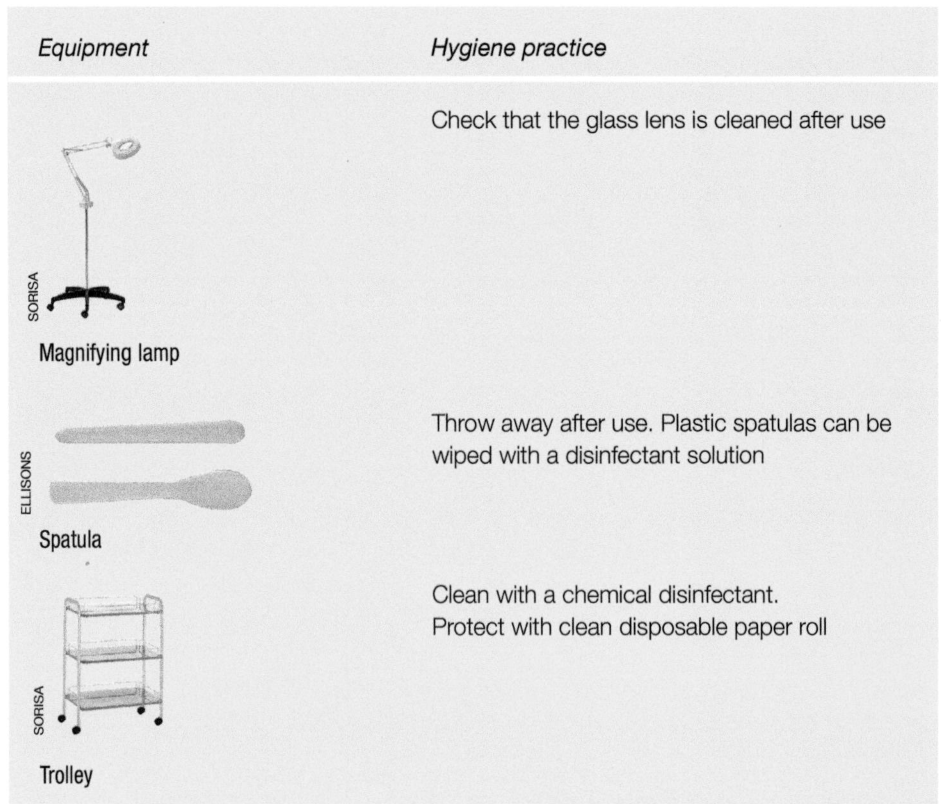

Equipment	*Hygiene practice*
SORISA Magnifying lamp	Check that the glass lens is cleaned after use
ELLISONS Spatula	Throw away after use. Plastic spatulas can be wiped with a disinfectant solution
SORISA Trolley	Clean with a chemical disinfectant. Protect with clean disposable paper roll

Preparation of the beauty therapist Ensure that the service area is warm and comfortable, ventilation is sufficient and that lighting is suited to assist client relaxation, and in order that the service is performed competently. Check that the area is free from any trip hazards that could cause a fall.

Wash the hands, to remove surface dirt preventing cross-infection, this will also show the client you have good hygiene practice.

Follow proper hygiene and personal presentation requirements to ensure a professional **personal appearance** at all times.

Preparing the work area Check the work area to make sure you have all the equipment, products and materials you require for the facial service. Use the checklist provided on pp. 139–142.

Prepare the beauty couch or chair following your salon's **workplace policies**.

Outcome 2: Consult, plan and prepare for facial services with clients

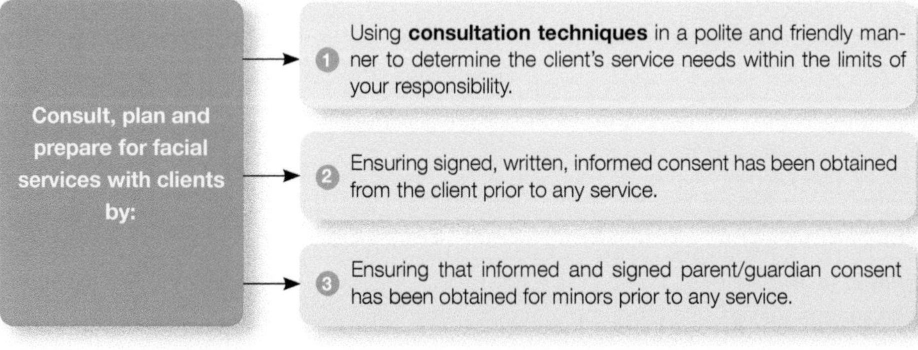

(Continued) Consult, plan and prepare for facial services with clients by:

4. Ensuring that a parent/guardian is present throughout the service for minors under the age of 16.
5. Encouraging clients to ask questions to clarify any points.
6. Asking your client appropriate questions to identify if they have any **contra-indications** to facial services.
7. Accurately recording your client's responses to questioning.
8. Ensuring client advice is given without reference to a specific medical condition and without causing undue alarm and concern.
9. **Preparing the client** to meet the needs of the agreed service and following any given instructions.
10. Ensuring the client is in a comfortable and relaxed position.
11. Effectively removing the client's make-up to meet the needs of the service.
12. Correctly performing a skin analysis on the client and accurately recording the **skin type**.
13. Referring clients with conditions that may affect the service to the relevant member of staff.
14. Selecting suitable products for the client's **skin type** based on the results of the skin analysis and instructions from the senior beauty therapist.

> If you see something that needs to be done, do it without having to be asked. This is called 'using your Initiative' and is an important employability skill.
>
> **Sally-Anne Braithwaite**

Preparing the client – the consultation

The consultation should be carried out in the privacy of the service work area. This takes place when the client first meets you at the start of the service and will take approximately 10 minutes. The consultation enables the beauty therapist to assess whether the client is suitable for service or whether service is contra-indicated in some way.

Ask the client specific questions about their current skincare routine and general health. The client's answers will suggest to the therapist what is required, and what is achievable, from a skincare programme. Listen to the client to find out sufficient information to make suggestions.

Contra-indications to service Certain skin and eye conditions prevent you from carrying out the basic facial service, these are known as **contra-indications**.

If, when looking at the client's skin and eyes before the service, you think you recognize any of the following conditions, a basic facial service must not be carried out. You will need to refer the client tactfully to the relevant person in the salon to get agreement as to whether the service can go ahead.

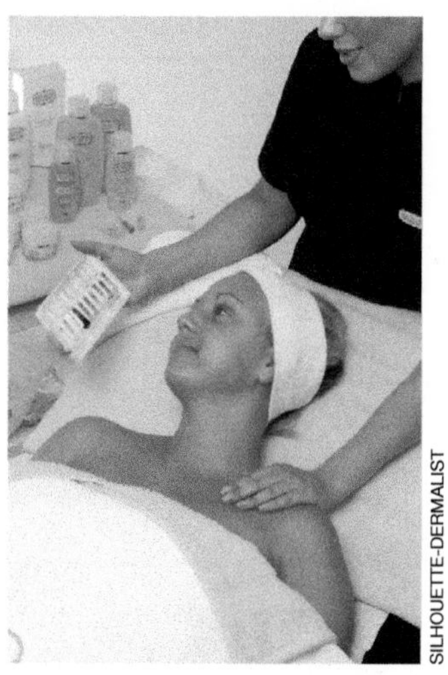
SILHOUETTE-DERMALIST

Consultation prior to a facial service

Conditions that prevent service All the skin and eye conditions listed below are contagious – they can be passed on to other clients. You must never treat a client with any of these conditions.

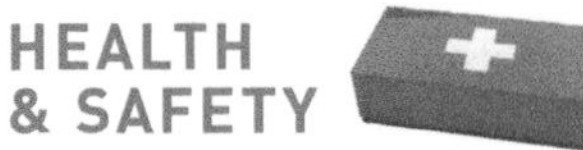

Contra-indication

Remember – you might be wrong when you think you have a client with a contra-indication.

Always check with the senior therapist if unsure – the client might be able to have the service after all.

Never diagnose (say what you think it is) and try to avoid causing the client embarrassment.

The senior therapist may recommend that the client seeks medical advice before the facial service goes ahead.

Name of contra-indication	*Cause*	*Appearance*
DR M H BECK Impetigo	A contagious **bacterial** infection caused by minute, single-celled organisms and which results in skin inflammation	The skin appears red and is itchy. Small blisters appear, which burst and then form honey coloured crusts
DR M H BECK Tinea corporis or body ringworm	A contagious infection of the skin caused by a **fungus**. Fungal diseases of the skin feed off the waste products of the skin	Small, scaly red patches spread outwards and then heal from the centre, leaving a ring. Found on the limbs
DR M H BECK Conjunctivitis or pink eye	A contagious **bacterial** infection of the mucous membrane that covers the eyelids	The skin of the inner conjunctiva of the eye becomes inflamed, the eye becomes very red and sore, and pus might appear leaving a sticky coating on the lashes
DR M H BECK Hordeolum or styes	A contagious **bacterial** infection of the sebaceous glands of eyelash hair follicles	Small lumps appear, usually containing pus. This is a sign that the skin around the base of the eyelash hair is infected

Name of contra-indication	*Cause*	*Appearance*
localised red lump surrounding a hair follicle indicating infection DR M H BECK Furuncles or boils	A contagious **bacterial** infection in the skin around the hair follicle	Red, painful lumps extend into the skin around a hair follicle. A central core of pus develops appearing as yellowish-whitish fluid in surrounding tissues
DR M H BECK Herpes simplex or cold sore	A contagious **viral** disorder of the skin. **Viruses** require living tissue to survive. They attack the healthy cell and multiply within the cell. Cold sores often appear when the skin's resistance is low due to stress or ill-health	Inflammation of the skin occurs in small areas. The skin becomes red and feels itchy, and small blisters appear. These are followed by a crust, which might crack and weep tissue fluid

Conditions that might restrict service The skin conditions below are non-contagious – they cannot be passed on to other clients. Clients with these conditions can be treated, but you might need to adapt your service application.

HEALTH & SAFETY

Cold sores

Clients who suffer from cold sores (herpes simplex) should be advised to avoid excessive UV light because this can stimulate production of the sores.

Name of contra-indication	*Cause*	*Appearance*	*Service*
DR M H BECK Skin eczema	Inflammation of the skin caused by contact with a skin irritant	The skin becomes red, swells and blisters can appear. The blisters burst, which causes scabs to form on the skin	Ensure you find out what irritants make the eczema worse and avoid contact with such products, e.g. it might be perfumed products The skin can benefit from cosmetic products that contain soothing ingredients such as lavender Do not treat if the skin is broken

Name of contra-indication	*Cause*	*Appearance*	*Service*
DR M H BECK Skin psoriasis	Cause unknown but becomes worse when the person is stressed Often hereditary (passed on from parents)	Itchy, red, flaky patches of skin, which can become infected if the skin is broken	The skin can benefit from cosmetic products that contain soothing ingredients such as lavender Do not treat if the skin is broken
WELLCOME PHOTO LIBRARY Broken bones	Injury – should be treated medically	The breakage might not be obvious. Therefore, if the client is new, check there have been no recent broken bones at the consultation	The broken bone must not be handled Always check first with the relevant person in the **workplace**

HEALTH & SAFETY

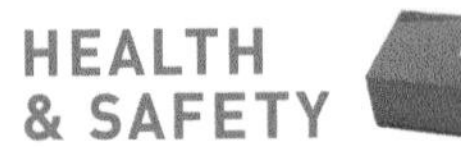

Skin disorders

If a client shows a skin disorder and you are at all unsure, check with the relevant person in the workplace before starting the service.

A client with a skin disorder is usually advised to visit their GP. This is relevant for all contra-indications that prohibit service and also for those that restrict service, mainly eczema and psoriasis.

HEALTH & SAFETY

Cuts, abrasions, bruising, redness and swelling

If the skin has been damaged but is no longer infected or at risk from **secondary infection**, you might be able to treat the skin. Check with the senior beauty therapist before you proceed.

COURSEMATE

For a video on home care products, see this book's accompanying CourseMate.

During the consultation the beauty therapist can also explain what is involved in the service, how long it takes and what **aftercare advice** home care is required. If the client is a minor, under the age of 16, it is necessary to have the permission of the parent/guardian for the facial service. The parent/guardian will also have to be present when the service is received.

Also during the consultation, the client will:

- find out what the beauty therapist can recommend to meet their treatment requirements
- ask questions and receive honest professional advice concerning the most suitable choice of skincare product
- confirm and agree the service aim.

All details should be recorded accurately on the client record card before, during and following the service. A sample record card follows.

Sample client record card

Date	Beauty therapist name	
Client name	Date of birth (Identifying client age group)	
Home address		Postcode
Email address	Landline telephone number	Mobile telephone number
Name of doctor	Doctor's address and telephone number	
Related medical history (Conditions that may restrict or prohibit service application.)		
Are you taking any medication? (This may affect the sensitivity of the skin to the service.)		

CONTRA-INDICATIONS REQUIRING MEDICAL REFERRAL
(Preventing **facial service** application.)

- ☐ bacterial infections (e.g. impetigo)
- ☐ viral infections (e.g. herpes simplex)
- ☐ fungal infections (e.g. tinea unguium)
- ☐ eye infections (e.g. conjunctivitis)
- ☐ systemic medical conditions
- ☐ severe skin conditions

SKIN GROUP

- ☐ oily
- ☐ dry
- ☐ combination

FACIAL PRODUCTS

- ☐ cleanser
- ☐ mask – non-setting
- ☐ toner
- ☐ moisturiser
- ☐ eye cleanser

CONTRA-INDICATIONS THAT RESTRICT SERVICE
(Facial service may require adaptation.)

- ☐ cuts and abrasions
- ☐ bruising and swelling
- ☐ recent scar tissue
- ☐ eczema
- ☐ skin allergies
- ☐ psoriasis

SKIN CONDITION CHARACTERISTICS

- ☐ sensitive
- ☐ milia
- ☐ dehydrated
- ☐ comedones
- ☐ broken capillaries
- ☐ papules
- ☐ pustules
- ☐ open pores

EQUIPMENT AND MATERIALS

- ☐ magnifying lamp
- ☐ spatulas
- ☐ consumables
- ☐ protective covering

Beauty therapist signature (for reference)

Client signature (confirmation of details)

Sample client record card (continued)

SERVICE ADVICE
Basic facial service – *This service will take 30 minutes.*

SERVICE PLAN
Record relevant details of your service and advice provided for future reference.
Ensure the client's records are up-to-date, accurate and fully completed following service. Non-compliance may invalidate insurance.

DURING
Find out:
- what products the client is currently using to cleanse and care for the skin of the face and neck
- how regularly the products are used
- satisfaction with their current skincare routine
- explain: how the products used should be applied and removed

Note:
- any unwanted reaction (contra-action), if any occur

AFTER
Record:
- results of service
- what products have been used in the basic facial service
- the effectiveness of service
- any samples provided (review their success at the next appointment)

Advise on:
- product application and removal in order to gain the best benefit from product use
- product application and removal in order to gain maximum benefit from product use
- use of make-up following facial service
- recommended time intervals between services
- the importance of a course of service to improve the skin condition

RETAIL OPPORTUNITIES
Advise on:
- products that would be suitable for the client to use at home to care for their skin
- recommendations for further facial services
- further products or services that you have recommended that the client may or may not have received before

Note:
- any purchase made by the client

EVALUATION
Record:
- comments on the client's satisfaction with the service
- record how you will progress the **service plan** to maintain and advance the service results in the future

HEALTH AND SAFETY
Advise on:
- avoidance of activities or product application that may cause an unwanted skin reaction (contra-action)
- appropriate action to be taken in the event of an unwanted skin reaction

Obtain the client's signature to confirm all details. This also enables continuity of the service and up-to-date tracking of services received.

At the end of the consultation the client should fully understand what the proposed service involves:

1 Check with the senior beauty therapist that your facial service plan meets their satisfaction.

2 Ask the client to remove jewellery from the service area, to prevent it becoming soiled by facial products. It may be necessary to remove contact lenses if worn. Place the jewellery in view of the client following your workplace policy, usually in a small, clean bowl.

3 Offer the client a gown to wear, allowing privacy for the client to change. Position the client into a comfortable and relaxed position for the service. The beauty couch or chair should offer back support and be comfortable. Cover the client. Place a small hand towel across their shoulders.

4 Fasten a clean headband around the client's hairline. Position the headband so that it does not cover the skin of the face and is comfortable for the client.

5 After preparing the client, wash your hands: this shows the client that you work hygienically.

TOP TIP

Communicating with your client

Communication includes talking with your client (verbal communication) and also what your body language is telling the client (non-verbal communication).

You might have given a client a great facial service but will you be asked to do it again if you are not interested, cheerful and helpful?

HEALTH & SAFETY

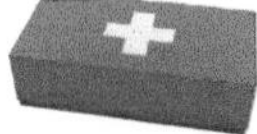

Posture

It is important that the client is positioned correctly on the couch. This will:

- check that the client is comfortable throughout the service and is supported properly
- prevent discomfort to the beauty therapist, which may lead to muscle injury and long-term postural problems
- enable the service to be carried out properly.

Outcome 3: Carry out facial services

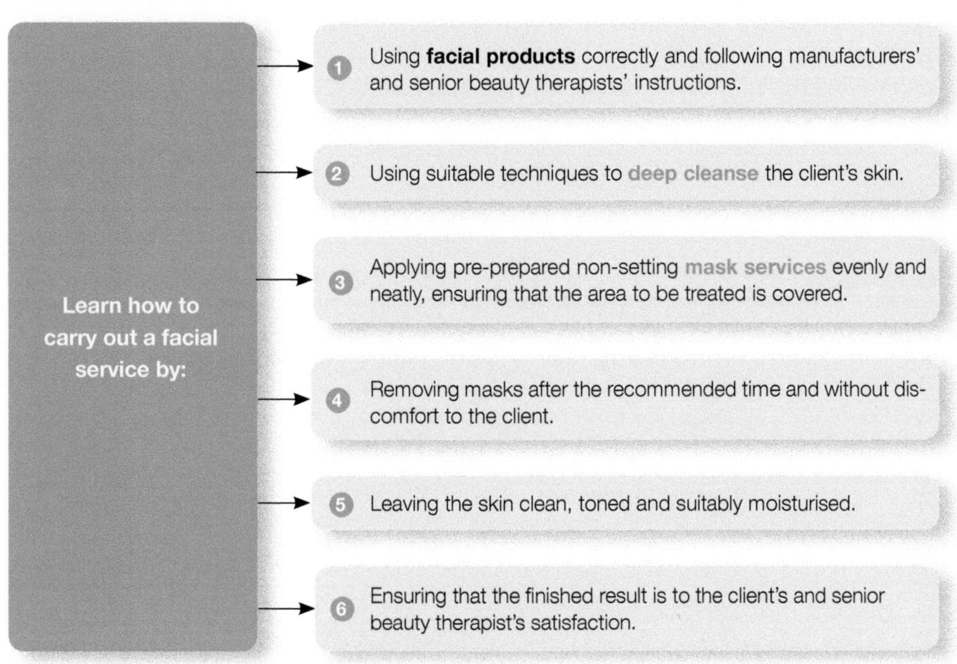

"A good team member has good listening and communication skills, respects their colleagues and is able to get their point across in the correct manner.

Sally-Anne Braithwaite

Basic facial service procedure

Briefly, the stages in the basic facial service procedure are:

- consultation
- skin analysis
- superficial cleanse
- deep cleanse
- skin toning
- mask application
- mask removal
- skin toning
- skin moisturising.

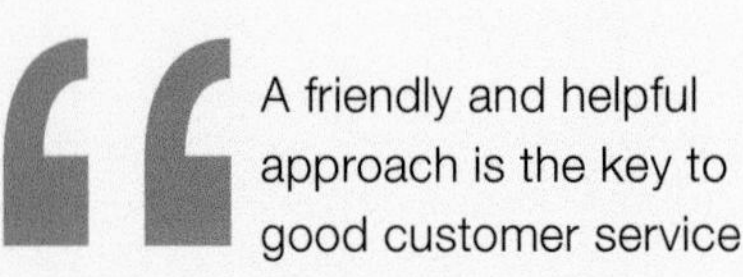

> A friendly and helpful approach is the key to good customer service.
>
> **Sally-Anne Braithwaite**

Skin cleansing service There are two parts in the cleansing routine:

1. The superficial cleanse uses lightweight cleansing preparations to soften and dissolve surface make-up if worn, dirt and grease.
2. The **deep cleanse** may use a heavier cleansing product – often a cream or balm – which allows **massage** movements to be applied to the skin without the cleansing product evaporating (disappearing) from the skin's surface. It must always be carried out using a product suitable for the skin type.

Superficial cleansing The face is cleansed in the following order:

1. the eye tissue and eyelashes
2. the lips
3. the neck, chin, cheeks and forehead.

BEST PRACTICE

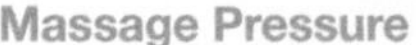

Massage Pressure

Reduce pressure when working over the neck.

Do not close the nostril openings when cleansing the nose.

Pressure must always be upwards and outwards to avoid stretching the delicate facial skin.

Deep cleansing The deep cleanse involves a series of massage movements using the hands and cleansing product. The skin becomes warm during the massage, which aids the absorption of the cleanser into the hair follicles and pores and increases the cleansing action.

ALWAYS REMEMBER

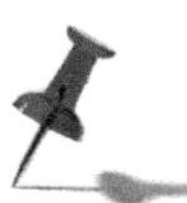

Use a cleansing skincare preparation formulated to care for the delicate skin tissue of the eye to avoid irritation and possible swelling of the skin.

TOP TIP

Choosing a cleansing product

Skin type	Cleansing product
Oily	Foaming cleanser/ Cleansing lotion
Dry	Cleansing milk/ Cleansing cream
Combination	Foaming cleanser/ Cleansing lotion/ Cleansing milk

Step-by-step: Superficial cleanse

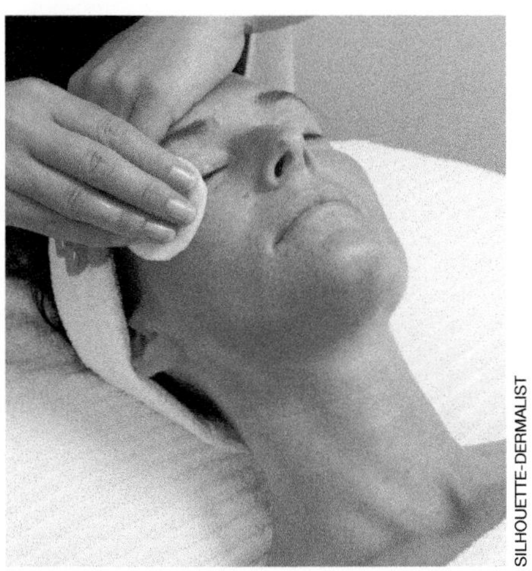
SILHOUETTE-DERMALIST

1 Wash your hands.

2 Cleanse the eye area using a suitable eye make-up remover.

3 Each eye is cleansed separately by supporting the delicate eye tissue with the non-working hand. Apply eye make-up remover (oily or non-oily) directly to clean, damp cotton wool. First, stroke down the length of the eyelashes, then cleanse the eye tissue in a sweeping circle, outwards across the upper eyelid, circling beneath the lower eyelashes towards the nose. Repeat, changing the cotton wool regularly until the eye area and cotton wool shows clean. Any make-up left along the eyelash line should be removed with a clean cotton bud.

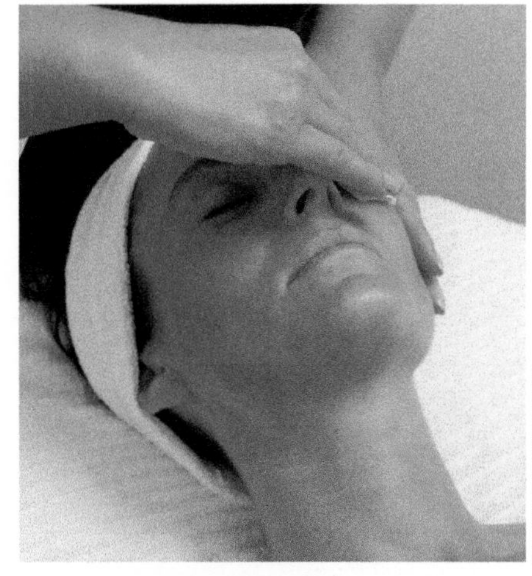
SILHOUETTE-DERMALIST

4 Cleanse the lips, preferably with a suitable make-up remover, i.e. cleansing milk or lotion. Apply a little product to a damp cotton wool. Wipe the cleanser across the lips. Support the corner of the mouth with the non-working hand. Repeat, changing the cotton wool regularly until the lip area and cotton wool shows clean.

5 Select a cleansing product to suit your client's skin type: Whichever cleanser is chosen, it should have the following qualities:

- it should cleanse the skin effectively without causing irritation
- it should remove all make-up and skin debris
- it should feel pleasant to use
- it should be easy to remove from the skin.

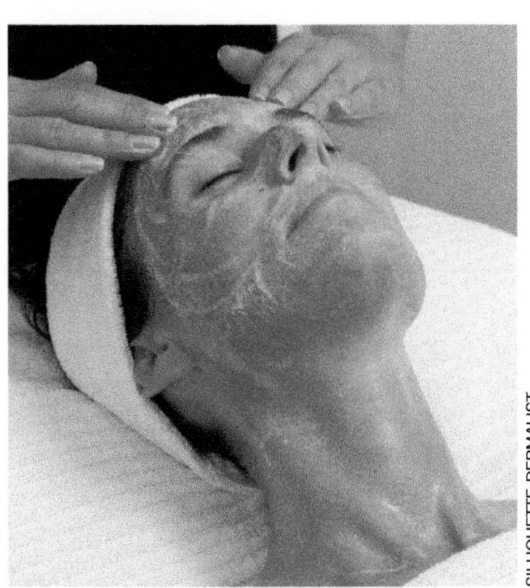
SILHOUETTE-DERMALIST

6 Apply the cleanser to the client's skin using your hands – enough to cover the face and neck – and massage gently over the surface of the skin. Using light, circular movements with the fingertips, gently massage the product into the skin, beginning at the bottom of the neck and finishing at the forehead.

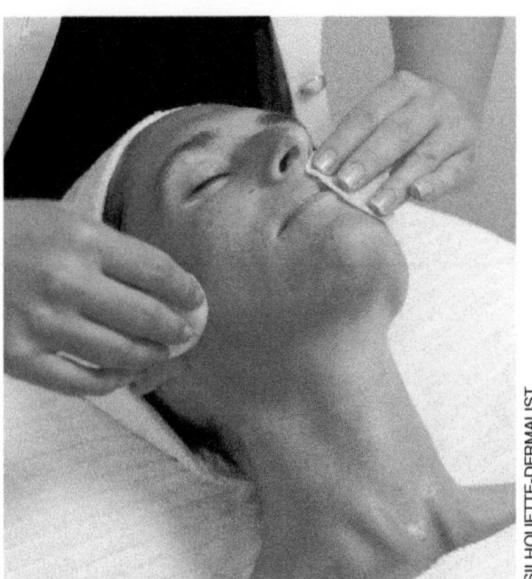
SILHOUETTE-DERMALIST

7 Remove the cleanser thoroughly, in an upwards and outwards direction, with clean damp cotton wool facial sponges dampened with clean, warm water or warm towels if preferred.

8 Repeat this process until all excess cleanser has been removed.

ALWAYS REMEMBER

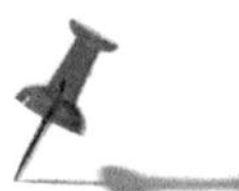

Skincare Ingredients

Skincare products may contain additional ingredients to treat and care for the skin.

The product shown contains lavender and camomile which are plant extracts which calm a sensitive skin type helping to reduce any red areas.

Never use a product that contains ingredients that are unsuitable for the skin type.

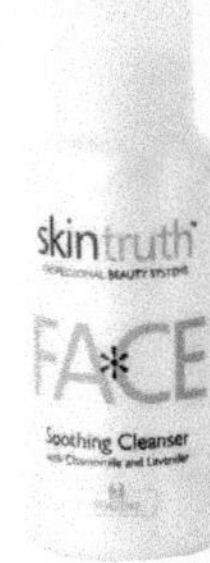

TOP TIP

Male client service

It is preferable to remove facial products with dampened sponges or hot towels rather than cotton wool, which can drag and collect on coarse facial hair.

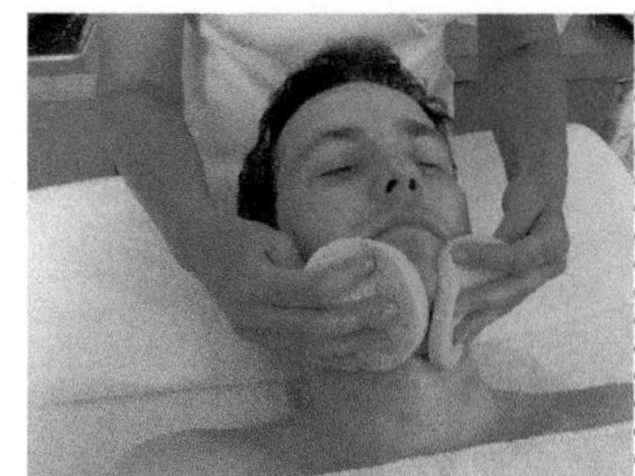

Male client service

Step-by-step: Deep cleanse

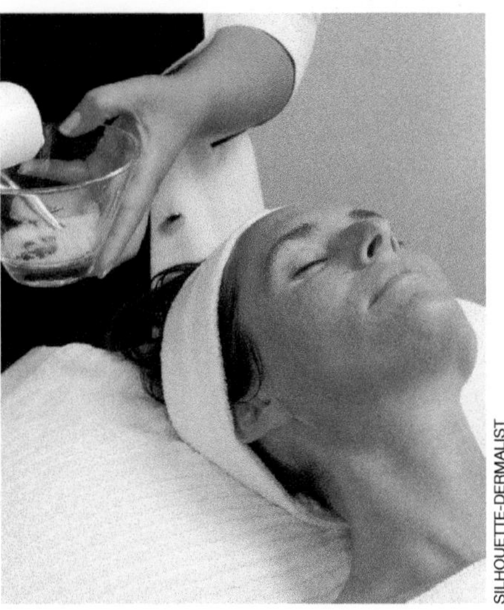

SILHOUETTE-DERMALIST

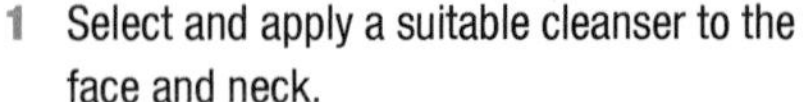

1 Select and apply a suitable cleanser to the face and neck.

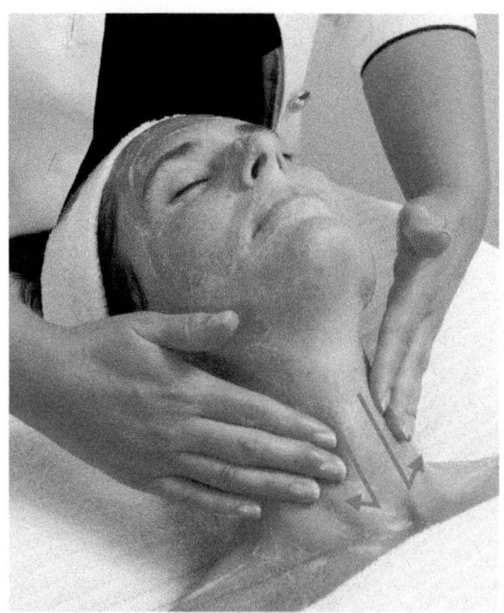

SILHOUETTE-DERMALIST

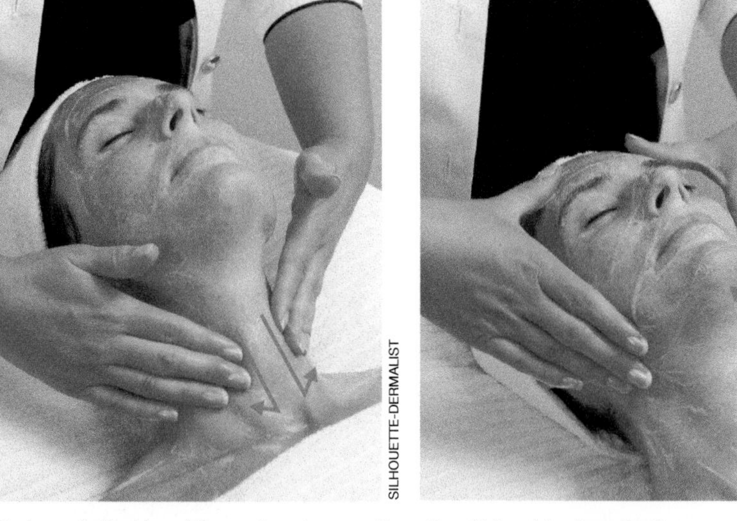

SILHOUETTE-DERMALIST

2 Stroke up both sides of the neck, using your fingertips. At the chin, draw the fingers outwards at the angle of the jaw and lightly stroke down to the neck to the starting position.

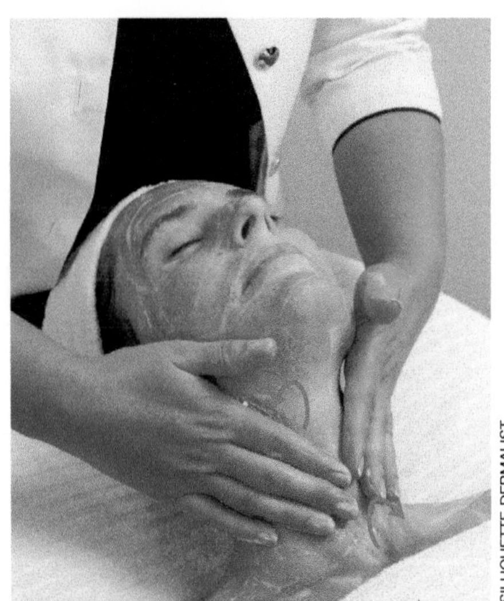

SILHOUETTE-DERMALIST

3 Apply small circular movements over the skin of the face and neck.

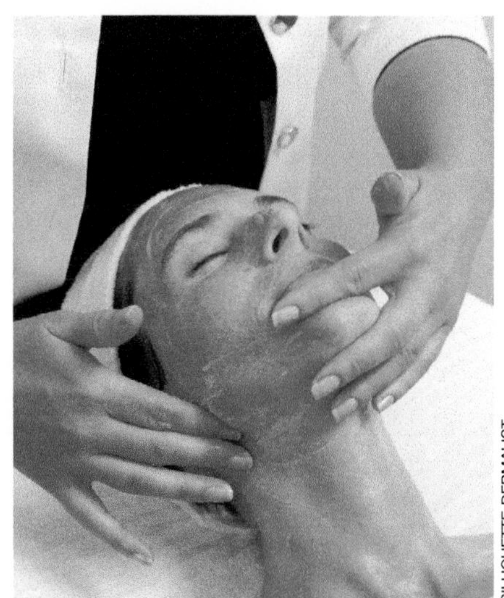

SILHOUETTE-DERMALIST

4 Draw the fingertips outwards to the angle of the jaw. Rest each index finger against the jaw bone. Place the middle finger beneath the jaw bone. Move the right hand towards the chin. When the index finger glides over the chin, return the fingers to the starting position beneath the jaw bone. Repeat with the left hand.

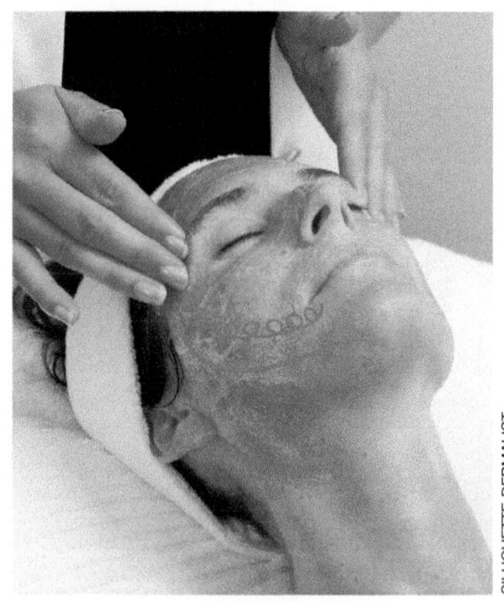

SILHOUETTE-DERMALIST

5 Apply circular movements, starting at the chin, working up towards the nose and finishing at the temples. Slide the fingers from the temples back to the chin, and repeat.

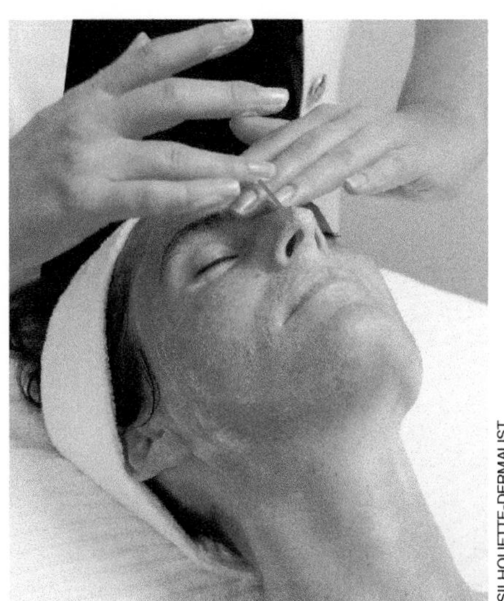

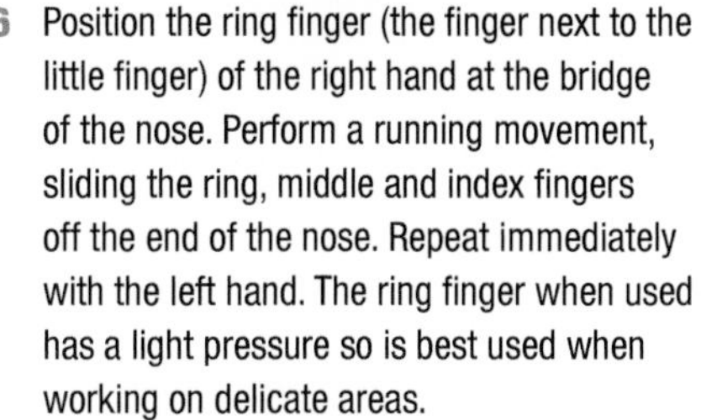

6 Position the ring finger (the finger next to the little finger) of the right hand at the bridge of the nose. Perform a running movement, sliding the ring, middle and index fingers off the end of the nose. Repeat immediately with the left hand. The ring finger when used has a light pressure so is best used when working on delicate areas.

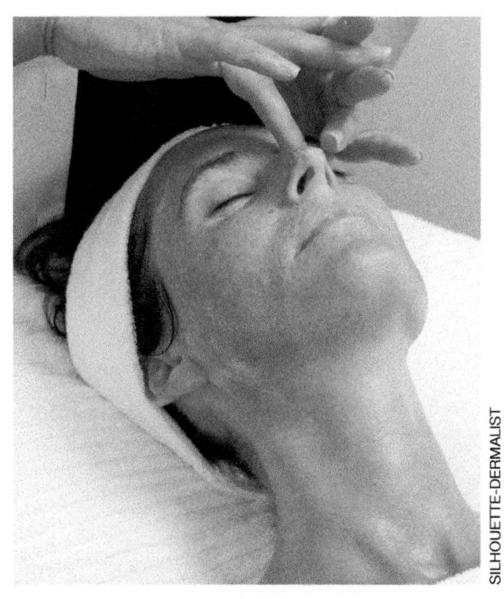

7 With the ring fingers of both hands trace a circle around the eye. Begin at the inner corner of the upper brow bone; slide to the outer corners of the brow bone, around and under the eyes, and return to the starting position.

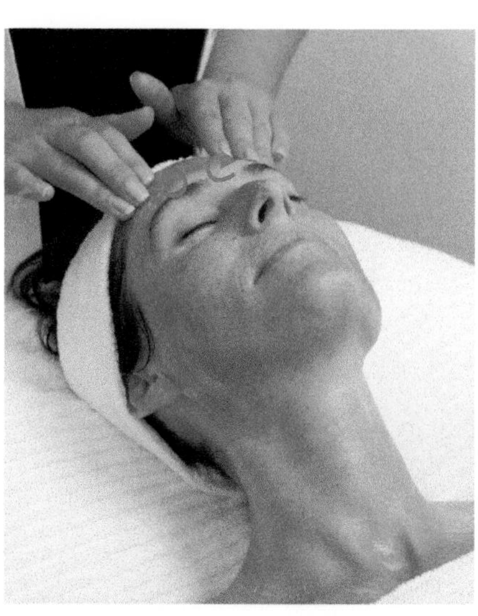

8 Using both hands, apply small circular movements across the forehead.

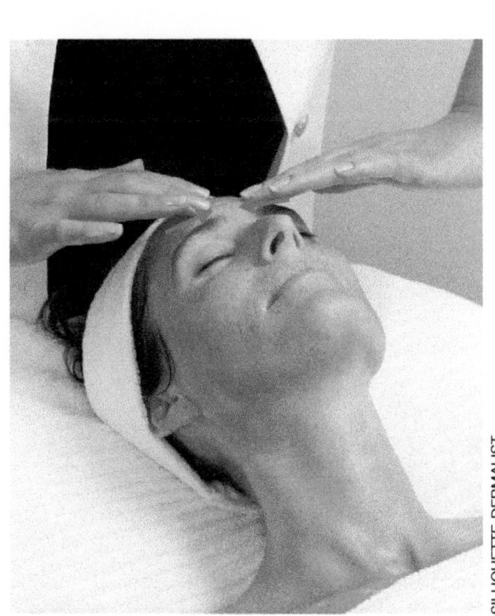

9 Open the index and middle fingers of each hand and perform a criss-cross stroking movement over the forehead.

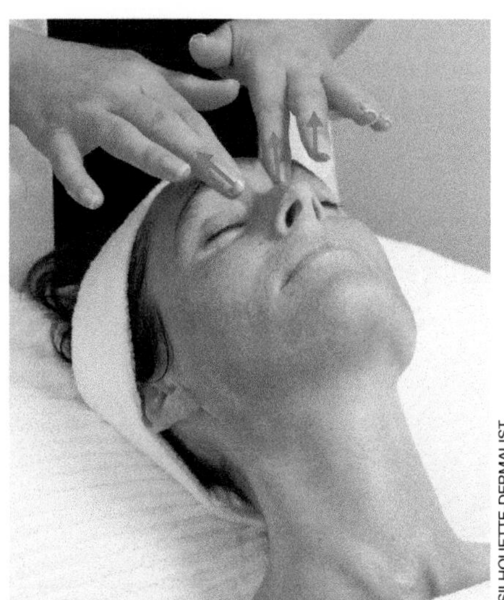

10 Slide the index fingers upwards slightly, lifting the inner eyebrow. Lift the centre of the the eyebrow with the middle finger. Finally, lift the outer corner of the eyebrow with the ring finger. Slide the ring fingers around the outer corner and beneath the eye.

11 With the pads of each hand, apply slight pressure at the temples. This indicates to the client that the cleansing sequence is complete.

12 Remove the cleansing product from the skin, using damp cotton wool or facial sponges.

TOP TIP

Combination skin

If preferred, different toning lotions can be applied to treat the different skin types of a combination skin.

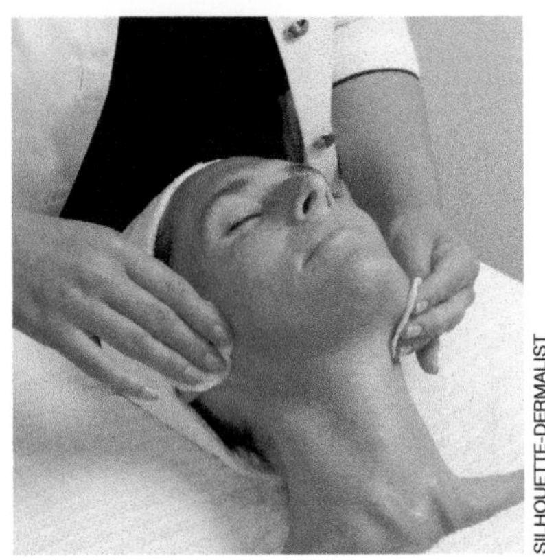

SILHOUETTE-DERMALIST

Applying toner

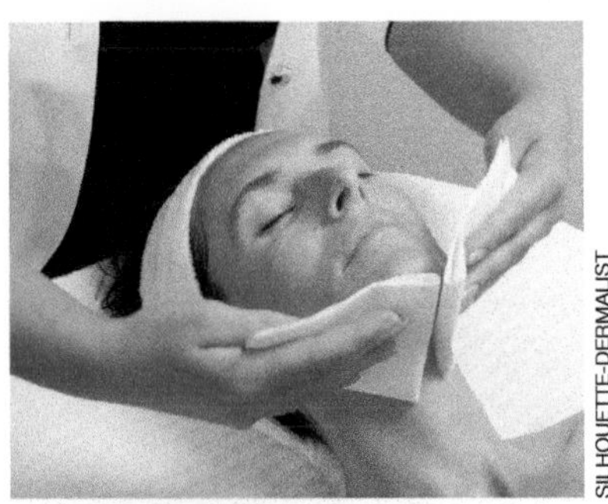

SILHOUETTE-DERMALIST

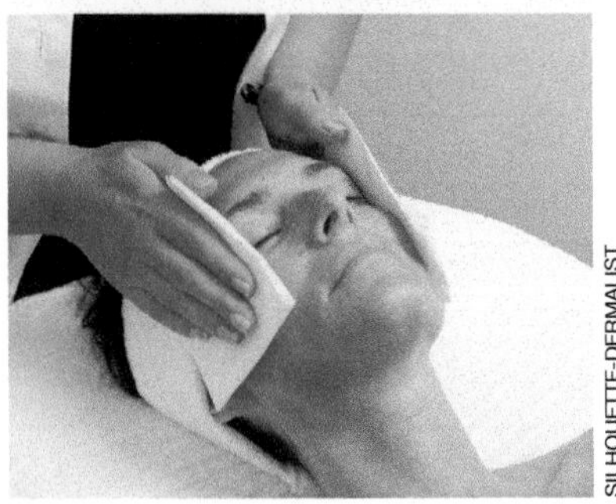

SILHOUETTE-DERMALIST

Blotting the skin

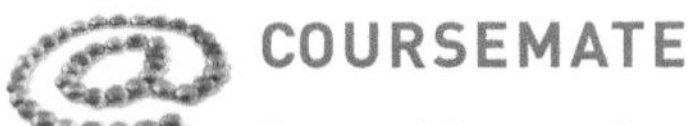

COURSEMATE

For a video on face mask application, please see this book's accompanying CourseMate.

Skin toning After the skin has been cleansed it is then toned with a suitable lotion. Whichever toning lotion is chosen it should have the following qualities:

- it should produce a cooling effect on the skin when the water or alcohol evaporates from the skin's surface
- it should create a skin-tightening effect on the skin. This reduces the flow of sebum and sweat onto the skin's surface
- it should remove skin products easily from the skin without causing any skin irritation.

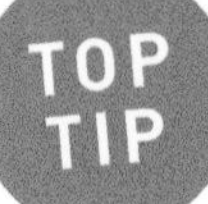

Choosing a toning lotion

Skin type	*Toning lotion*
Oily	**Astringents**, the strongest toning lotions with a high alcohol content to stimulate and promote skin healing
Dry	Skin bracers and **skin fresheners**, the mildest toning lotions, contain little or no alcohol They consist of mainly purified water and floral extracts for their toning properties
Combination	**Skin tonics**, slightly stronger toning lotion that braces and freshens. Might contain a little of an astringent agent

How to apply toner

1. Apply the selected toner to two pieces of clean damp cotton wool, which are wiped gently upwards and outwards over the surface of the skin.
2. The toner can be applied under pressure as a fine spray, using a vaporizer. This produces a fine mist of the toning lotion over the skin. Protect the eye tissue with damp cotton wool if using this technique.
3. After toner application, blot the skin dry with a soft facial tissue. Place the tissue over the face and neck and mould it to the skin to absorb excess moisture.

The skin can be inspected at this stage using a magnifying lamp to enlarge the skin's surface to help you identify further facial skin characteristics.

Mask service

The face mask is applied when the skin has been thoroughly cleansed and toned. It is usually applied as the final facial service because of its cleansing, tightening, refining and soothing effects upon the skin. Select the appropriate mask ingredients to treat the skin type. There are two types of mask:

- setting masks: are applied in a thin layer over the skin's surface and are then allowed to dry before removal
- non-setting masks: stay soft on application; they do not tighten like a setting mask.

You are required to competently apply a non-setting mask.

Non-setting mask These are pre-prepared and have a softening and moisturising effect on the skin. Each mask contains various plant extracts or chemical substances to treat different skin conditions. Instructions will be provided with the mask, stating how the product is to be used professionally.

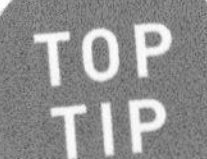

TOP TIP

Pre-prepared mask

This type of mask is often available for retail sale to the client and will enable the client to continue to care for the skin at home.

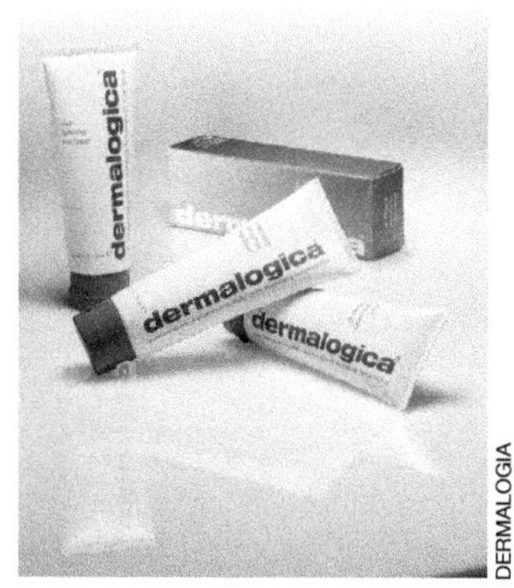

Pre-prepared service mask

How to apply a non-setting mask The method of mask preparation, application and removal are different for the various mask types. The guidelines below are for a non-setting, pre-prepared mask.

TOP TIP

Maintaining the working area

It is important to work in a hygienic, organized manner, leaving the work-station neat and tidy and removing all waste materials both during and at the end of the service.

1 Select the non-setting mask suited to the client's skin type. Always read the manufacturer's instructions before applying.

2 Discuss the service procedure with the client, especially:

- what the mask will feel like on application
- what sensation the client is likely to feel
- how long the mask will be left on the skin.

Generally, the mask will be left in place for 10–20 minutes.

3 Using a clean mask brush, begin to apply the mask. Apply the mask evenly and quickly so that it has maximum effect on the whole face. Don't apply it too thickly; as well as making mask removal difficult it is wasteful as only the part that is in contact with the skin has any effect. Keep the mask clear of the nostrils, the lips, the eyebrows and the hairline.

4 Apply dampened cotton wool pads over the eyes to relax the client.

5 Leave the mask for the recommended service time and according to the effect required.

6 Wash your hands.

7 When the mask is ready for removal, remove the eye pads.

8 Remove the mask using mask removal sponges or warm towels as shown, which should be damp – not wet – for client comfort and so that water does not run into the client's eyes, nose or hairline.

9 When the mask is thoroughly removed, apply the appropriate toning lotion. Blot the skin dry with a facial tissue. Moisturiser application follows.

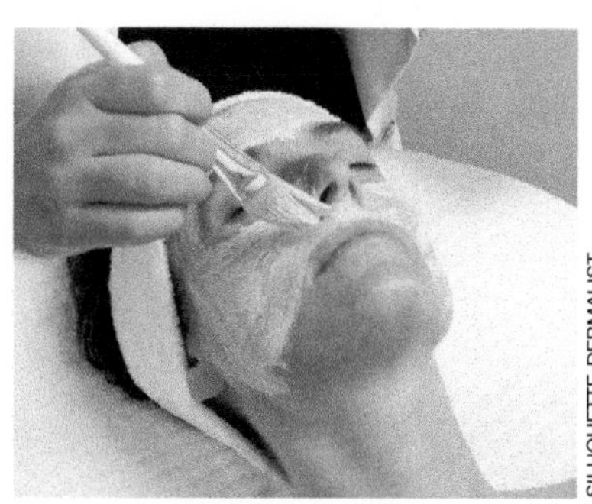

Mask application

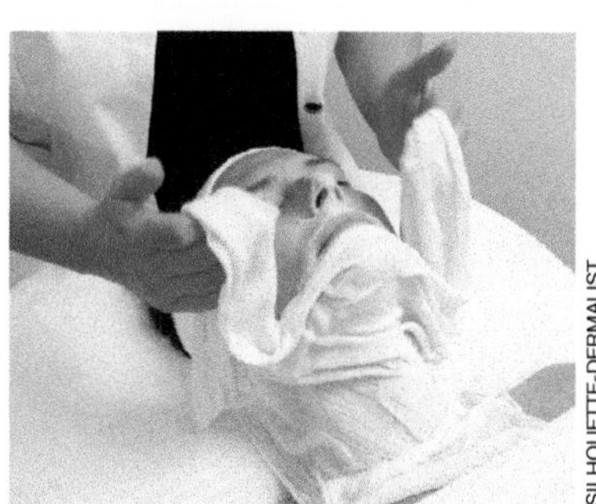

Mask removal with hot towels

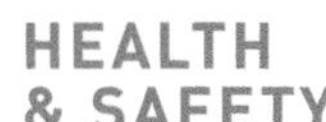

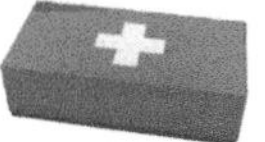

Sensitive skin

It is important to discuss normal skin reactions and sensations with a client who has a sensitive skin so that the client can tell you if there is a contra-action, an unwanted skin reaction to the mask.

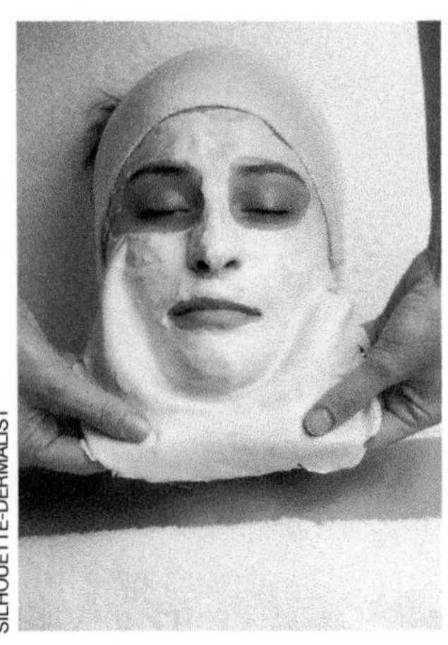

A setting face mask

TOP TIP

Moisturiser ingredients

Many moisturisers contain ingredients that improve the condition of the skin, such as vitamin E – an excellent skin conditioner – or UV filters to protect the skin from the premature ageing effects of sunlight.

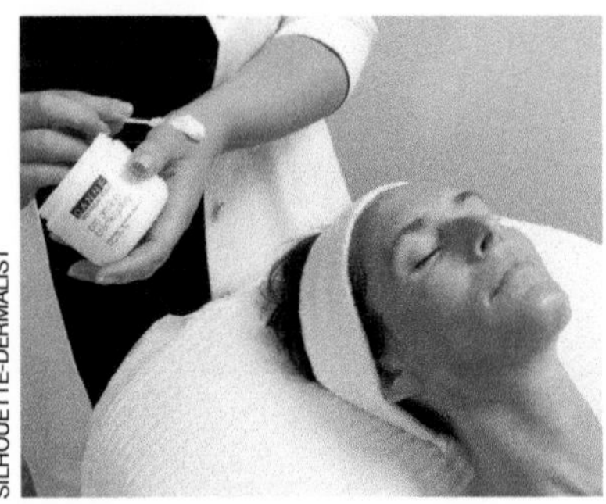

Applying moisturiser

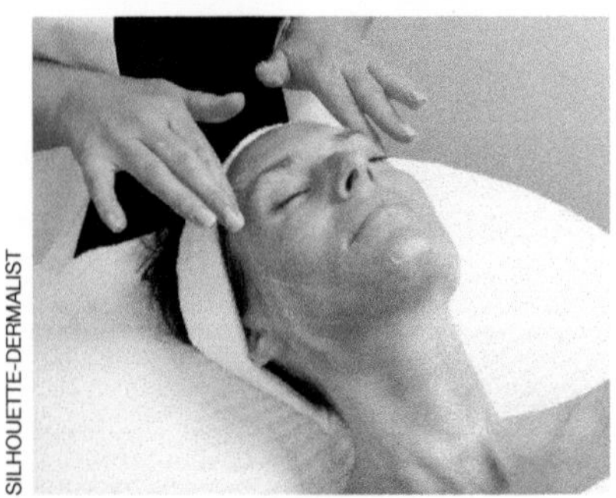

Spreading moisturiser evenly to the face and neck

TOP TIP

Choosing a moisturiser

Skin type	*Moisturiser*
Oily	Moisturising lotion
Dry	Moisturising cream
Combination	Moisturising lotion

Skin moisturising The basic formulation of a moisturiser is oil and water. The water content helps to return lost moisture to the surface layers of the skin; the oil content prevents moisture loss from the surface of the skin.

Often, a **humectant** (moisture holding) ingredient is included, such as **glycerine**, which attracts moisture from the surrounding air and stops the moisturiser from drying out.

Moisturisers are available for wear during the day or night and are available in different formulations to suit different skin types. Select a moisturising day product to suit your client's skin type.

Whichever moisturiser is chosen, it should have the following qualities:

- it should soften the skin and relieve skin tightness and sensitivity
- it should plump out the skin's tissues with moisture, minimizing the appearance of fine lines.
- it should reduce moisture loss from the skin surface.

TOP TIP

Moisturiser formulations

Moisturising lotions contain 85–90 per cent water and 10–15 per cent oil. Moisturising creams contain 70–85 per cent water and 10–15 per cent oil. Hypo-allergenic moisturisers are available for clients with sensitive skins. These are screened for all known common sensitizing agents such as lanolin and perfume.

How to apply moisturiser Moisturiser is applied after the final application of toning lotion.

1. Place a small amount of moisturiser in the palms of the hands. If the product is in a jar, remove the moisturiser with a clean spatula.
2. Apply moisturiser in small dots to the neck, chin, cheeks, nose and forehead. Spread it quickly and evenly in a fine film over the face, using light upwards and outwards stroking movements.
3. Blot excess moisturiser from the skin using a facial tissue.

The work area should be in a good state ready for further services.

Completing facial services

Check that the finished result is to the client's and the senior beauty therapist's satisfaction.

Make sure the client's records are up-to-date at the end of the service. This is important when you need to refer to them in the future. Record all details from the service accurately including retail sales on the client record card. Follow up the success of the service, home-care routine at the next service. The record should then be stored securely.

The client should be given home-care advice so that the skin can be cared for at home. This will be different for each client, depending on individual needs.

Outcome 4: Provide aftercare advice

Learn how to provide aftercare advice which supports and meets the needs of your client's service by:
1 Giving **advice** and recommendations accurately and constructively.
2 Giving your clients suitable **advice** on basic facial skincare.

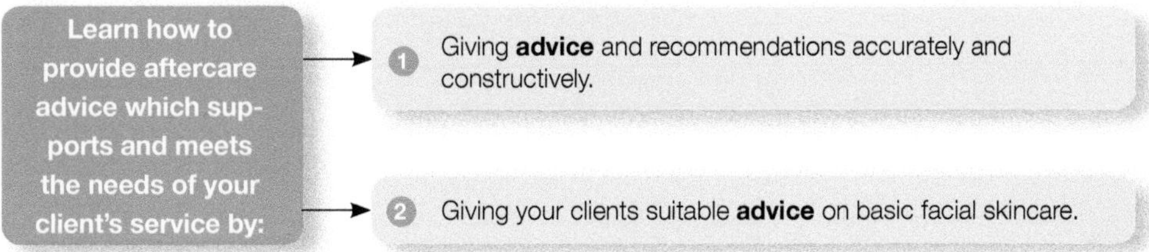

TOP TIP

Advise the client on skincare preparations to use and help to maintain good skin condition.

1. **Cleanse the eye area using a suitable eye make-up remover. Cleanse each eye separately to avoid cross-infection.**
2. **Apply cleansing products in an upwards and outwards direction to avoid damaging the skin.**
3. **Apply toning lotion to damp cotton wool and wipe gently upwards and outwards over the neck and face or if in a spray, spray onto the skin's surface.**
4. **Apply moisturiser in small dots to the neck and chin and cheeks, nose and forehead evenly spreading in a fine film over the face, using light upwards, outwards stroking movements.**

TOP TIP

Mineral make-up

Mineral make-up is increasingly being applied following a facial so the skin is still able to breathe.

Basic home-care advice

- Discuss the use of make-up if to be worn following the service. Generally, only lip and eye make-up should be worn directly after a facial service.
- Warn the client that a few blemishes might be experienced. These are caused by the cleansing action of the facial.
- If a client is given a sample of a service product, explain its correct use in terms of application and removal so that the client can gain maximum benefit from the product.
- Recommend the skin is cleansed and toned, twice a day, morning and night. Advise on the correct products to use.

- A moisturiser should be applied for day use and a separate moisturiser applied for night use. Each is formulated to achieve a different effect. Advise on the correct products to use.
- The skin should be toned and moisturised following mask application.
- Advise the client on a service plan to improve the facial skin condition as necessary and what other professional services you could recommend within your responsibility. This may be provided in written form, make sure your instructions are clear.
- Advise the client that the correct time space between facial services is usually 14–28 days. Assist the client to re-book for a further service.

ACTIVITY

Client satisfaction

It is important that the client enjoys their facial service as they will then most probably book to receive further services, and long-term improvements to the skin will become noticeable.

However, the client may not have enjoyed the service because of how you performed it. With a colleague think of reasons why a client may not have been happy with the facial service.

Promoting products Providing advice also gives you the opportunity to recommend retail products. This improves the salon's retail sales and overall profits.

Contra-actions Ask clients to contact the salon immediately and speak with the senior beauty therapist if any unwanted reaction to the service occurs. Such contra-actions (e.g. an allergy, recognized by redness, swelling and inflammation) should be noted on the client's record card for future reference.

Ensure the client's service card is completed accurately with all details of the service recorded. Store the record card securely in compliance with the Data Protection Act 1998.

GLOSSARY OF KEY WORDS

Acid mantle acid film on the skin's surface created by a combination of sweat and sebum. The acid mantle is protective and discourages the growth of bacteria and fungi.

Aftercare advice recommended advice given to the client following a service to continue the benefits of the service.

Allergen a substance that the skin is sensitive to and which causes an allergic reaction.

Allergic skin if the skin is sensitive to a particular substance an allergic skin reaction will occur. This is recognized by irritation, swelling and inflammation.

Aseptic a situation described as trying to destroy bacteria. One which you should try to achieve in the workplace.

Blood nutritive liquid circulating through the blood vessels; transports essential nutrients to the cells and removes waste products; transports other important substances such as oxygen and hormones.

Blood vessels tubular structures in the body that carry blood.

Cell the smallest and simplest unit capable of life.

Cleanser a skincare product that removes dead skin cells, excess sweat and oil (sebum), make-up and dirt from the skin's surface to maintain a healthy skin appearance.

Consultation assessment of a client's needs using different assessment techniques, including questioning and natural observation.

Contra-action an unwanted or negative reaction occurring during or after service application.

Contra-indication a problematic condition present that means that service might not go ahead or may restrict the service requiring it to be adapted in some way.

Cross-infection the transfer of contagious microorganisms.

Data Protection Act 1998 legislation designed to protect client privacy and confidentiality.

Deep cleanse uses a heavier-than-usual cleansing product – often a cream – that allows massage movements to be applied to the skin without the cleansing product evaporating.

Dermis the inner portion of the skin, situated underneath the epidermis.

Disinfection the removal of microorganisms by chemical or physical means which slows the growth of disease.

Epidermis the outer layer of the skin.

Facial a service to improve the appearance, condition and functioning of the skin and underlying structures.

Fibres found in the dermis and give the skin its strength and elasticity. Yellow elastin gives the skin its elasticity, white collagen gives skin its strength.

Fungus microscopic plants that in humans, are parasites. Fungal diseases of the skin feed off the waste products of the skin. They are found on the skin's surface or they can attack deeper tissues.

Hair follicle an appendage (structure) in the skin formed from epidermal tissue. Cells move up the hair follicle from the bottom (the hair bulb), changing in structure, to form the hair.

Hygiene the recommended standard of cleanliness necessary in the workplace to prevent cross-infection and secondary infection. The standard expected, as laid down in law, industry code of practice or written procedures specified by the workplace.

Lymph a clear, straw-coloured liquid circulating in the lymph vessels and lymphatics of the body, filtered out of the blood plasma.

Mask service a skin-cleansing preparation applied to the skin. It might contain different ingredients to have a deep cleansing, toning, nourishing or refreshing effect. It can be applied to the hands, feet and/or face. It may be of a setting or non-setting formulation.

Massage manipulation of the soft tissues of the body, producing heat and stimulating the muscular, circulatory and nervous system.

Melanin a pigment in the skin that contributes to skin colour.

Melanocytes cells that produce the skin pigment melanin, which contributes to skin colour.

Moisturiser a skincare preparation (formulation of oil and water) that helps maintain the skin's natural moisture by locking moisture into the skin, giving protection and hydration.

Muscle tissue responsible for movement of the body.

Nerve a collection of single neurons surrounded by a protective sheath through which impulses are transmitted between the brain or spinal cord and another part of the body.

Organizational requirements beauty therapy procedures issued by the workplace management.

Papillae projections near the surface of the dermis, which contain nerve endings and blood capillaries. These supply the upper epidermis with nutrition.

Personal appearance the standard expected as laid down in industry codes of practice or written procedures specified by the workplace.

Sebaceous gland a minute sac-like organ usually attached to the hair follicle. The cells of the gland break down and produce the sebum. Found all over the body except the soles of the feet and the palms of the hands.

Sebum the skin's natural oil, which keeps the skin supple.

Secondary infection bacterial activity causing infection.

Service plan the plan you intend to perform to carry out a particular service to meet the client's needs.

Skin analysis assessment of the client's skin type and condition.

Skin appendages structures within the skin including sweat glands (that excrete sweat), hair follicles (that produce hair), sebaceous glands (that produce sebum) and nails – a horny substance that protects the ends of the fingers.

Skin tone the strength and elasticity of the skin.

Skin type the different way each skin functions provides the skin type. Skin types include dry (lacking in oil), oily (too much oil) and combination (a mixture of the other two skin types).

Sterilization the total destruction of all microorganisms.

Subcutaneous tissue a layer of fatty tissue situated below the epidermis and dermis.

Superficial cleanse uses lightweight cleansing products to remove surface make-up, dirt and grease.

Sweat glands small structures in the skin of the dermis and epidermis that excrete sweat. Their function is to regulate body temperature through the evaporation of sweat from the skin's surface.

Toning lotion a skincare preparation to remove all traces of cleanser from the skin. It produces a cooling effect on the skin and has a skin tightening effect.

Virus virus particles attack healthy body cells and multiply within the cell. Eventually the virus kills the cell – the cell walls break down and the virus parts are freed to attack further cells.

Workplace the word used to describe the environment in which you carry out your work. Normally, this will be your salon.

Workplace policies the documentation prepared by an employer on the procedures to be followed in the workplace.

Working practices activities and procedures, working techniques used to perform your job.

ASSESSMENT OF KNOWLEDGE AND UNDERSTANDING

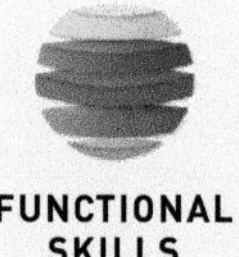

Assist with facial skincare services

Having covered the learning objectives for assisting with facial skincare services – test what you need to know and understand by answering the following short questions below.

The information covers:

- organizational and legal requirements
- how to work safely and effectively when assisting with facial services
- anatomy and physiology
- client consultation and service planning
- facial services
- aftercare advice for clients.

Organizational and legal requirements

1 Why it is important when treating minors to have a parent/guardian present during the facial service?

2 Why is it necessary to follow a senior therapist's instructions when assisting with facial services?

3 What may be the consequences of not referring to the senior therapist when assisting with facial services?

4 What condition should the work area be left in following the facial service and why is this important?

5 What is your salon's service time for completing a basic facial service?

6 Why is it important to complete services in a commercially viable time?

How to work safely and effectively when assisting with facial services

1 What is the difference between sterilizing and disinfecting equipment?

2 What is the importance of personal presentation and hygiene when carrying out facial services?

3 List the essential equipment, and materials required to set up the work area for facial services.

4 What are the necessary environmental conditions for facial services that must be checked for before every service application?

5 Why is it important to check equipment used before every facial service?

6 How should the client be prepared and positioned for a facial service?

Anatomy and physiology

1 Name three functions of the skin.

2 How many layers of the epidermis are there?

3 What is the dermis and where is the dermis situated?

4 How would you recognize the following skin conditions:

- sensitive?
- comedone?
- milia?
- pustules?
- papules?

5 Label the features of the cross-section of the skin shown below:

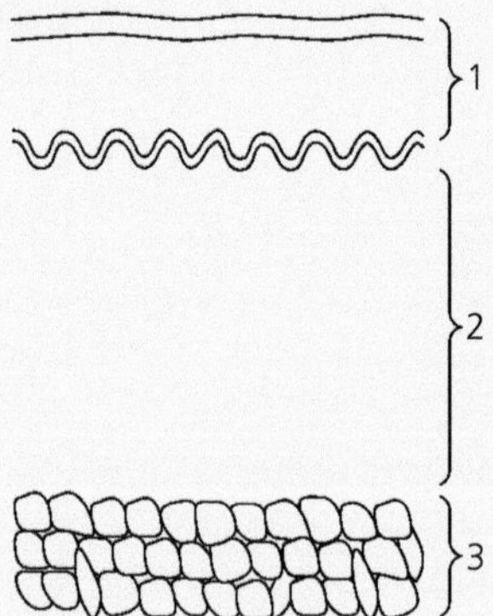

6 Why is it important to recognize the skin characteristics of different ethnic client groups?

Client consultation and service planning

1 What is the purpose of the consultation?

2 What details should be recorded on the client's record card?

3 What questions and listening skills are essential in order to find out the information required to inform planning?

4 At the consultation you notice a client has a crusty blemish by her lip. What action do you take?

5 How do you identify a client's skin type and service requirements?

6 How should all client records be stored to comply with the Data Protection Act 1998?

7 Name four facial conditions that would contra-indicate service.

8 How can you ensure client comfort when preparing the facial service area?

Facial services

1 How long would you allow for a complete basic facial service?

2 Design a facial service, for a client with a dry skin type. Describe:

- the aim of the facial service
- the facial skin products you are going to use
- the aftercare advice to be given to maintain the skin condition.

Consider what products the client should be recommended to use at home and how to use them.

3 Why is it important to keep accurate records of the client's service?

4 What is the purpose of the following skincare products?

- cleanser
- toning lotion
- moisturiser
- face mask.

5 What contra-actions could occur during a facial service and what action would you take?

Aftercare advice for clients

1 What skincare products would you recommend that a client use as part of her home-care routine?

2 How would you explain to the client the correct application and – where relevant – removal of the following products for home use?

- cleansing milk
- toning lotion
- non-setting face mask.

3 How often would you recommend a basic facial service?

4 How should the work area be left following each service, and why?

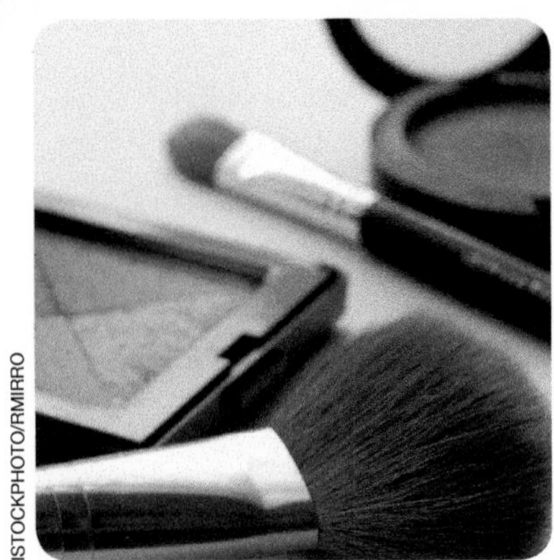
ISTOCKPHOTO/RMIRRO

7 Assist with day make-up

Learning Objectives

This chapter covers the **Assist with day make-up** unit.

This unit is all about the skills you will need to assist with and carry out a basic day make-up in the workplace. This will be under the care or supervision of the senior beauty therapist. You will learn how to prepare the make-up work area, carryout a skin analysis and use consultation techniques to select and apply the most suitable skincare and make-up products for different clients.

These will include: foundation, concealer, powder, eye products, cheek and lip products. The finished look should be to the satisfaction of the client and senior beauty therapist. Aftercare advice should be given to the client on products used and how to maintain (keep the look fresh) and how best to remove the make-up products when required.

There are **four** learning outcomes which you must achieve competently:

1. **Maintain safe and effective working methods when providing day make-up**
2. **Consult and prepare for make-up**
3. **Apply day make-up**
4. **Provide aftercare advice**

Your assessor will observe your performance on **at least three occasions** which will be recorded. Each must be performed on a different client.

From the **range** statement, you must show that you have:

- used all **consultation techniques**
- identified all **skin types**

(continued on the next page)

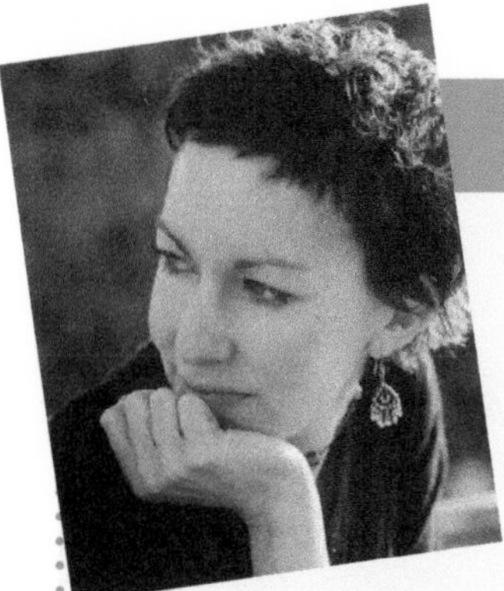

ROLE MODEL

Julia Francis

Make-up artist and body painter
www.juliafrancis.co.uk

"I have been a make-up artist for over 10 years working with some of the industry's leading photographers, advertising agencies, directors, musicians and actors. For film and TV my credits include *Star Wars, Hitchhiker's Guide to the Galaxy, Wimbledon* and *Eastenders*. My Celebrity clients include Sir Tom Jones, Colin Firth and Jonathan Ross. Agencies and brands that I have worked with include Bacardi, Pantene, Olay, Gillette and Saatchi & Saatchi.

I am also an experienced teacher and make-up consultant and have been conducting workshops for many years. Monthly workshops offer students a unique opportunity to find out how to move forward in a career as a make-up artist.

To find out more about these workshops, please email me at: workshops@juliafrancis.co.uk.

(continued)

- carried out all types of **preparation of the client**
- used all types of **make-up products**
- given all types of **advice**.

When providing day make-up service it is important to use the skills you have learnt in the following units:

Health and Safety

Developing positive working relationships

Preparing and maintaining the salon treatment work area

Facial skincare

Practical skills, knowledge and understanding

The table here will help you to check progress in gaining the necessary practical skills, knowledge and understanding for **Assist with day make-up**.

Tick (✓) when you feel you have gained the practical skills, knowledge and understanding in each of the following areas:

	Practical skills, knowledge and understanding checklist	✓
1	The aim of a basic day **make-up**.	
2	Contra-indications that prevent or restrict day make-up service.	
3	**Equipment** and materials needed.	
4	How to prepare the service area.	
5	How to prepare yourself before the day make-up.	
6	Client consultation to decide what the make-up service will include.	
7	How to prepare the client for the service.	
8	How to carry out a basic day make-up.	
9	**Aftercare advice** to be given to the client following the make-up service.	
10	Contra-actions (unwanted reaction) to look for during or following the day make-up service.	

When you have ticked all the areas you can ask your assessor to assess you on assisting with day make-up. After practical assessment, your assessor might decide that you need to practice further to improve your skills. If so, your assessor will tell you how and where you need to improve to gain competence.

After assessment of what you need to know and understand there may be 'gaps' that require you to study further. Your assessor will tell you what you need to study to achieve the required level of knowledge and understanding.

Make-up services

Make-up is applied to improve the appearance of the skin and our facial features, i.e. the nose, lips, eyes, etc. This can make us feel more confident as imperfections are disguised – made less obvious, i.e. spots and dark circles under the eyes while our best features are emphasized – made more obvious, i.e. lip gloss applied to enhance the lips.

Each client is different and will have different make-up application needs. This will be chosen and suited to their skin tone, facial features, hair colouring and the type of **make-up occasion** it is to be worn for.

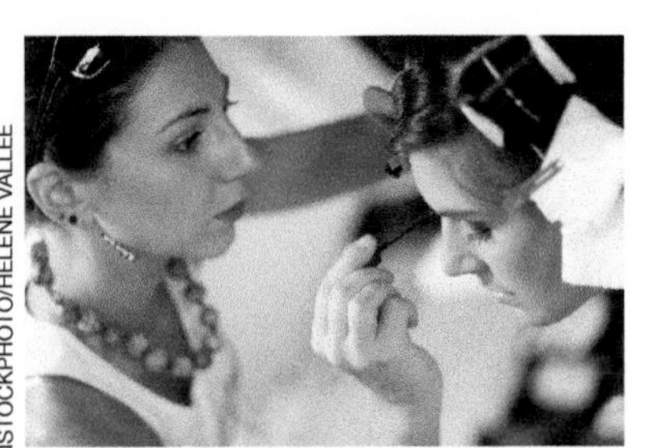
ISTOCKPHOTO/HELENE VALLEE

Each client is different and will have different make-up application requirements

For this chapter, day make-up application is discussed.

The day make-up service includes:

- **consultation** and **skin analysis** to decide the client's **skin type** and make-up application requirements
- skin cleansing and toning to remove surface dirt, make-up and skin debris
- **moisturiser** application to protect and hydrate (add moisture to) the skin
- make-up application to suit the client's skin type, age and skin colouring or tone.

Anatomy and physiology of the skin

You need to know about the skin, its structure and function (how it works) as this will allow you to recognize the appearance of each skin according to its skin type, age and racial characteristics. This will enable you to make the correct choice of skincare and make-up products to ensure the make-up will look its best and suit the client's skin.

Refer to Chapter 6 **Facial skincare** p. 127 to learn what you need to know about:

- the basic structure of the skin, e.g. epidermis and dermis
- the basic function of the skin, i.e. sensation, protection, temperature control, sensitivity
- different racial skin characteristics
- how the skin changes as it ages.

The structure and function of our skin provides our skin type, this is discussed in Chapter 6: **Facial skincare** p. 134.

Make-up is made to suit the skin type for which it is to be applied, to get the best possible results, so it is important to correctly identify the skin type at the consultation.

Making an appointment for day make-up

When giving **assistance** with reception duties you may be required to make a make-up service appointment, the following will help you in your job role.

When a client makes an appointment for a basic day make-up, the receptionist should ask a few basic questions:

- What is the client's name and telephone number? This will help you to get the client record cards ready before they arrive for the service. The telephone number is important in case you need to contact the client for any reason, e.g. to cancel or rearrange an appointment.
- Which beauty therapist does the client want to book with? If a particular beauty therapist is asked for you will have to check on availability.
- When does the client want the make-up, i.e. day/date and time? If any of these are not available, suggest another time or day as near to this as possible.
- Explain that contact lenses, if worn, will need to be removed before make-up application is applied. This will avoid make-up entering the eye which could lead to eye irritation and watering eyes.
- Has the client had the make-up service before? This allows you to discuss any questions about the make-up service from their previous experience.

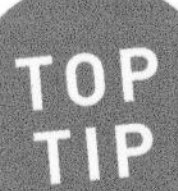

Booking appointments

- **If the client is having her hair styled before the make-up, advise her that it will be necessary to move it away from the facial area briefly while the skin is prepared before make-up application. A large hair clip is usually used to avoid spoiling the hair.**
- **Check if she has any known allergies to any make-up products.**
- **Is the client used to wearing make-up – remember this is a day make-up so the colours will not be too strong and a more subtle result is generally required, explain this.**
- **If the client wants a facial before the make-up, this would not be recommended as the make-up generally will not last as the skin is stimulated, it becomes warmer, produces more oil and is also oilier because of the products used during the facial. However, mineral make-up is increasingly used following facials as its formulation does not cause clogging, called congestion of the pores.**
- **Recommend that the client does not shape her eyebrows before make-up service as the skin will become redder or darker dependent upon the skin tone. This will affect the appearance of make-up colour in the area. The skin could also become infected in the area as it is open following hair removal.**

ALWAYS REMEMBER

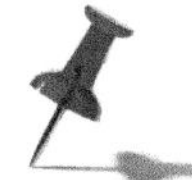

Being productive

When booking an appointment this provides an opportunity to link sell – check if the client would like another service. You have linked one service to another. You can do this when carrying out the make-up service, the client may wish to buy a product such as the lipstick used.

You may have targets for selling, so this will help you meet them.

When booking the appointment allow 30 minutes for a basic day make-up. This does not allow consultation and preparation time.

When preparing for the make-up service you will need to prepare the work area, yourself and client.

Outcome 1: Maintain safe and effective working methods when providing day make-up service

Learn how to maintain safe and effective working methods when providing day make-up by:

1. Setting up the work area to meet salon procedures and any given instructions.
2. Making sure that environmental conditions are suitable for the client and the service.
3. Ensuring your personal hygiene, protection and personal appearance meets accepted industry and organizational requirements.
4. Ensuring all tools and equipment are cleaned using the correct methods.
5. Effectively disinfecting your hands prior to applying make-up.
6. Maintaining accepted industry hygiene and safety practices throughout the service.
7. Positioning equipment and materials for ease and safety of use.
8. Ensuring your own posture and position minimizes fatigue and the risk of injury while working.
9. Disposing of waste materials safely and correctly.
10. Ensuring that the service is cost-effective and is carried out within a commercially viable time.
11. Leaving the work area in a condition suitable for further services.
12. Ensuring the client's records are up-to-date, accurate, easy to read and signed by the client and practitioner.

ALWAYS REMEMBER

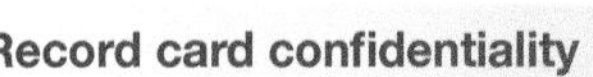

Record card confidentiality

When preparing the area for day make-up collect the client record card. If it is a new client the necessary details will need to be completed first. All details are confidential and should only be seen with those who have permission to do so. When finished with, the client records should be stored securely. This is your legal responsibility to comply with the **Data Protection Act (1998)**.

HEALTH & SAFETY

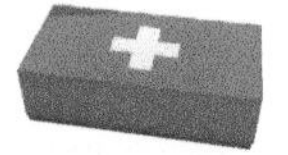

Selecting products

Always check with the senior beauty therapist that you are selecting the correct products for the client's skin type and make-up preferences (wishes).

Equipment materials and products used in a basic day make-up service

It is important that you understand the purpose of the different equipment, materials and products and any related health and safety practice related to their use.

Item	*Use*	*Health and safety practice*
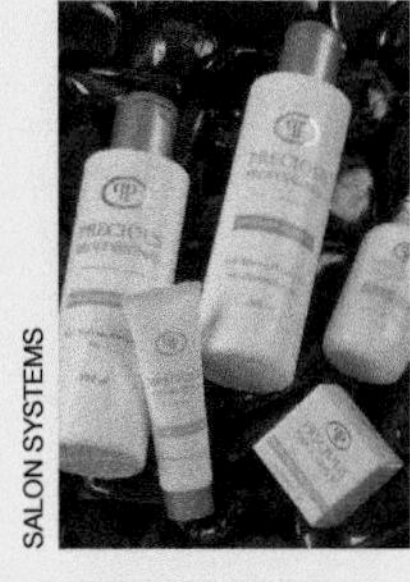 ELLISONS Bowls – various sizes	Can be used to hold client jewellery; skincare preparations and cotton wool	Clean after use with a detergent, disinfectant, rinse and dry If using to hold water, keep on a stable surface to avoid spillage
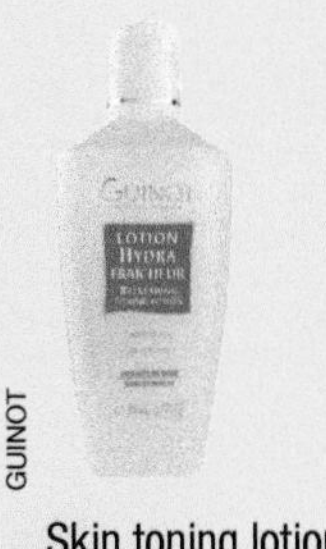 SALON SYSTEMS	Usually a combination of oil and water that will remove oil, make-up and other substances from the skin's surface Different cleansing preparations are available to the beauty therapist whose formulations are designed to treat the different skin types and conditions	If a client has a sensitive skin a product should be used that has any possible skin sensitizers removed, this is called hypo-allergenic Use the correct cleansing product for the skin type to avoid skin irritation or sensitivity Avoid too much pressure which could cause the skin to become too stimulated and warm affecting skin colour, make-up effect and its lasting properties Avoid using too much **cleanser** around the eye area to avoid it entering the eye causing eye irritation
GUINOT Skin toning lotion 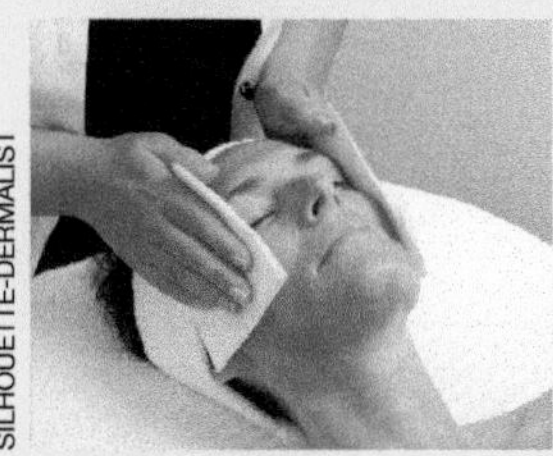 SILHOUETTE-DERMALIST Skin blotting	Applied after the skin has been cleansed **Toning lotions** remove any remaining cleanser from the skin's surface, they can also have a skin tightening effect, making the pores smaller Various toning preparations are available in formulations for the different skin types and conditions	If the client has a sensitive skin use a hypo-allergenic product. Use the correct toning product for the skin type to avoid skin irritation or sensitivity Replace lids immediately to avoid spillage Gently blot the skin dry following toning lotion application with a soft facial tissue to avoid over-stimulation of the skin as the toner evaporates or disappears from the skin's surface If irritated the skin will become warm and reddened or darkened dependent upon skin colour affecting the final make-up appearance. It may also have to be removed!
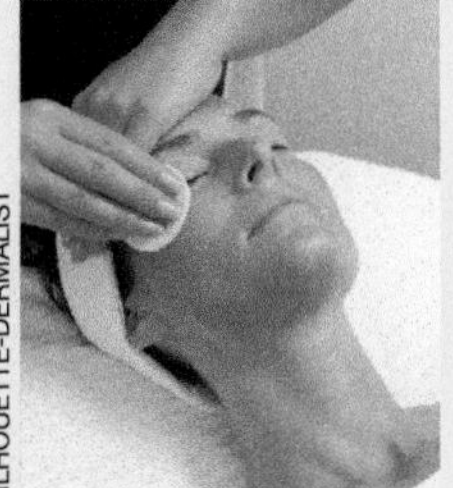 SILHOUETTE-DERMALIST Eye make-up removal	Eye make-up remover cleanses the eyelids and lashes, gently dissolving oils, dirt and make-up if worn. It can also condition the delicate skin Formulated as a lotion or gel, it is made to remove either water-based or oil-based products or both	If a client has a sensitive skin use a hypo-allergenic product Support the delicate eye tissue with the hand when cleansing the eye area to avoid stretching the skin Avoid using too much eye make-up remover as it may enter the eye causing irritation Never apply pressure over the eyeball when cleansing the eye area

Item	*Use*	*Health and safety practice*
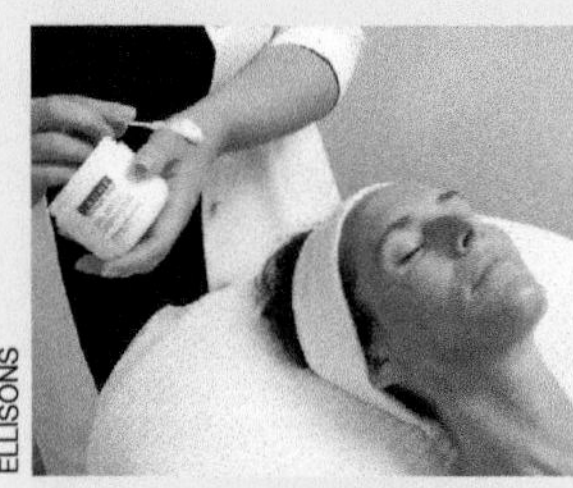 ELLISONS Moisturiser application	The skin needs water to keep it soft and supple. Moisture is constantly being lost. The application of a moisturiser helps to maintain the natural oil and moisture balance by locking moisture into the skin, providing protection and hydration The basic formulation of a moisturiser is oil and water	If a client has a sensitive skin use a hypo-allergenic product Always use a spatula to remove moisturiser if in an open container to prevent contamination Return lids immediately after use for hygiene and to prevent the quality of the product spoiling
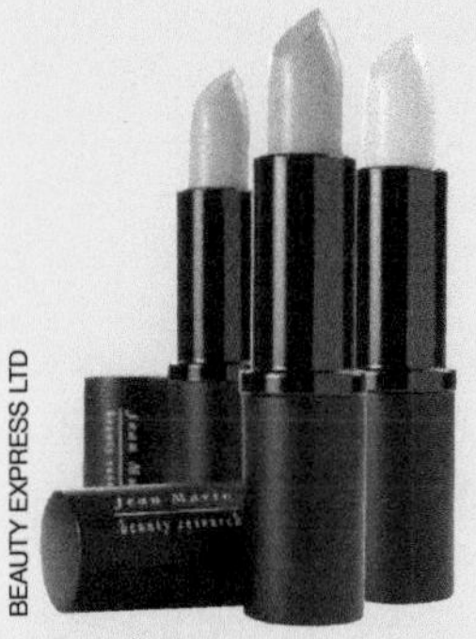 BEAUTY EXPRESS LTD Concealer	A make-up product used to disguise any imperfections These are formulated to be used in different areas, such as those for use around the eyes that are lighter in texture	**Concealer** formulated for covering blemishes such a spots are unsuitable for use around the eye as they are heavier in texture and can stretch the skin when applied If the concealer is in a container use a clean disposable spatula to remove. If it has a brush applicator attached to the product, for hygiene reasons this cannot be used. Use a disposable brush or clean make-up brush to apply
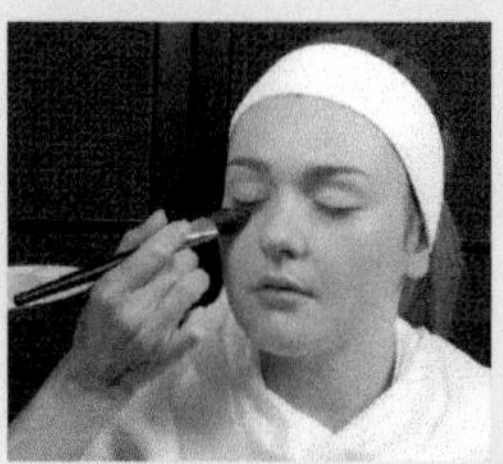 Foundation	**Foundation** is applied to produce an even skin tone and disguise blemishes Special ingredients may be included in foundations for the skin type to achieve the best result They are available in cream, liquid, compact, stick, gel, cake, mousse, mineral-based and tinted moisturisers	Apply foundations to suit the skin type. The correct choice will ensure that the make-up lasts all day If the foundation is in a container, remove some from its container using a clean disposable spatula. Place it onto a clean make-up palette Use either clean sponges, fingers or a foundation brush to apply it evenly to the skin If the client has any ingredient allergies these can be checked from the material safety data sheet (MSDS) which lists ingredients used in the product. This ensures you choose products safely
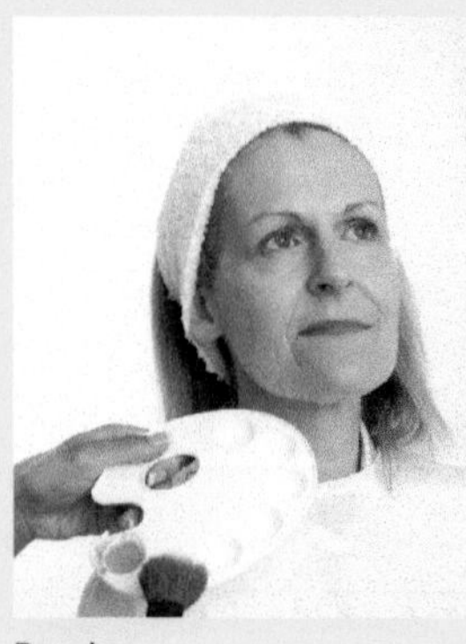 Powder	**Powder** is applied to set the foundation, disguising minor blemishes and making the skin surface appear smooth Powder products can also be used to change the shape of the face. Blushers are used to add warmth and draw attention to the face shape	Powder products should be removed from their containers using a disposable spatula and placed onto a clean make-up palette Use clean cotton wool or a velour puff to apply face powder and clean make-up brushes to remove excess powder from the face and to apply **blusher**

Item	*Use*	*Health and safety practice*
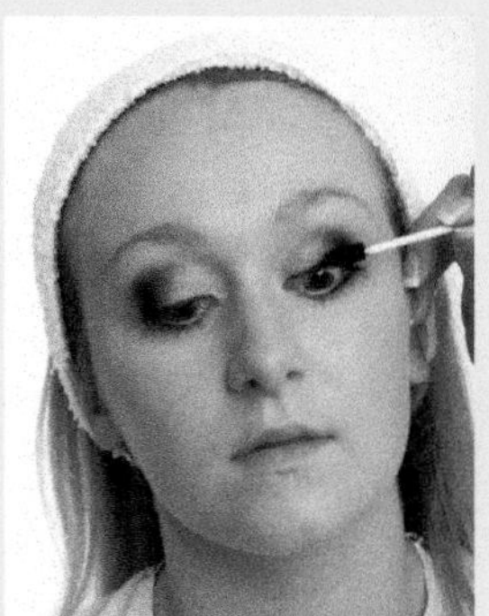 Eye products	Eye products include eyeshadows pencils and mascara	Powder eyeshadows should be removed from their containers and placed onto a clean make-up palette. They should be applied using disposable make-up eyeshadow applicators or clean brushes Eye pencils should be sharpened using a pencil sharpener before use to expose a clean surface for each client Mascara should be applied using a disposable brush or make-up brush that can be cleaned following use
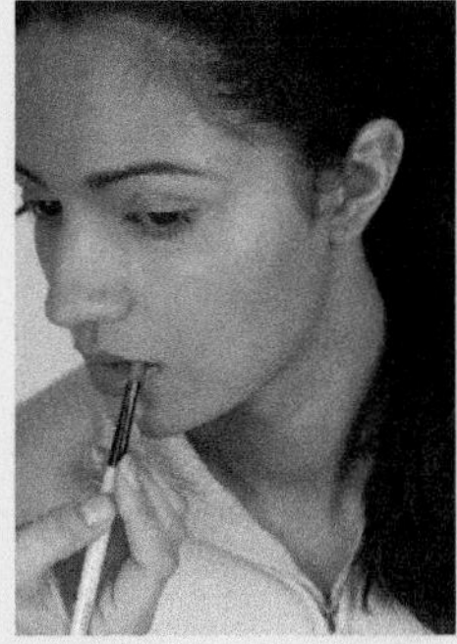 Lip products	Lip products include lip pencils, lip balms, lip stains and lipsticks, and lip glosses	Lip pencils should be sharpened using a pencil sharpener before use to expose a clean surface for each client Other lip products should be removed from their container and applied using a disposable brush or make-up brush that can be cleaned following use Lip stain may be applied using a disposable make-up sponge

HEALTH & SAFETY

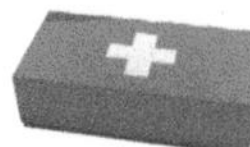

Make-up shelf life

Make-up can only be kept for a certain length of time its 'shelf life', i.e. mascara requires replacement every 6 months once opened. Inform the responsible person if a product requires replacement.

Know your products

You will always be asked advice on the best products for people. You will only be able to answer questions within your job responsibility. Any advice should be accurate to meet the needs of the client. It is essential that you have a good knowledge of all the products that you apply. This will inspire client confidence in you.

Julia Francis

Equipment and materials

Before carrying out the basic day make-up, check that you have the necessary equipment and materials at hand. Refer to the equipment and materials checklist to make sure that you have all that is required to perform a basic day make-up service. Tick next to each item on the checklist to help as you prepare the work area.

ALWAYS REMEMBER

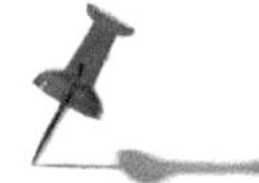

Workstation

You may have a fixed work station for applying make-up. This should be prepared according to your workplace policy. Keep it clean and tidy at all times.

EQUIPMENT AND MATERIALS CHECKLIST FOR BASIC DAY MAKE-UP

SORISA

Couch

Couch or **beauty chair** with sit-up and lie-down positions and an easy-to-clean surface ☐

SORISA

Trolley

Trolley on which to place everything required for the make-up service ☐

ELLISONS

Disposable tissue

Disposable tissue to cover the work surface and the couch or beauty chair ☐

ELLISONS

Headband

Headband or **hair clips** to protect the client's hair while cleansing the skin and keeping the hair away from the face during make-up application ☐

Towels

Towels (2) clean for each client – one to be placed at the head end of the couch or chair if used. The other to be placed over the client's chest and shoulders to protect their clothing. Alternatively a make-up cape may be worn ☐

ELLISONS

Dry/damp cotton wool

Dry cotton wool may be used to apply powder ☐
Damp cotton wool to use during skin preparation, i.e. cleansing

SORISA

Cotton buds

Cotton buds are useful as a disposable tool to soften the application effect of products such as eyeliner and to correct any accidental mistakes ☐

ELLISONS

Large facial tissues

Large facial tissues to blot the skin dry after facial toning, and to protect the skin during make-up application. Also to absorb any client perspiration if this occurs during application ☐

ELLISONS

Bowls

Bowls to hold facial and make-up products and materials ☐

ELLISONS

Lined pedal bin

Lined pedal bin for waste materials ☐

Eye make-up remover

Facial skin cleansing products to suit all skin types, including eye make-up remover, cleanser and toner to prepare the skin ☐

GUINOT

Moisturiser

Moisturiser (lightweight) or **skin primer** to help make-up application and protect the skin from absorbing the make-up ☐

SORISA

Bright lighting/magnifying lamp

Bright lighting/magnifying lamp to look at the skin after cleansing to check for areas requiring attention, i.e. broken capillaries and dark eye circles – these may need concealing ☐

Make-up brushes (assorted) to apply different make-up products to the different facial areas ☐

BEAUTY EXPRESS LTD

Large face powder

Large face powder to remove excess face powder ☐

BEAUTY EXPRESS LTD

Foundation brush

Foundation brush to apply foundation ☐

BEAUTY EXPRESS LTD

Blusher brush

Blusher brush to apply powder colour to the face ☐

BEAUTY EXPRESS LTD

Small flat angle-edged eyeshadow brush

Small flat angle-edged eyeshadow brush to apply and blend powder eye make-up products in the socket area of the eye (above the eyelid) ☐

BEAUTY EXPRESS LTD

Small rounded-edged eyeshadow brush

Small rounded-edged eyeshadow brush to apply eyeshadow, blend and shade ☐

BEAUTY EXPRESS LTD

Medium firm eyeshadow blending brush

Medium firm eyeshadow blending brush to blend powder eye colours and soften harsh lines and colour ☐

BEAUTY EXPRESS LTD

Small concealer brush

Small concealer brush for exact placement of concealing product in areas such as around the nose and mouth ☐

BEAUTY EXPRESS LTD

Eyebrow brush

Eyebrow brush to remove excess make-up from the brow hair and to add colour, blend eyebrow pencil and brush the brow hair into shape ☐

BEAUTY EXPRESS LTD

Eyeliner brush

Eyeliner brush a fine brush creating a precise line used to apply make-up colour to surround the eyes ☐

BEAUTY EXPRESS LTD

Mascara wand/comb

Mascara wand/comb to apply mascara and remove excess mascara to separate the eyelashes ☐

BEAUTY EXPRESS LTD

Lip brush

Lip brush to apply lip products and ensure a definite, balanced outline to the lips ☐

Disposable applicators

Disposable applicators and brushes these are ideal to prevent cross-infection, for example eyeshadow, mascara applicators and lip brushes ☐

ELLISONS

Cosmetic sponges

Cosmetic sponges for applying foundation ☐

Make-up palette

Make-up palette for preparing and placing make-up products onto ☐

Velour puff

Velour puff to apply powder to set the foundation ☐

Pencil sharpener

Pencil sharpener for exposing a new surface, preventing cross-infection when using cosmetic pencils and to sharpen the point to achieve defined make-up effects, i.e. lining the lips ☐

ELLISONS

Small plastic spatulas Orange sticks

Small spatulas and **orange sticks** to remove make-up products from their containers ☐

ELLISONS

Brush cleaner

Brush cleaner to care for and keep brushes in a hygienic condition ☐

ELLISONS

Make-up (a range)

Make-up (a range) to suit different skin types, tones and age groups ☐

Hand mirror

Hand mirror to show the client the make-up results if a large make-up mirror is not available ☐

Foundation
Powder
Eyebrow colour
Browbone
Socket
Eyelid
Blusher
Contour
Mascara
Eyeliner
Lip liner
Lip product

Client record card

Client record card to record the client's personal details, products used and details of the service ☐

Sterilization and disinfection

It is important that good hygienic practice is considered before and throughout the client service. This will help prevent cross-infection – the transfer of harmful bacteria/microorganisms from one person to another.

All equipment should be sterilized, or disinfected using the most suitable method before use on each client.

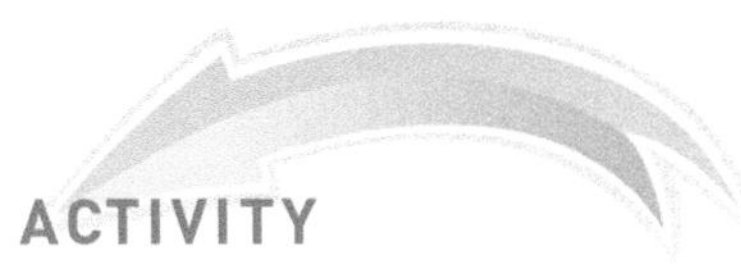

ACTIVITY

Hygiene equipment
Look at the equipment and material check list and state what method of sterilization or disinfection you would use to prevent cross-infection. Remember some items are disposable so do not include.

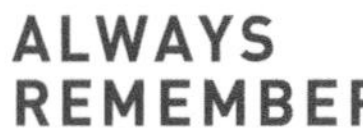
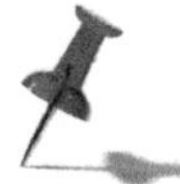

ALWAYS REMEMBER

Work area appearance
The work area should be kept clean at all times always ready for the next service to be carried out.

Hygiene checks

- ensure that all tools and equipment are clean and sterile before use
- disinfect work surface regularly
- use disposable items whenever possible. Throw away immediately after use in a covered, lined waste container
- follow hygienic practices at all times
- maintain a high standard of personal **hygiene** at all times.

HEALTH & SAFETY

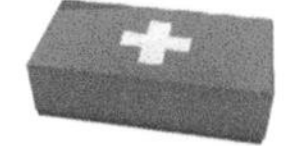

Hygiene make-up brushes
Wash brushes in warm water and mild detergent after use. Rinse in disinfecting solution, rinse and dry naturally. Once dry place in a UV cabinet ready for use.

An alcohol-based cleanser may be used to clean make-up brushes after cleaning in warm water and detergent first.

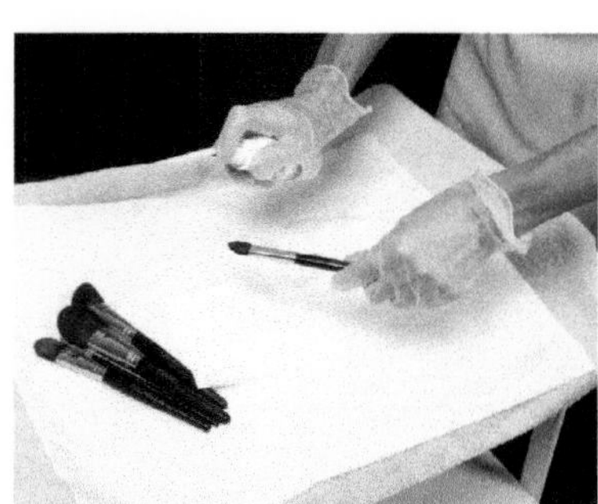

Application of a professional brush cleaner

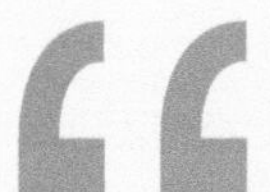

Preparing your work area
Have all products to hand and position them to allow you to work efficiently avoiding discomfort and injury to yourself.

Julia Francis

Preparation of the beauty therapist

Wash the hands to remove surface dirt preventing cross-infection, this will also show the client you have good hygiene practice. Hand gel disinfectant may be used as required.

Follow the correct **salon requirements** for hygiene and personal presentation to ensure a professional image at all times.

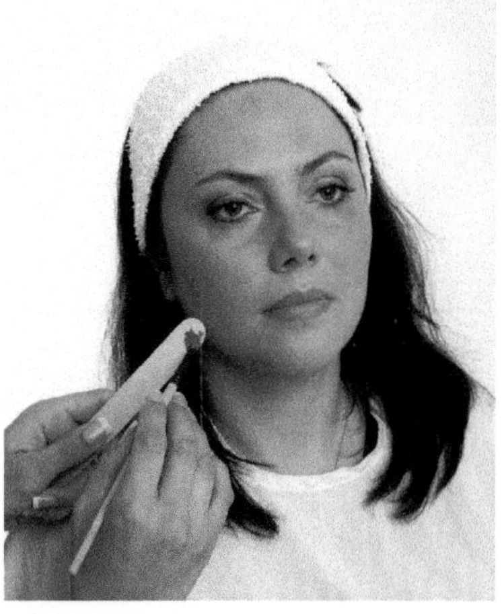

A beauty therapist applying day make-up

Preparing the work area

The make-up area should be well lit, ideally with the kind of light the make-up will be seen in so in this case natural light, **white light** as it is a day make-up.

Check the work area to make sure that you have all the equipment and materials for the make-up service. Use the checklist provided on pp. 172–176

Prepare the work couch or beauty chair following the salon policy.

ALWAYS REMEMBER

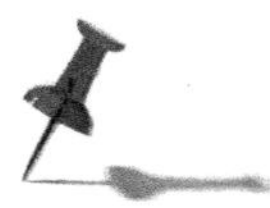

Day make-up

Make-up worn in white light (natural daylight) needs to be subtle (not too obvious) and neutral colours should be chosen as daylight intensifies colours making them appear more obvious. Fluorescent light also sharpens colours, dark colours are intensified so natural, neutral colours should be chosen. This must be considered as it may also be seen in this type of lighting.

All equipment should be placed on the trolley or work surface, in front of the make-up mirror. Good ventilation is important so that the client's skin does not become too warm. It is easier to apply make-up to cool skin and it will last longer.

Keeping the work area tidy presents a professional image and prevents time being wasted looking for products.

The work area at the end of the service should always be in a condition to provide further make-up services.

Outcome 2: Consult and prepare for make-up

Learn how to consult and prepare for make-up by:

1. Using **consultation techniques** in a polite and friendly manner to determine the client's preferences within the limits of your responsibility.
2. Ensuring that informed and signed parent/guardian consent is obtained for minors prior to any service.
3. Ensuring that a parent/guardian is present throughout the service for minors.
4. Obtaining signed, written informed consent from the client prior to carrying out the service.
5. Asking your client appropriate questions to identify if they have any **contra-indications** to day make-up.
6. Accurately recording your client's responses to questioning.
7. Encouraging clients to ask questions to clarify any points.
8. Ensuring client advice is given without reference to a specific medical condition and without causing undue alarm and concern.
9. Ensuring the client is in a comfortable and relaxed position.
10. **Preparing the client** to meet the needs of the agreed make-up plan following the senior beauty therapist's instructions.
11. Ensuring the skin is clean, toned and suitably moisturised prior to the application of make-up.
12. Accurately recognizing and recording the client's **skin type**.

(Conitnued) Learn how to consult and prepare for make-up by:

13 Referring clients with conditions that may affect the service to the senior beauty therapist.

14 Selecting suitable **make-up products** to suit the client's **skin type** and their preferences following the senior beauty therapist's instructions.

Preparing the client – the consultation

The consultation should be carried out in the privacy of the service work area. This takes place when the client first meets you at the start of the service and will take approximately 10 minutes. The consultation enables the beauty therapist to:

- Ask the client specific questions about their general health and current skincare and make-up routine. The client's answers will inform the beauty therapist what is required and what is achievable from the make-up service.
- Listen to the client to find out sufficient information to make suggestions.
- Assess whether the client is suitable for the service or whether the service is contra-indicated in some way.

TOP TIP

Consultation questioning technique

At the consultation you will be asking questions using verbal communication, speaking face-to-face with the client. Use open questions to ensure you get as much information as possible from the client, these questions start with 'who', 'what', 'when', 'where', and 'why'.

ACTIVITY

Questions to ask the client

Think of five questions you could ask the client to make sure that the make-up effect, colours and products selected suited the client.

HEALTH & SAFETY

Contra-indications referral

Never say what you think a contra-indication is, you are not qualified to know the limits of your authority. Refer the client to the senior beauty therapist who will recommend that the client sees her GP for professional advice, without causing the client any anxiety. Make a note of this on the client's records.

ACTIVITY

Day make-up application

What is the main purpose of day make-up application?

Collect examples of different looks. Remember fashion techniques, make-up products and colours can influence the required look.

Keep yourself up-to-date and knowledgeable in order to meet your clients' needs and requirements.

It is important to fully understand the effect the client wishes to achieve. Good communication is essential.

Contra-indications to service

Certain skin and eye conditions prevent you from carrying out basic day make-up service, these are known as contra-indications.

- If when looking at the client's skin and eyes before the service, you think you recognize a contra-indication basic day make-up must not be carried out. You will need to tactfully refer to the relevant person usually the senior beauty therapist for her to confirm whether the service can go ahead.

Conditions that prevent service These conditions are contagious – they can be passed on to other clients. You must never treat clients with these conditions, see

ALWAYS REMEMBER

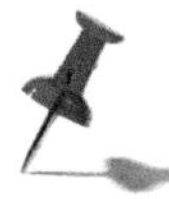

Direction from named responsible person

Know who is the person responsible for supervising you during any given task or service, or the person whom you are required to report things to. Seeking guidance means tasks are completed as to plan and things run smoothly.

pp. 146–147 for more information. However, when the condition is healed and clear such as conjunctivitis and herpes simplex the service can go ahead.

Conditions that restrict service These conditions are non-contagious – they cannot be passed on to other clients. Clients with these conditions can be treated, but you may need to adapt your make-up application. These include redness, bruising and mild skin irritation in the area which is not painful and would not cause any harm to the client. Discuss what you need to do with the senior beauty therapist, see Chapter 6 pp. 147–148.

TOP TIP

Sensitive skin

Redness and skin irritation can follow cleansing and toning procedure on sensitive skin.

Apply a calming soothing moisturiser before make-up application, the skin will become less red and irritated. Hypo-allergenic products would be best to choose.

Understand the client's make-up needs

It is essential that a make-up artist is able to create a look based on the client's needs and that the choice of products meets the client's requirements. You will need to know how long certain looks will take to create and what you need to have available in order to make them happen.

Julia Francis

During the consultation the beauty therapist can explain what is involved in the service, how long it will take and any aftercare advice to be followed.

If the client is a minor under the age of 16, it is necessary to have the parent/guardian permission for the make-up service. The parent/guardian will also have to be present when the service is received.

Discuss the make-up plan with the client to ensure that the day make-up will meet their needs. You may need to ask questions to help you:

- 'Do you normally wear make-up?'
- 'Are there any colours that you particularly like or dislike?'
- 'Are there any products you do not want applied?'

During the consultation the client will:

- discover what the beauty therapist can provide
- ask questions and receive honest professional advice concerning the most suitable make-up products to be applied and how to make the most of their features and skin appearance
- confirm and agree the service aim.

All details should be recorded accurately on the client record card before, during and following the service. A sample record card follows:

Sample client record card

Date	Beauty therapist name	
Client name	Date of birth (Identifying client age group.)	
Home address	Postcode	
Email address	Landline telephone number	Mobile telephone number
Name of doctor	Doctor's address and telephone number	
Related medical history (Conditions that may restrict or prohibit service application.)		
Are you taking any medication? (This may affect skin sensitivity.)		

CONTRA-INDICATIONS REQUIRING MEDICAL REFERRAL
(Preventing the application of make-up.)

- ☐ bacterial infections (e.g. impetigo, conjunctivitis)
- ☐ viral infections (e.g. herpes simplex)
- ☐ fungal infections (e.g. tinea corporis)
- ☐ parasitic infestations (e.g. pediculosis and scabies)

SKIN TYPE
☐ oily ☐ dry ☐ combination

CONCEALER
☐ cream ☐ stick ☐ liquid

FOUNDATION
☐ liquid ☐ compact
☐ stick ☐ cream
☐ mineral ☐ tinted moisturiser

POWDER
☐ loose ☐ compact ☐ mineral

BRONZING PRODUCTS
☐ powder ☐ gel ☐ liquid

EYE PRODUCTS FOR EYE AREA
☐ cream eyeshadow ☐ liquid eyeliner
☐ pencil eyeliner ☐ powder eyeshadow
☐ kohl eyeliner ☐ mineral and pigment eyeshadows
☐ cake eyeliner ☐ gel eyeshadow

EYE PRODUCTS FOR EYEBROW AREA
☐ pencil ☐ liquid
☐ shadow ☐ eyebrow mascara

EYE PRODUCTS FOR EYELASHES
☐ waterproof mascara ☐ non-waterproof mascara

CONTRA-INDICATIONS WHICH RESTRICT SERVICE
(Service may require adaptation.)

☐ cuts and abrasions ☐ bruising and swelling
☐ recent scar tissue ☐ eczema
☐ skin allergies ☐ vitiligo
☐ styes ☐ hyper keratosis
☐ watery eyes

MAKE-UP CONTEXT
☐ day

CHEEK PRODUCTS
☐ highlighter ☐ shader
☐ blusher

LIP PRODUCTS
☐ pencil lip liner ☐ lip gloss
☐ lipstick ☐ lip balm

Foundation
Powder
Eyebrow colour
Browbone
Socket
Eyelid
Blusher
Contour
Mascara
Eyeliner
Lip liner
Lip product

Record of make-up products applied

Beauty therapist signature (for reference)
Client signature (confirmation of details)

Sample client record card (continued)

SERVICE ADVICE

Make-up service – allow 30 minutes

SERVICE PLAN

Record details of your service and advice given for future reference.

Ensure the client's records are up-to-date, accurate and fully completed following service. Non-compliance may invalidate insurance.

DURING

Find out:

- what products the client is currently using to cleanse and care for the skin of the face and neck

Discuss:

- the importance of a good skincare routine for good make-up application
- how satisfied the client is with their current make-up look
- tips and explain each stage of the make-up application to ensure client understanding

Note:

- any contra-action (unwanted reaction), if any occurs

AFTER

Record:

- what skincare products have been used
- what products have been used in the make-up service
- how and where the make-up products have been applied
- any samples provided (check their success at the next appointment)

Advise on:

- how to reapply products to achieve/maintain (keep) the make-up look
- correct make-up removal

RETAIL OPPORTUNITIES

Advise on:

- products that would be suitable for the client to use at home to care for their skin
- the benefits of each make-up product during application
- recommendations for further make-up services
- further products or services that the client may or may not have received before

Note:

- any purchase made by the client

EVALUATION

Record:

- comments on the client's satisfaction with the service
- if poor results are achieved, the reasons why

HEALTH AND SAFETY

Advise on:

- avoiding activities or products that may cause a contra-action
- correct necessary action to be taken in the event of an unwanted skin reaction

The record card should be signed and dated following the consultation to confirm the suitability and agreement to the make-up service.

At the end of the consultation the client should fully understand what the make-up service involves.

Check with the senior beauty therapist that your make-up plan meets their satisfaction.

Clean your hands using an approved hand-cleansing technique in front of your client who will see that you are hygienic in your work.

Preparing the client

Ask the client to remove jewellery from the service area, to prevent it becoming soiled by skincare and make-up products and to avoid interference with application, i.e. necklaces and facial piercings. It may be necessary to remove contact lenses. Follow your workplace policy regarding handling and storage of client jewellery when removed.

The client needs only to remove their upper outer clothing, usually to their underwear. Offer the client a gown or place a clean towel or make-up cape across their chest and shoulders. A headband or hair clip should be used to keep hair away from the face.

Position the client in a comfortable and relaxed position for the make-up service.

Check that the client is comfortable. The client's back and neck should be adequately supported.

After preparing the client and before touching the skin, clean your hands again.

Now cleanse and tone the skin using products appropriate to their skin type and condition. The cleansing routine is found in Chapter 6 on pp. 153–155 and moisturiser application on p. 158.

ALWAYS REMEMBER

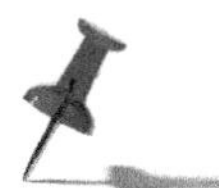

Posture

Check that the client is positioned at the correct height for you to work without straining which could lead to muscle injury and long-term postural problems. You need to be able to apply the make-up with the least possible effort.

BEST PRACTICE

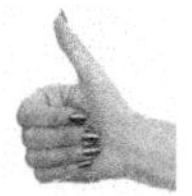

Thoroughly remove existing make-up

Do not be careless in make-up removal. Remove thoroughly, stubborn make-up using the correct products without irritating the skin. You are not competent if old make-up remains before applying new make-up. However, remember make-up can be permanently applied by a tattooing process, i.e. eyeliner and lip liner so check this with your client at consultation.

Avoid too much pressure and stimulation of the skin when cleansing and preparing the skin for make-up application. The skin will become too warm causing the skin to redden which will require correction and the make-up will not last.

Inspect the skin using a magnifying light if necessary when cleansed, this will show any areas that you may need to disguise.

HEALTH & SAFETY

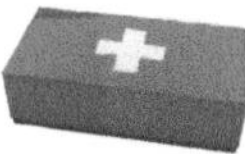

Client records

It is important that accurate records are kept and stored to meet the requirements of the Data Protection Act (1998) and referenced at each service.

HEALTH & SAFETY

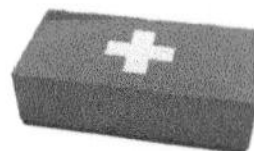

Washings hands

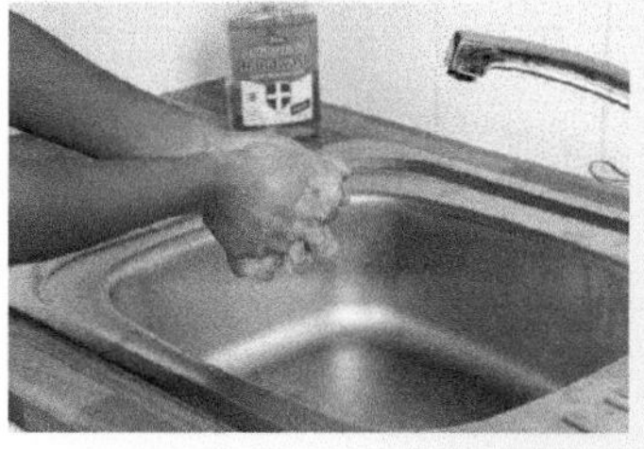

Remember when washing hands, follow Habia recommended guidelines shown in Chapter 2, pp. 27–28.

ACTIVITY

Cleansing preparations

When preparing the skin for make-up, what cleanser and toner would you choose for the following skin types?

- oily
- dry
- combination
- sensitive.

Be calm under pressure

Always remain calm and professional even in situations where you are running out of time. An employable make-up artist is always a calm make-up artist.

Julia Francis

ALWAYS REMEMBER

Areas that may require to be disguised.

This will be achieved using a concealer or foundation make-up product.

Broken capillaries, often found on sensitive skin	ISTOCKPHOTO/EKSPANSIO
Pustules inflamed spot with a yellow centre indicating infection If excessive this will contra-indicate make-up i.e. sebaceous gland disorder acne vulgaris p. 36	MARK LEES, SKINCARE, INC
Papules inflamed spot which is red and hard and may become infected	LORRAINE NORDMANN Papule present on the forehead LORRAINE NORDMANN Concealer is applied to disguise the papule
Dark circles	LORRAINE NORDMANN Concealer is applied to disguise dark circles under the eyes
Areas of lighter skin colouring called **hypo-pigmentation**	
Areas of darker skin colouring called **hyper-pigmentation**	MURAD MEDICAL GROUP

Finally apply a light textured moisturiser or a skin **primer**, this has the following benefits:

- it prevents the natural secretions of the skin, i.e. oil and sweat changing the colour of the foundation
- it forms a barrier between the skin and the make-up preventing the skin from absorbing the make-up which can cause the pores to clog
- it makes it easier to apply the make-up to the skin's surface.

Record the skincare products used on the record card.

Make-up is then applied in a specific order so that:

- products are applied correctly – the rule is cream on cream, powder on powder
- the client understands how and when the make-up products are applied
- a balanced look is created – your features are not all the same size so some correction may be required.

Basic day make-up procedure

The stages in the basic day make-up service procedure are:

1. conceal any blemishes
2. apply foundation
3. apply powder
4. apply blusher
5. apply eye products
6. apply lip products.

Outcome 3: Apply day make-up

Learn how to apply day make-up by:
1 Using make-up products correctly and following senior beauty therapists' and manufacturers' instructions.
2 Applying any necessary foundation and concealer to create an even skin tone.
3 Applying a suitable powder to achieve the desired finish.
4 Applying eye products to enhance the eye area, eyebrows and eyelashes.
5 Applying cheek products to enhance the client's natural colouring.
6 Applying lip products to enhance the client's lips.
7 Ensuring that the finished result and look is to the client's and senior beauty therapist's satisfaction.

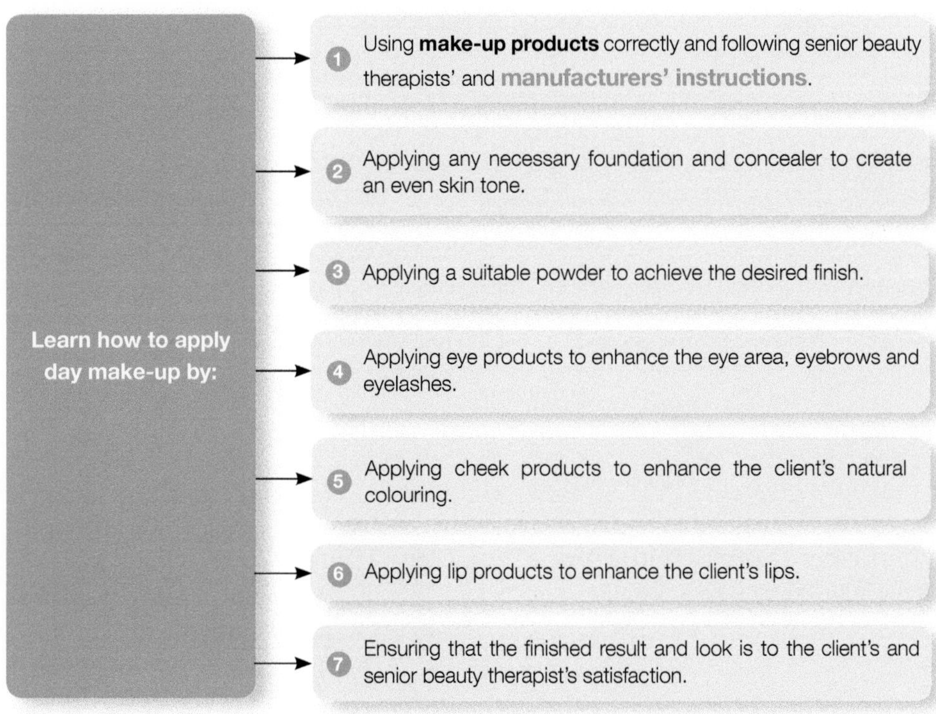

TOP TIP

If the client has a very oily skin, oil control lotions can be applied containing powder which absorbs the skin's natural oil, reducing shine.

TOP TIP

Creating balance in the face

The lips below are uneven so to correct and achieve a balanced (even) look, a lip liner is used to draw a new line and lip colour applied to achieve balance and to make the lips even.

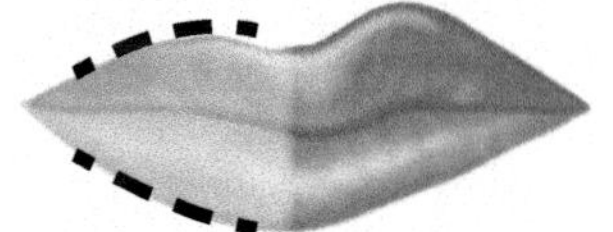

Uneven lips

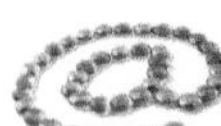

COURSEMATE

For a video on selecting and applying foundation, see this book's accompanying CourseMate.

ACTIVITY

Body language

Remember non-verbal communication – communicating using the body including the eyes called body language.

During the make-up application give examples of how you could tell if the client was not happy with the make-up look being achieved by their **body language**.

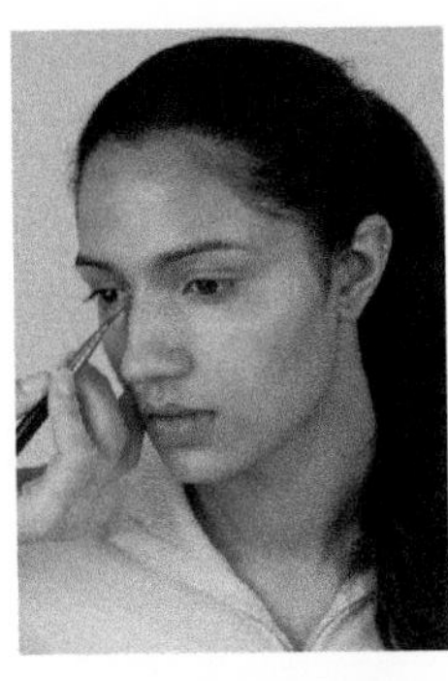
Concealer application

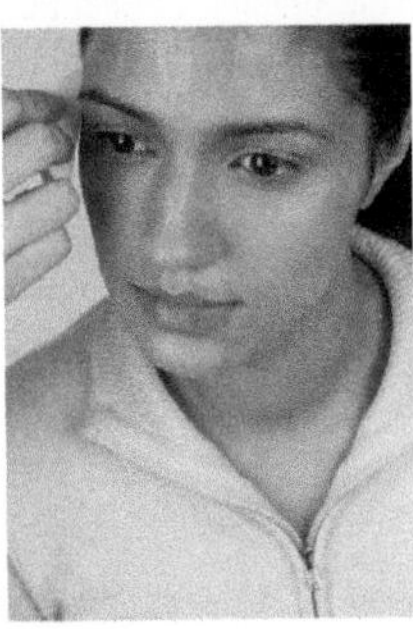
Foundation application

Concealer Apply concealer to:

- disguise imperfections such as blemishes, dark circles under they eyes, uneven skin colour, achieving a more even skin tone.

Select the concealer colour to suit and correct the skin tone and the facial area to which it is to be applied.
Apply with a make-up brush or sponge and blend to match the skin.

Available in a range of consistencies, i.e. liquid/cream, which affects the coverage which can be achieved. This may be used before or after foundation application.

Our client has had concealer applied to disguise dark circles under the eyes.

Foundation Apply foundation to:

- produce an even skin tone
- disguise small skin blemishes.

Test the colour on the jawline to obtain the correct colour.

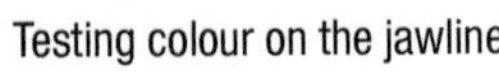
Testing colour on the jawline

Mix colours together to obtain the correct tone to suit the skin if necessary and immediately follow with the test colour.

Apply using a foundation brush or sponge. The foundation should be blended without disturbing any concealer that you may have applied underneath. Blend carefully including at the jawline and the hairline.

Available in cream, liquid, compact stick, gel, cake, mousse, mineral base and tinted moisturiser formulations.

TOP TIP

Mineral powder is applied to provide an even skin tone and achieve the effects of foundation so may be applied as an alternative.

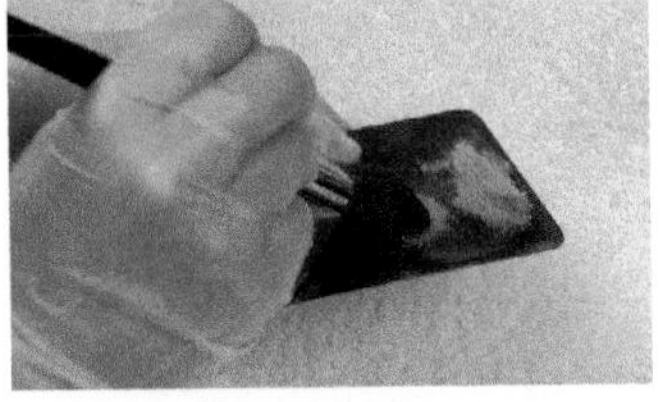
Mineral powder placed on a palette before application

Powder Apply powder to:

- set the foundation
- disguise small skin blemishes, the pores can appear smaller after application
- provide a base to help the application of further powder products such as powder blusher
- absorb the skin's oil and perspiration making the make-up last longer.

Apply loose powder to the skin using a clean piece of cotton wool or velour puff. Brush off excess loose powder with a powder brush. Brush in upwards and downwards strokes over the face.

Available in loose and powder compact formulations.

Our client has loose powder applied to set the foundation helping the look to last longer.

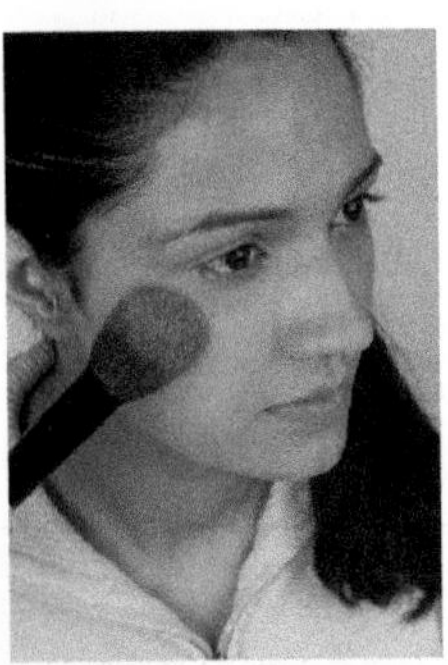
Powder application

ALWAYS REMEMBER

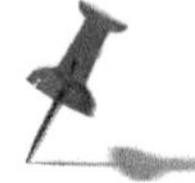

Powder compact is used and can be recommended to the client to remove shine from the skin during the day. They provide a heavier coverage.

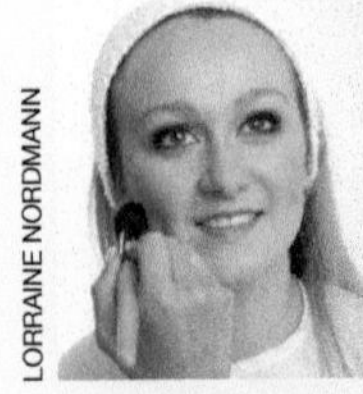
LORRAINE NORDMANN

Applying bronzing product
Bronzing powders are popular powder products applied to create a healthy, tanned appearance to the skin.

Blusher Apply blusher to:

- add colour to the face
- draw attention to the cheekbones
- alter the appearance of the face shape when applied in the cheek area.

If a powder blusher is used apply after face powder with a blusher brush.

If cream or liquid is used apply after foundation with a sponge.

Available in powder, cream and liquid formulations.

Our client has powder blusher applied.

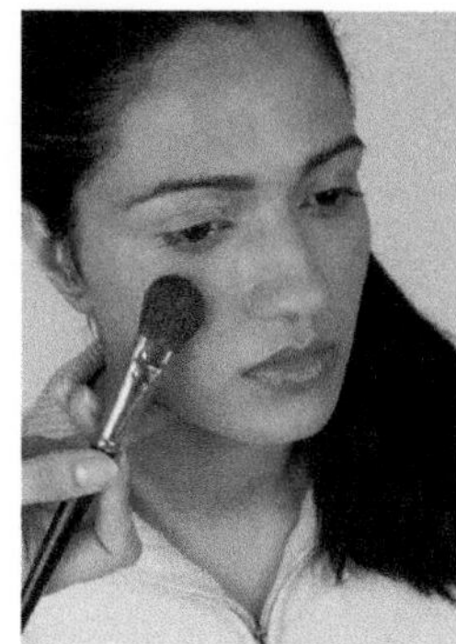

Powder blusher application

Eye products Apply eye products to:

- emphasize – draw attention to the eyes and their shape
- alter the shape and appearance of the eyes
- lengthen the eyelashes
- make sparse eyebrows appear fuller and define their shape.

Eye products include **eyeshadow**, **eyeliner**, **eyebrow colour** and **mascara**.

Complementary colours shown are chosen in a purple range applied to the eyelid. Light purple on the lid and a darker shade in the socket, this is called **shading**. A lighter ivory shade is applied to the eyebrow bone drawing attention to it, this is called **highlighting**.

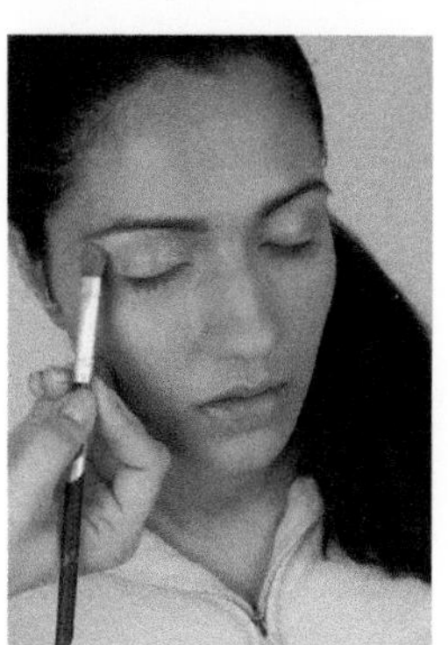

Eyeshadow is applied to emphasize the eye area, the colour is chosen here to match the client's clothing

Sponge applicators and brushes apply eye make-up products and are selected according to the type of product being applied.

Available in powder, liquid, cream, wax and crayon formulations.

Our client has powder products applied to the eye, a highlighter is used on the brow bone area.

ALWAYS REMEMBER

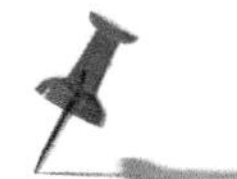

Waterproof mascara

A waterproof formulation is available which means it can withstand the eyes watering and will stay in place. A special eye make-up remover is required to remove this thoroughly.

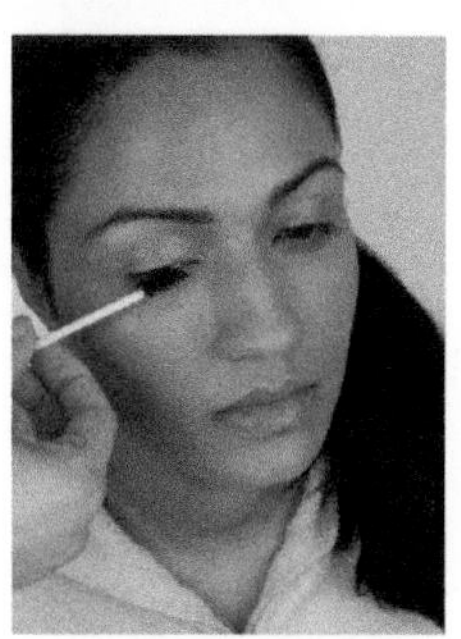

The upper and lower eyelashes are lengthened and made darker using a black mascara

A brush is used to apply the mascara.

Available in liquid, cream and block formulations.

Our client has liquid, lash lengthening mascara applied.

Apply colour shaping the natural brow hair using colour with a stiff small-angled brush and eyebrow brush.

Available in powder, pencil, liquid, mascara and wax formulations.

Our client has powder shadow applied.

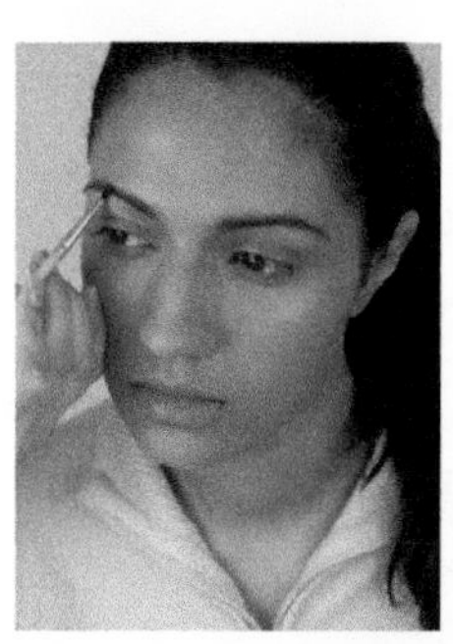

The appearance of the eyebrows is made stronger and thicker by filling in any gaps with a colour

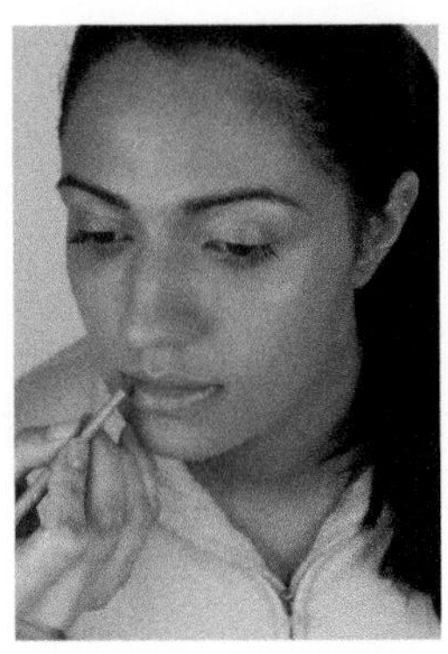
The lips are lined to the required shape in a colour to match the lipstick and suit the eyeshadow colours

Lip products Apply lip products to:

- emphasize – draw attention to the lips and their shape
- Alter the shape and appearance of the natural lips.

Lip products include **lip liner, lipstick, lip stain, lip balm** and **lip gloss.**

Outline the lips by using a sharpened lip pencil or lip liner brush using lipstick product.

Apply lip product by using a lip brush.

Our client has her lips outlined with pencil and then a lipstick applied with a non-glossy, matt formulation.

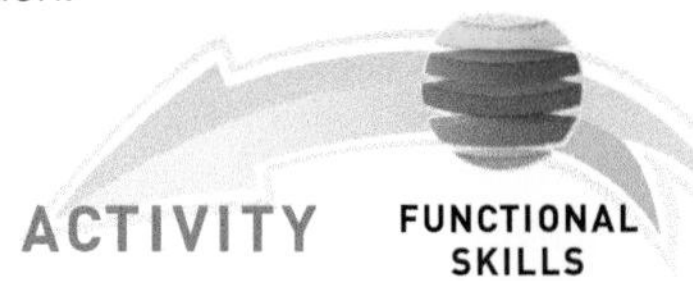

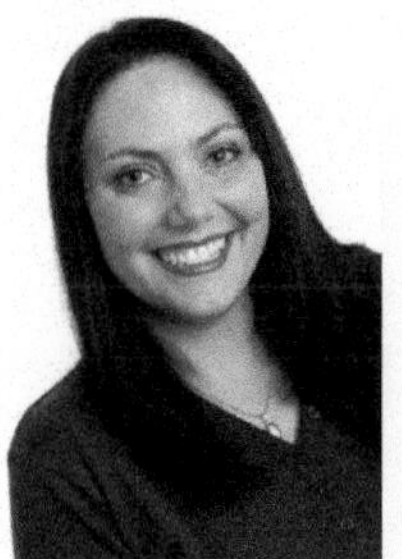
Make-up look

Day make-up look
Write down how the above day make-up look was created.
Alternatively collect images yourself and explain:
What color and make-up products have been used and how they have been applied to achieve each final look?

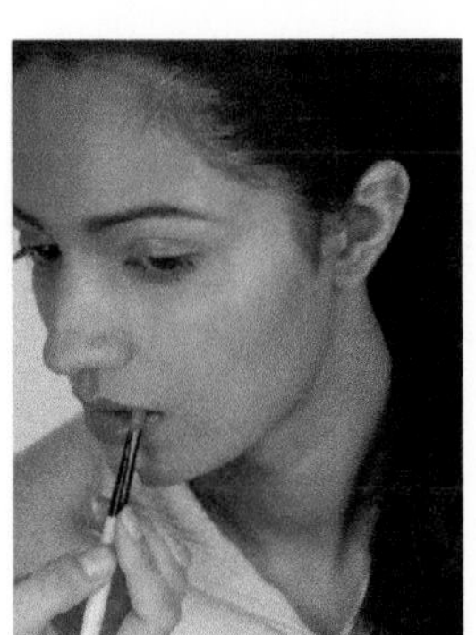
The chosen lipstick is applied

When you have finished ... Fix the client's hair and then discuss the final make-up look in front of the mirror. Explain again how each product has been applied to create the final result.

Check that the final look is to the client's and senior beauty therapist's satisfaction and meets the agreed service plan.

Make sure that the client's records are updated at the end of the service. This is important and you may need to refer to them in the future. The record card should then be stored securely.

The client should be given advice so that the make-up look can be maintained for the rest of the day and she knows how to remove it correctly.

At the end of the make-up service the work area should be in a good state ready for further make-up services. Waste should be disposed of in accordance with waste disposal legislation and workplace policy.

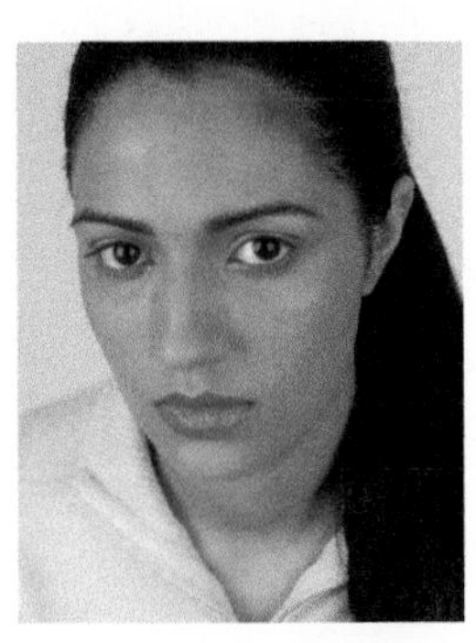
The final day make-up look

COURSEMATE
For a video on day make-up, please see this book's accompanying CourseMate.

Outcome 4: Provide aftercare advice

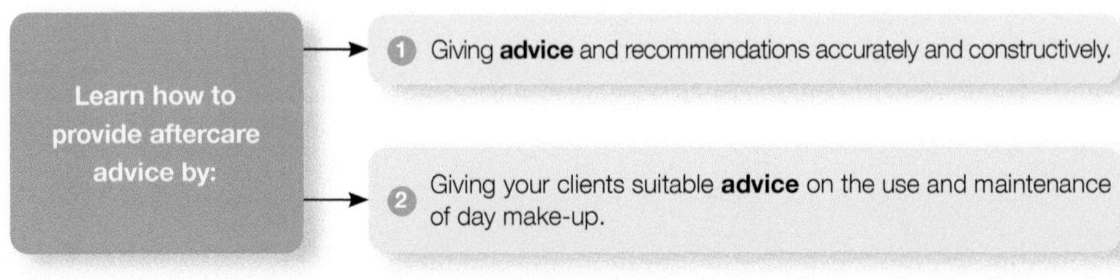

> **Clean your brushes**
> Always work with clean brushes and a clean make-up. Never use the same brushes on more than one person and always maintain high levels of health and hygiene standards.
>
> **Julia Francis**

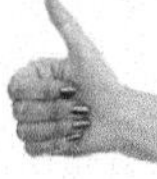

BEST PRACTICE

Make-up chart
Provide the client with a make-up chart which illustrates what make-up products you have applied and where on the face to achieve the result.

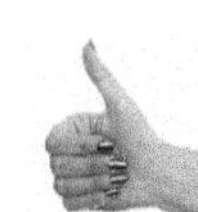

BEST PRACTICE

Share tips
Tell the client how they can get the best result out of any products purchased.

Basic home-care advice

- Advise the client on the skincare preparations and make-up products she can use at home.
- Make-up maintenance – advise the client on application procedures to maintain the basic day make-up effect: use of pressed powder to remove shine; lip liner to keep lip colour in place; re-application of blusher to add warmth.
- Eye cleansing: cleanse the eye by using a recommended eye make-up remover. Support the outer corner of the eye with one hand to avoid stretching the skin. Remove waterproof mascara with an oily eye make-up remover.
- Skin cleansing advice: apply cleansing preparations to remove facial make-up with the recommended cleanser type in an upwards and outwards direction.

  Remove according to manufacturer's instructions.
- Apply the recommended toner according to manufacturer's instructions to re-move excess cleanser.
- Skin moisturising: apply day or night moisturiser dependent upon when the make-up is removed. Apply in small dots to the neck, chin, cheeks, nose and forehead. Spread quickly a thin film over the face, using light upward, outward stroking movements. Blot the skin with a soft facial tissue to remove excess moisturiser.

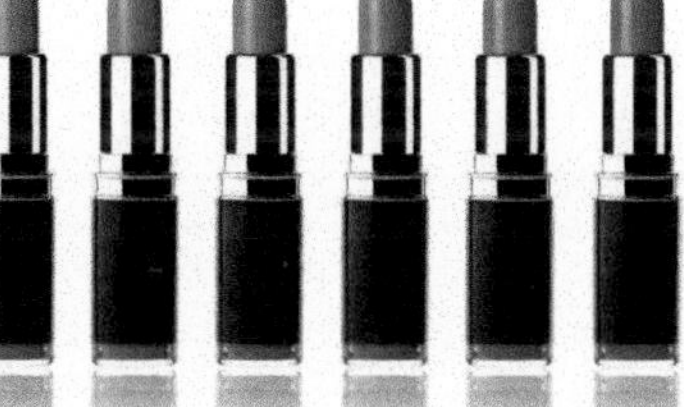

Retail make-up product such as lipstick which can be purchased following ap-plication - useful for the client to maintain their make-up look

Promoting products

Providing advice gives you the opportunity to recommend related retail products. Have products and equipment available to use that you have used, i.e. skincare preparations, make-up and make-up brushes.

Explain what action to take in the event of a **contra-action**. This may occur during or following service.

Contra-actions

Contra-actions include:

- An allergy, recognized by redness, swelling and inflammation.

  If this occurs remove product from the skin, apply a soothing lotion. The product should not be used again.
- Watery eyes, if the client's eyes continuously water during make-up application, remove make-up and stop the service.

- Excessive perspiration, some clients may perspire which will affect the make-up application and the result. Blot the skin dry with a facial tissue and apply more loose powder to absorb perspiration. If this continues stop the service.
- Ask clients to contact the salon immediately and speak with the senior beauty therapist if any unwanted reaction occurs following the service.
- Record any contra-action and action taken, advice recommended on the client record card.

GLOSSARY OF KEY WORDS

Aftercare advice recommended advice given to the client following the service to continue the benefits of the service.

Assistance providing help and support.

Blusher make-up product applied to add warmth to the face and draw attention to the cheekbones.

Body language communication involving the body.

Cleanser a skincare preparation that removes dead skin cells, excess sweat and oil (sebum), make-up and dirt from the skin's surface to maintain a healthy skin appearance.

Communication the exchange of information and understanding between people.

Concealer make-up product used to disguise small skin imperfections such as blemishes, uneven skin colour and dark circles under the eyes.

Consultation assessment of the client's needs using different assessment techniques including questioning and visual inspection of the service area.

Contra-action an unwanted reaction occurring during or after service application.

Contra-indication a condition present that means the service may not go ahead or may require it to be adapted in some way.

Equipment tools used within make-up service.

Eyeshadow make-up applied to the eye to suit the natural eye colour, and enhance the eyes.

Eyebrow colour make-up applied to emphasize the eyebrows, it can make the eyebrows look stronger and thicker by filling in any gaps with colour.

Eyeliner make-up applied to outline and emphasize the eye area.

Foundation make-up product applied to produce an even skin tone, to disguise small blemishes.

Hygiene the recommended cleanliness necessary in the workplace to prevent cross-infection and secondary infection. The standard expected, as laid down in law, industry codes of practice or written workplace procedures.

Hyper-pigmentation increased or darker skin colouring in an area.

Hypo-pigmentation loss of colouring in an area.

Limits of your authority your level of responsibility as written in your own job description and workplace policies.

Lip balm a lip moisturiser which may contain colour.

Lip gloss make-up applied to the lips to provide a moist, shiny look.

Lip liner make-up used to outline the lip shape creating a balanced shape to suit the face.

Lip stain make-up product which adds intense colour to the lips.

Lipstick make-up applied to the lips to add colour and keep the lips in good condition.

Make-up cosmetics applied to enhance the skin of the face and features and create balance to the face.

Make-up occasion the event the make-up is to be applied for, i.e. day, evening, special occasion.

Make-up products different cosmetics available to suit skin type, colour and condition, i.e. sensitive, oily, mature. Make-up products include concealer, foundation, powder, blusher, eye products and lip products.

Manufacturers' instructions guidance issued by manufacturers or suppliers of products or equipment, concerning their safe and efficient use.

Mascara make-up that enhances the natural eyelashes making them appear longer, changed in colour and/or thicker.

Mineral make-up make-up created from finely ground minerals which are used in different make-up products.

Moisturiser a skincare preparation (formulation of oil and water) that helps maintain the skin's natural moisture by locking moisture into the skin, giving protection and hydration.

Opportunity a situation that makes it possible to do something that you have to do or want to do.

Organizational requirements beauty therapy procedures or work rules provided by the workplace management.

Personal appearance expected standards of workplace appearance.

Powder make-up applied to set the foundation, disguise minor skin blemishes and make the skin look smoother and oil free. Powder may also hold colour such as powder eyeshadow and blusher.

Primer provides a base for make-up and acts as a barrier preventing the absorption of the products into the skin.

Relevant person an individual responsible for supervizing you during a given task or service, or the person whom you are required to report things to.

Salon requirements any salon procedures or work rules issued by the workplace management.

Skin analysis assessment of the client's skin type and condition.

Skin tone the strength and elasticity of the skin.

Skin type the different way each skin functions provides their skin type. Skin types include dry (lacking in oil), oily (too much oil) and combination (a mixture of the two skin types).

Toning lotion a skincare preparation to remove all traces of cleanser from the skin. It has a cooling and tightening effect on the skin.

Verbal communication occurs when you talk directly to another person either face-to-face, directly or indirectly, over the telephone.

ASSESSMENT OF KNOWLEDGE AND UNDERSTANDING

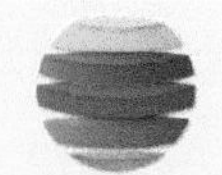

FUNCTIONAL SKILLS

Having covered the learning objectives for **Assist with day make-up** answer the following short questions below.

The information covers:

- organizational and legal requirements
- how to work safely and effectively when providing day make-up
- consultation and service planning
- anatomy and physiology
- contra-indications and contra-actions
- make-up application
- aftercare advice for clients.

Organizational and legal requirements

1. What information will need to be recorded on the client's record card before, during and following a day make-up service?
2. What is your salon pricing structure for a basic day make-up? Why is it important to know the different prices of services in the salon?
3. How long should you allow when booking a basic day make-up? Why is it important to complete this service in the time allowed?
4. What environmental conditions should be checked for suitability of make-up service?

How to work safely and effectively when providing day make-up

1. Why is it important to identify the client's skin type at consultation before skin cleansing, toning, moisturising and make-up application?
2. If you identified during the skin consultation a skin condition that may prevent or restrict make-up application, who would you refer this to?
3. Give **four** examples of good hygiene practice that will prevent cross-infections during make-up application.
4. How is the client's skin prepared for make-up application?

Consultation and service planning

1. What type of questions would you need to ask if you needed to get more information from a client when carrying out the consultation?
2. Why should you record the answers on the record card to questions that you ask the client?
3. What is body language and why must this be observed? How could you recognize if a client was nervous through their body language who has not received the service before? How could you reassure her in the way you carry out the service and check her satisfaction throughout the service?
4. All clients are different, how can your consultation technique questioning, looking at the client's skin tone, facial features, hair colouring and previous client service records, help you plan the make-up service?

Anatomy and physiology

1. List **four** things that would help you identify the skin types listed below:
   - oily
   - dry
   - combination.

2 Find out how the following skin conditions can be recognized when looking at the skin and what causes them:
- sensitive
- comedone
- milia
- dehydrated
- broken capillaries
- pustules
- papules
- open pores
- dark circles.

3 How do the following structures in the dermis affect the surface appearance of the skin:
- sebaceous (oil) gland
- sweat gland
- blood capillary.

Contra-indications and contra-actions

1 Name **three** contra-indications to make-up service.

2 Bruising, redness and skin irritation restrict make-up application. What does 'restrict' mean and how would you adapt your make-up application for each of these conditions?

3 Give **two** examples of possible contra-actions that may occur during the make-up service and the correct action you would take.

Make-up application

1 Research the different types of powder, foundation, eye products, cheek products and lip products that would be suitable for a teenage skin with a few 'spots' – pustules and papules and a mature, dry skin with high colouring 'redness'.

2 Look for an image of a teenage person and a mature person without make-up on. On the charts provided design a make-up plan for each person and record what products you would use to achieve the look.

You may carry out this practical task on a real person taking a picture before and after your make-up application.

On the charts below show what products you would use and design a make-up plan for each client.

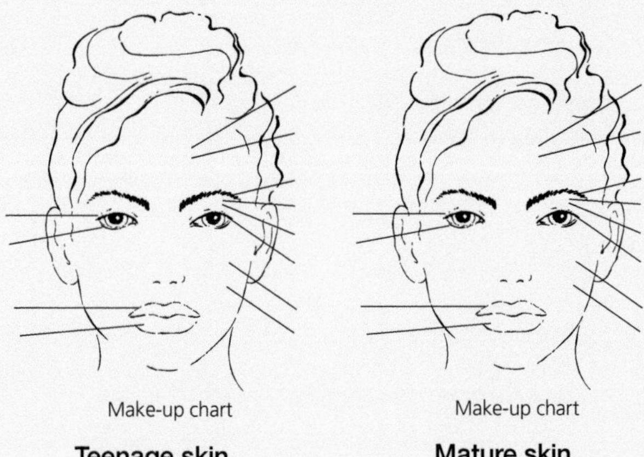

Teenage skin **Mature skin**

3 Why is make-up applied in a particular order or sequence?

4 How can minor imperfections be disguised with make-up?

5 What products would you use for this and give examples of how you would disguise **two** different imperfections explaining the product you would use and how it would be applied.

Aftercare advice for clients

1 What make-up products would you recommend for the client to use to maintain the appearance of the make-up following a basic day make-up application?

2 Why is it important to explain to a client the action to take if she had a contra-action following the make-up service? Give an example of a possible contra-action and the action to be taken by the client.

3 What make-up removal advice should be given to a client following the service?

4 What is the benefit of providing the client with written instructions on the make-up and skincare used following the make-up service?

8 Nail services

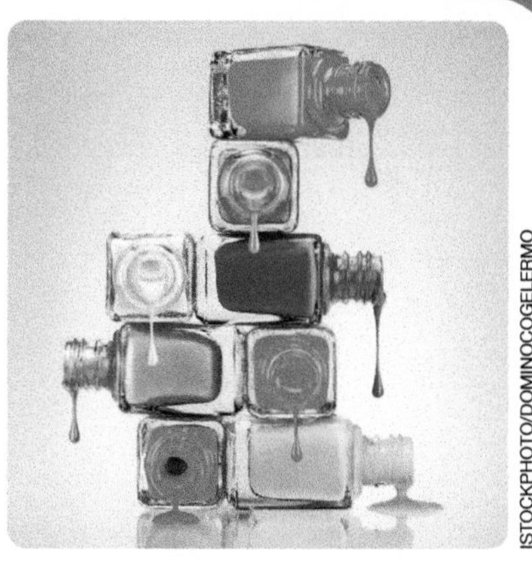
ISTOCKPHOTO/DOMINOCOGELERMO

Learning Objectives

This chapter covers the **Assist with nail services** unit.

This unit is all about the skills you will need to assist with nail services in the workplace.

There are **four** learning outcomes which you must achieve competently:

1. **Maintain safe and effective methods when assisting with nail services**
2. **Consult, plan and prepare for nail services with clients**
3. **Carry out nail services**
4. **Provide aftercare advice**

Your assessor will observe your performance on **at least three occasions** one of which will be performed on the feet.

From the **range** statement, you must show that you have:

- used all **consultation techniques**
- applied three of the four **nail finishes***
- given all types of **advice**.

*However, you must prove to your assessor that you have the necessary knowledge, understanding and skills to be able to perform competently in respect of all the items in this range.

When providing nail services it is important to use the skills you have learnt in the following units:

Health and Safety

Developing positive working relationships

Preparing and maintaining the salon treatment work area

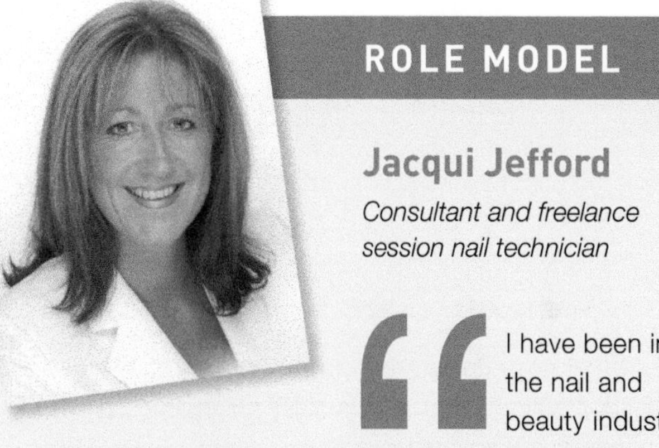

ROLE MODEL

Jacqui Jefford

Consultant and freelance session nail technician

"I have been in the nail and beauty industry for over 25 years, and I am one of the leading figures in the industry in the UK and internationally. My work has taken me to many countries as a consultant, educational advisor and presenter in competition work (winning, designing and judging them) and working in Marketing, TV and with the press. I also have my salon, school and delivery company and work with many colleges as a tutor, assessor and internal verifier. I have particularly enjoyed working at London and Paris Fashion Weeks as well as decorating the covers of top magazines such as Vogue. I have written four successful books and been involved in five DVDs. My passion has always been good education and I have worked alongside Habia on many projects over the last 10 years.

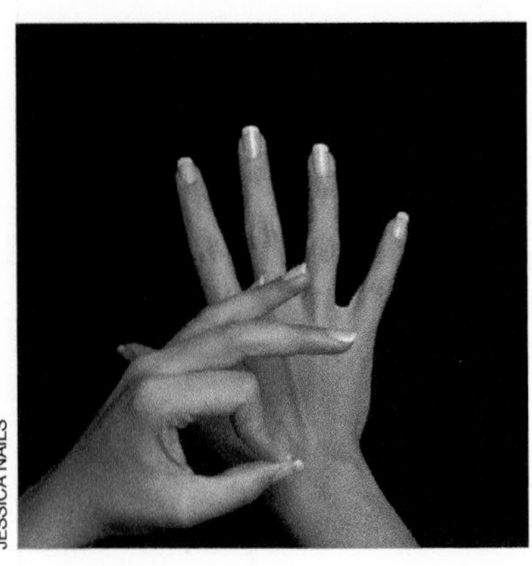

JESSICA NAILS

Healthy hands, healthy nails

Practical skills, knowledge and understanding

The table shown here will help you to check your progress in gaining the necessary practical skills, knowledge and understanding for **nail services**.

Tick (✓), when you feel you have gained the practical skills, knowledge and understanding in each of the following areas:

	Practical skills, knowledge and understanding checklist	✓
1	The aim of a basic nail service.	
2	Contra-indications that prevent or restrict a nail service.	
3	Equipment and materials needed.	
4	How to prepare the nail service area.	
5	How to prepare yourself before the nail service.	
6	Client consultation to decide what the nail service will include.	
7	How to prepare the client for the service.	
8	How to carry out the basic nail service to the hands and feet.	
9	Aftercare and advice to be given to the client following the nail service.	
10	Contra-actions (unwanted reaction) to look for during or following the nail service.	

> Never stop learning. Education is the key to knowledge. Knowledge is power.
>
> **Jacqui Jefford**

When you have ticked all the areas you can, ask your assessor to assess you on **Nail services**. After practical assessment, your assessor might decide that you still need to practice further to improve your skills. If so, your assessor will tell you how and where you need to improve to gain competence.

After assessment of your understanding there may be knowledge gaps that require you to study further. Your assessor will tell you what you need to study to achieve the required level of knowledge and understanding.

ALWAYS REMEMBER

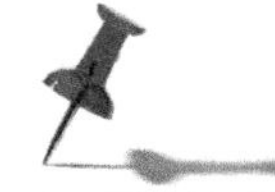

The skin

You need to have a knowledge of the basic structure of the skin. Refer to p. 127 Anatomy and physiology of the skin to learn more about its structure and function.

Basic nail services

Basic **nail** services aim to improve the instant appearance or look of the hands or feet by treating the:

- skin
- **cuticles**
- nails.

The skin

Healthy hands have soft, smooth skin. Wear and tear, or neglect, where the skin is not cared for can make the skin become dry, chapped, irritated, rough and even broken.

Healthy feet do not have a build-up of hard dry skin which may eventually crack which is uncomfortable and may lead to infection.

When carrying out a basic nail service, your aim is to maintain (keep) or return the skin, nails and cuticles to a healthy condition and appearance. This might take more than one service and you will need to advise the client on how to care for the hands and feet at home; this is called aftercare and advice.

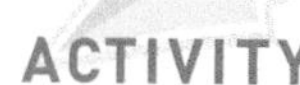

ACTIVITY

Healthy nails and skin

Find images for the hands and feet that show healthy, cared for skin, nails and cuticles.

Then look for images that show where the skin has become less healthy. Look for images of, for example, dry, chapped and irritated skin. This will help you to recognize the needs of the skin and nails, choose products and advise clients about products they could use at home to care for their hands and feet.

The cuticles

The cuticle is the part of the skin found around the base of the nail. When in a good condition, the cuticle is soft and loose (not tight). However, it can easily become tight, dry, split and overgrown at the base of the nail.

When carrying out the basic nail service, your aim is to soften and moisturise the cuticles. **Aftercare advice** must always be given so that clients know how to care for the cuticles themselves.

The cuticle is shown in more detail on pp. 196–197

The nails

The nails should be smooth, supple and have a healthy pink appearance. The edge that is filed (the **free edge**) should be even in shape. The nails of the hands can be shaped to suit the nail/hand shape or preference (client choice).

The nails of the feet are best kept short, cut neatly straight across as shaping can lead to a painful nail disorder called ingrowing nails see p. 213. The nails can lose their healthy pink colour and become ridged, pitted, brittle and bruised, and the free edge on the nails of the hand is easily split and broken. This can occur through poor health, lifestyle, effects of medication taken and neglect.

When carrying out the basic nail service, your aim is to maintain or improve the healthy pink colour of the nail, improve the smoothness and suppleness or flexibility of the nail and file the free edge to a suitable even shape and length.

Aftercare advice must always be given so that clients know how to care for the nails themselves.

You need to know about the different parts of the nail if you are to be able to improve its appearance, care properly for the nail and recognize an unhealthy nail that may require referral to a senior therapist.

The different parts are discussed on pp. 196–197.

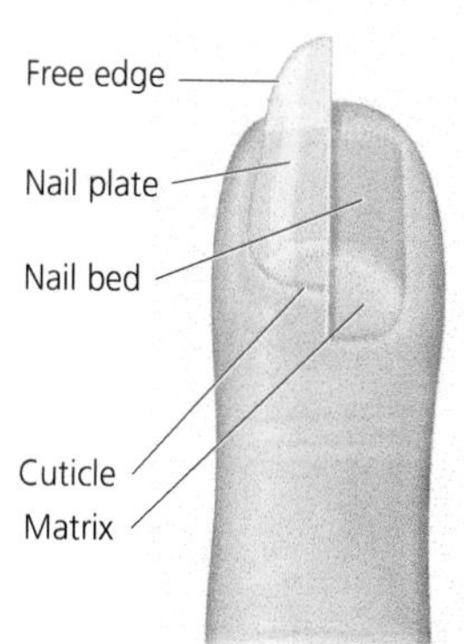

Parts of the nail

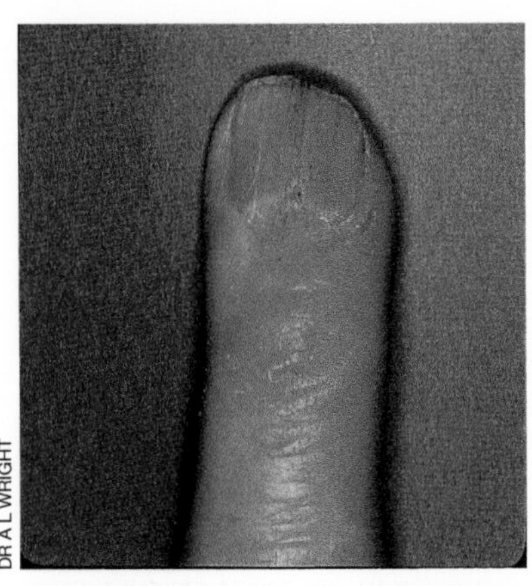

A nail showing ridges in the nail plate due to damage to the matrix

Anatomy and physiology

Nail parts and functions

The basic nail unit Nails grow from the ends of the fingers and toes and their main purpose is to form a hard protective shield. When healthy the nails appear a pink colour with a smooth even surface.

ALWAYS REMEMBER

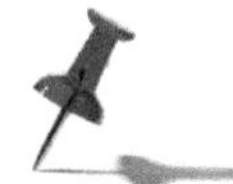

Damage to the matrix

If damage occurs to the **matrix** it can affect the health and appearance of the nail. For example, if the matrix is injured due to accidental damage such as a blow to the nail, permanent furrows or ridges might appear on the nail plate. The appearance of these ridges can be improved by the application of a ridge-filling base coat. If injury is serious the nail plate can be lost, and might never grow back.

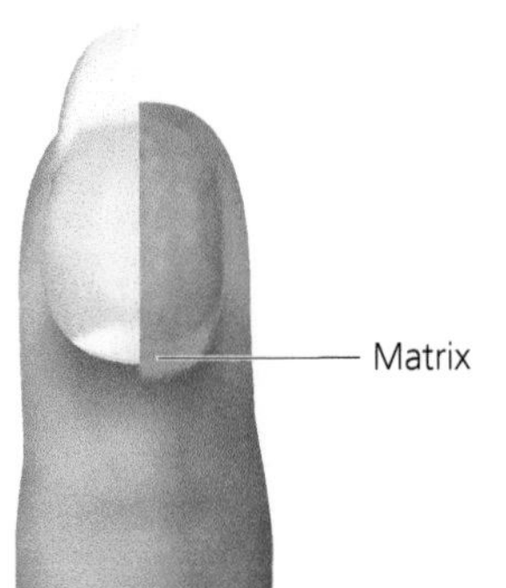

The matrix: the growing area of the nail that forms the nail plate

Matrix The matrix is found at the bottom of the nails and is the growing area of the nail. It is made up of **cells** – tiny particles that make up all living things. The cells in this area divide continuously to produce the nail plate.

Function: to produce new cells.

The nail plate The nail plate is the correct name for the part of the nail that covers the **nail bed**, the part of the skin on which the nail plate rests. The cells here are clear and have hardened. These hard cells act to protect the nail bed below and, because they are clear, allow you to see if the living nail bed is a healthy pink colour.

Function: to protect the nail bed.

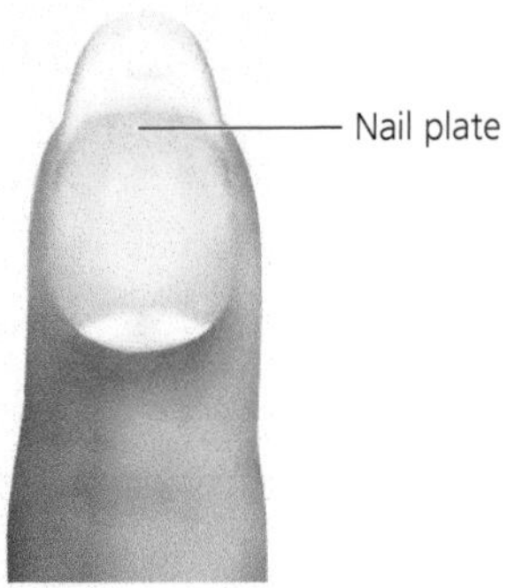

Nail plate: covers and protects the nail bed

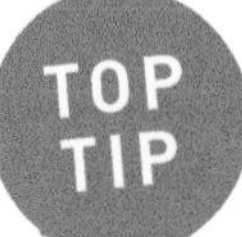

TOP TIP

Nail growth

The nails on the hands grow forward slowly over the nail bed, at a rate of 0. 5 mm to 1. 2 mm per week, this may differ from person to person. It takes between 4 and 6 months for a nail plate to grow fully from cuticle to free edge.

Fingernails grow more quickly than toenails, usually twice as fast.

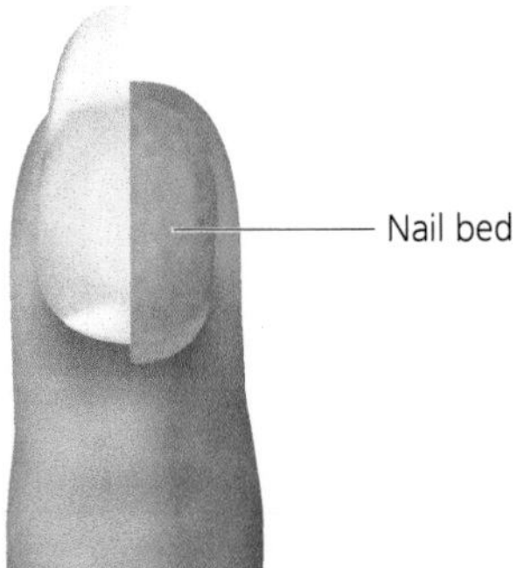

The nail bed: provides nourishment and protection

The nail bed The nail bed is the part of the skin covered by the nail plate. The nail plate and nail bed separate at the free-edge end of the finger. The nail bed is made up of living cells and contains many **blood vessels**, which carry blood that provides the nourishment necessary for healthy nail growth and repair; the nail bed also contains **nerves** that enable you to sense pain, heat, etc. providing protection from harm.

Function: to supply nourishment and protection.

Cuticle The cuticle is the overlapping skin at the bottom of the nail plate that grows forward onto the nail plate. When overgrown, it can grow high up onto the nail plate and will often split, which can then become infected. It is important to keep the cuticles soft and loose. The cuticle protects the matrix and nail bed from infection by preventing dirt and bacteria getting underneath the nail plate. This could lead to the bacterial infection paronychia see p. 213.

Function: to protect the matrix and nail bed from infection.

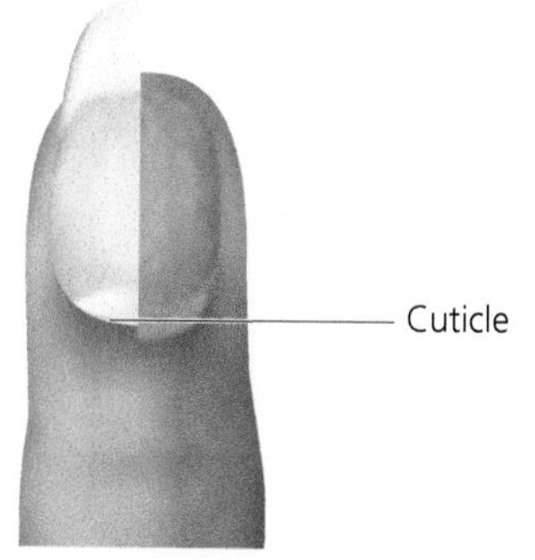

The cuticle: protects the nail bed from infection

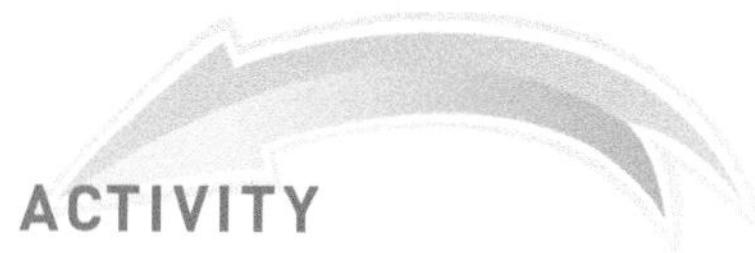

ACTIVITY

Recognizing nail structure
With a colleague identify the structural parts of each other's nails (on either the hands or feet).

Look for the free edge, nail plate, nail bed and cuticle. What part can you not see that you have learnt about?

Free edge The free edge is the part of the nail that grows beyond the tip of the fingers and toes. It is usually white, as it does not have the pink nail bed below it. It is the part of the nail that is filed.

Function: to protect the tip of the fingers and toes.

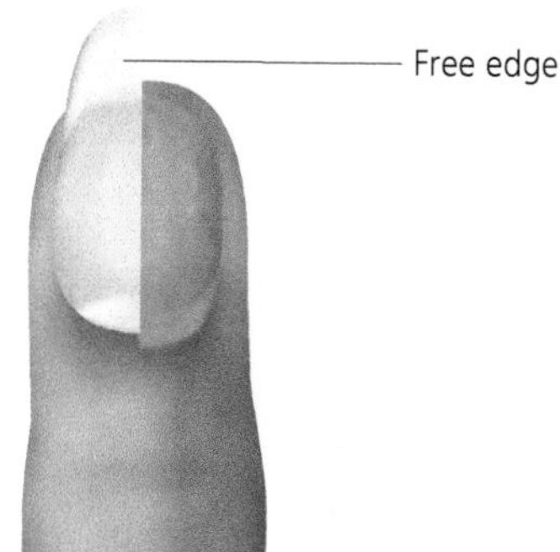

The free edge: protects the fingertip

Nail shapes

As stated previously the toenails should be kept short, cut straight across and filed smooth without shaping at the corners which could lead to ingrowing toenails. However, the nails of the hands are usually shaped, unless kept short due to client preference and usually when performing a male nail service.

ALWAYS REMEMBER

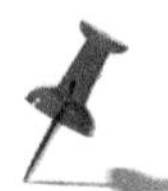

Checking the health of the skin on the feet
Always check between the toes where the skin can become sore and cracked and possibly suffer from a skin disorder such as tinea pedis - (athletes foot) see p. 212.

ALWAYS REMEMBER

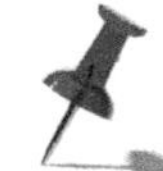

Factors affecting nail growth
Nails grow faster in summer than in winter; faster in young people than in older people; faster on the hand that is most often used, i.e. if you are right handed this will be the one on which the nails grow quickest. Illness and medication can affect nail growth, speeding it up or slowing it down.

Each client's hand size, finger length and nail shape is unique to them. It is important that the nail shape and length selected suits the client's hands and fingers. The free edge can be shaped to improve the appearance of the hands and fingers. Nail shapes include:

- Oval: the sides of the free edge are curved. This is an ideal shape for short, stubby fingers as it makes the fingers appear slimmer and longer.
- Square: the free edge is filed straight across. This nail shape will improve the appearance of thin, long fingers, making the fingers appear shorter and fuller.
- Squoval: a combination of oval and square nail shape. The nail is filed to a square finish at the free edge and is then gently curved at the corners.
- Round nails: the free edge is rounded and is an ideal shape for short nails. This style is popular with male clients.

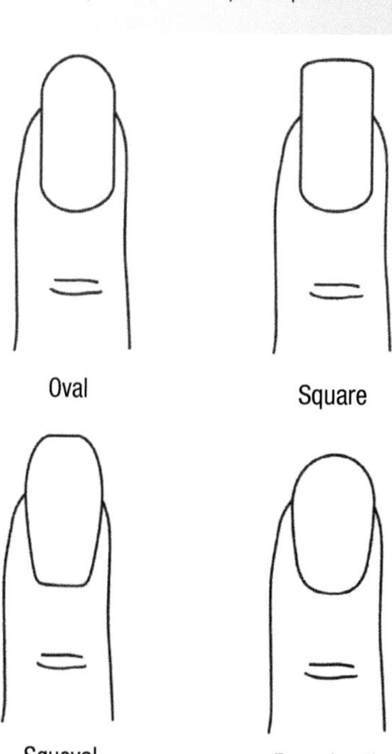

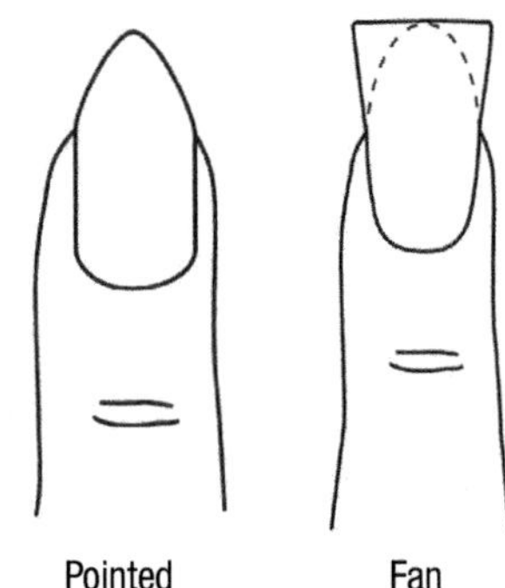

- Pointed: pointed nail shapes have a disadvantage in that the shape weakens the nail at the sides and it can then break easily.
- Fan: the nail becomes broader as it grows towards the free edge, appearing as a fan shape. The wider sides of the nail at the free edge can be shaped to achieve an oval shape.

ALWAYS REMEMBER

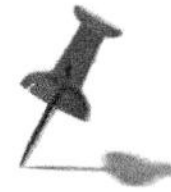

Pain

There are no blood vessels or nerves in the nail plate and free edge: this is why it can be cut without pain or bleeding.

TOP TIP

Nail shapes

- When filing the nail ensure the finished shape suits the client's nail/hand.
- If the fingers are long and thin, select a rounded shape/square shape and keep the length short.
- If the fingers are short and fat, the nails should be filed into an oval shape and the nail length should be longer to give an appearance of length to the fingers.

Outcome 1: Maintain safe and effective methods of working when assisting with nail services

Learn how to maintain safe and effective working methods when assisting with nail services by:

1. Setting up the work area in accordance with instructions.
2. Making sure that environmental conditions are suitable for the client and the service.
3. Ensuring your personal **hygiene** and appearance meets accepted industry Code of Practice for nail services and organizational requirements ensuring your personal hygiene and appearance meets accepted industry Code of Practice for nail services and **organizational requirements**.
4. Wearing suitable personal protective equipment (PPE) for the work that conforms to the **industry Code of Practice** for nail services.
5. Ensuring all tools and equipment are cleaned using the correct methods.
6. Effectively disinfecting your hands prior to nail service.
7. Maintaining accepted industry hygiene and safety practices throughout the service.
8. Positioning equipment and materials for ease and safety of use.
9. Ensuring your own posture and position minimizes fatigue and the risk of injury while working.
10. Disposing of waste materials safely and correctly.

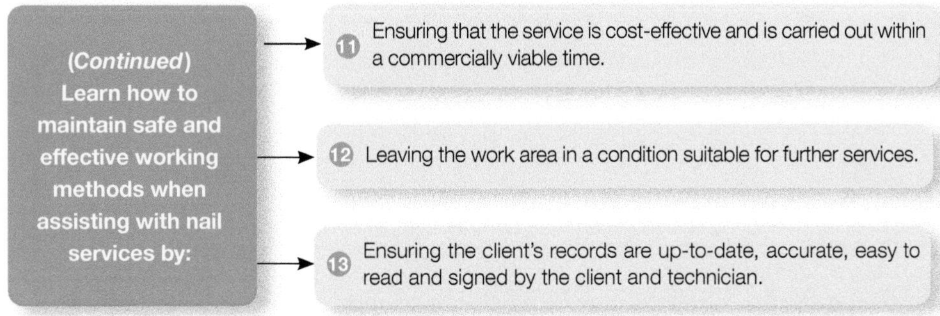

Making an appointment for nail services

When giving assistance with reception duties you may be required to make an appointment for nail services. The following will help you in your job role.

When a client makes an appointment for a basic nail service, the receptionist should ask a few basic questions:

- What is the client's name and telephone number? This will help you to get the client record card ready before they arrive for the service. The telephone number is important in case you need to cancel the service for any reason, or rearrange an appointment.
- Which beauty therapist does the client want to see? If a particular beauty therapist is asked for you will have to check on availability.
- When does the client want the nail service, i.e. day/date and time? If any of these are not available, suggest another time or day as near to this as possible.
- Has the client had the nail service before? This allows the client to ask you questions about the nail service. You may explain what a basic nail service includes.
- Inform the client if receiving a foot nail service where polish is to be applied that it would be a good idea to allow time for the polish to dry. Alternatively, they may wear footwear which will not smudge the newly painted toenails.
- Does the client require any other services in addition to the basic nail service? Always look at opportunities to increase service bookings, the salon needs to keep busy!

Remember, when making an appointment it is important to allow enough time to complete the service properly. It is also important for the beauty therapist to be able to complete the service in a commercially acceptable time. Allow 30 minutes for a basic nail service. This does not include consultation and preparation time.

The Data Protection Act 1998 All the clients' personal details are recorded on their record card.

These details are confidential or private. All information relating to a client should be stored securely either in a locked filing cabinet or electronically on a computer database. Only those staff with permission to access it can do so. Therefore, as soon as all service details have been recorded on the record card, the client's details should be stored securely.

It is important that all details are accurate and up-to-date.

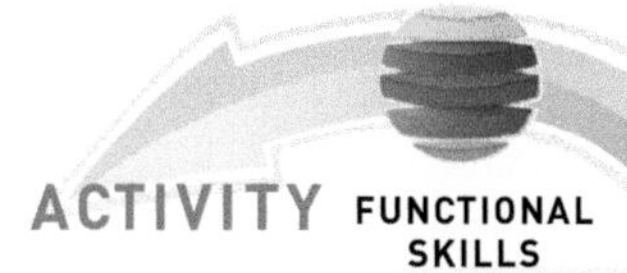

ACTIVITY FUNCTIONAL SKILLS

Recognizing service requirements

Collect images of different hand, feet and nail shapes from magazines.

Identify the nail shapes – do they suit the fingers and hands of the person?

What parts of a manicure service would benefit the skin, nails or cuticles for the images you have collected?

Select three and complete a service plan for each.

ALWAYS REMEMBER

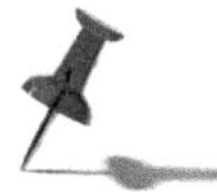

Timing

Allow 30 minutes for a basic nail service.

ACTIVITY

Service times

What is the time allowed for a basic nail service?

Why is it important to complete the service in this time?

Think of three reasons for both questions.

> An employer will always want someone with ideas and who shows passion in all they do.
>
> **Jacqui Jefford**

TOP TIP

Pedicure stations

Some pedicure bowls are permanently fixed in place at a pedicure work station. This equipment is increasingly popular with some chairs providing vibratory back massage at the same time!

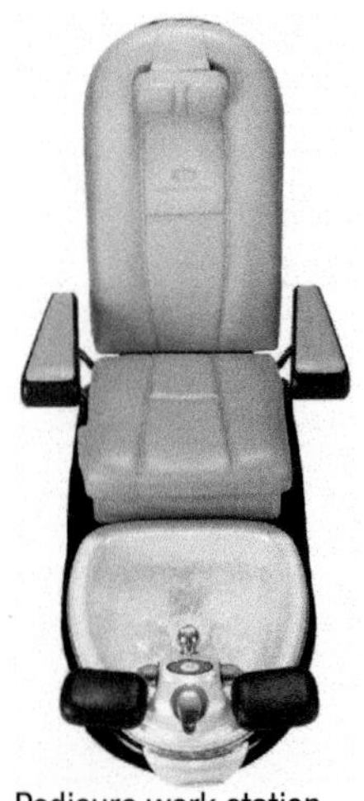

Pedicure work station

A basic nail service to the hands and feet includes:

Hands		*Feet*
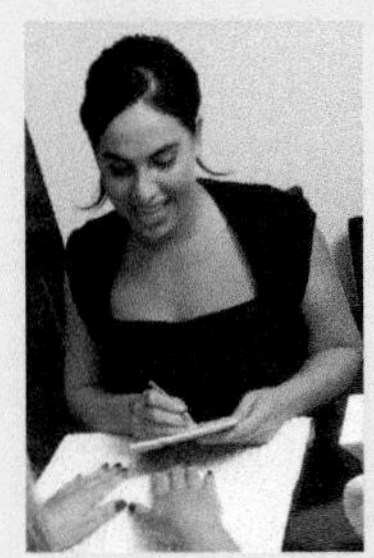	Consultation	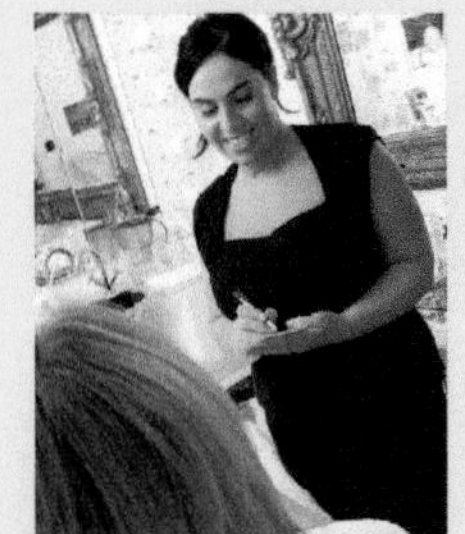
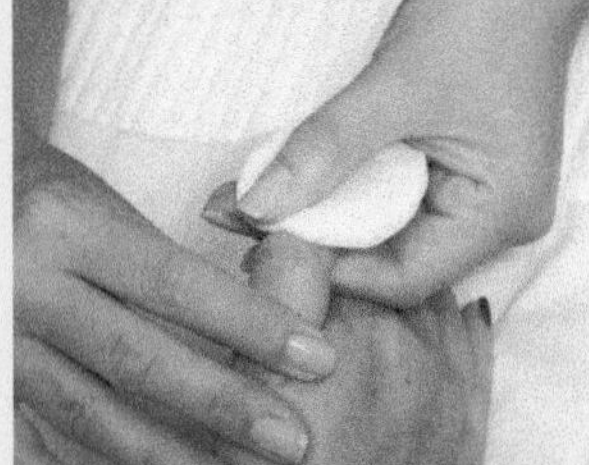	Nail polish removal (if worn)	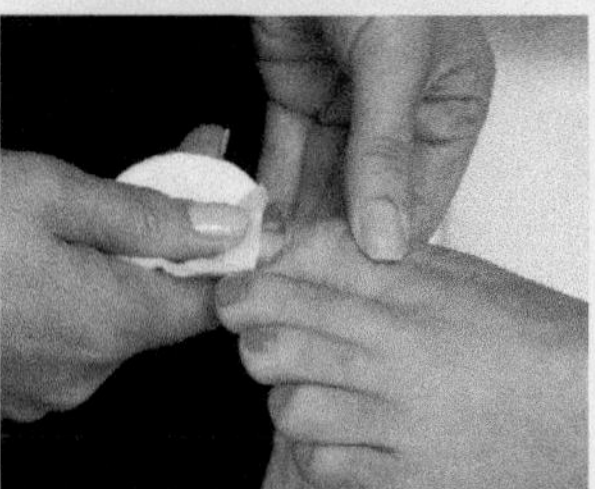
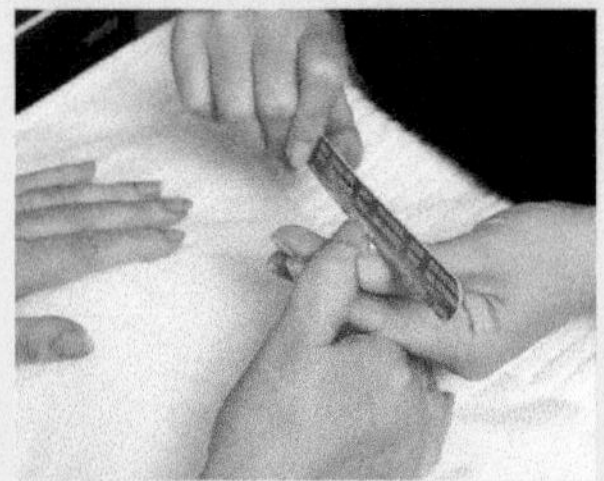	File	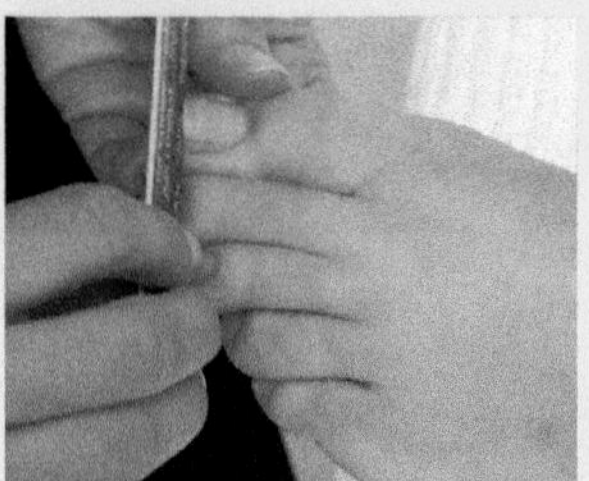
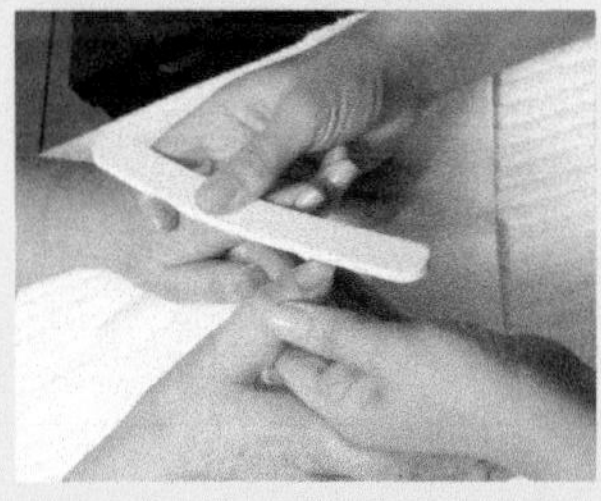	Buff	The toenails are not normally buffed for healthy nail growth but can be to reduce the appearance of ridges on the nail plate
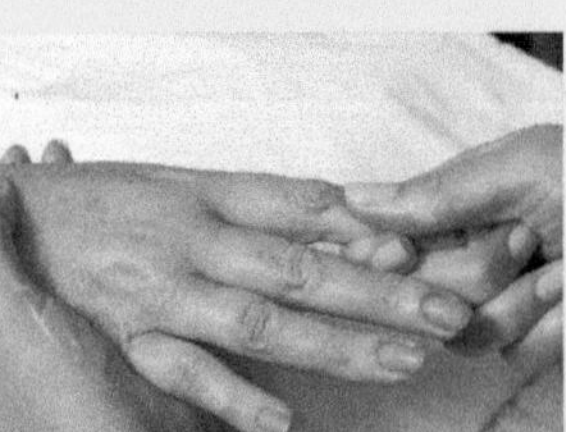	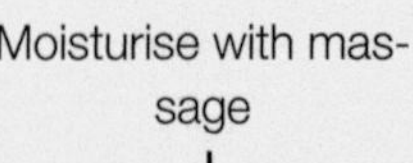 Moisturise with massage	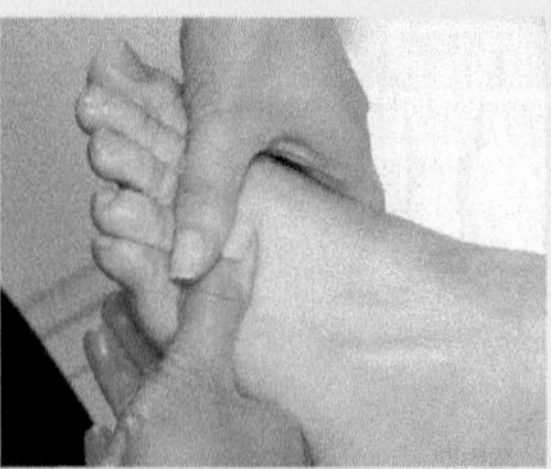
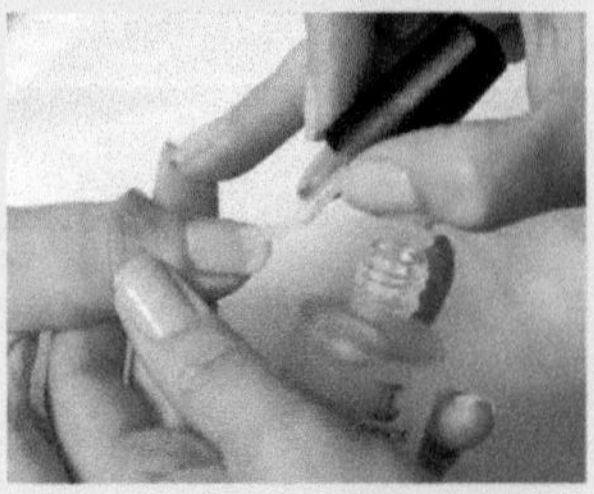	Nail polish application	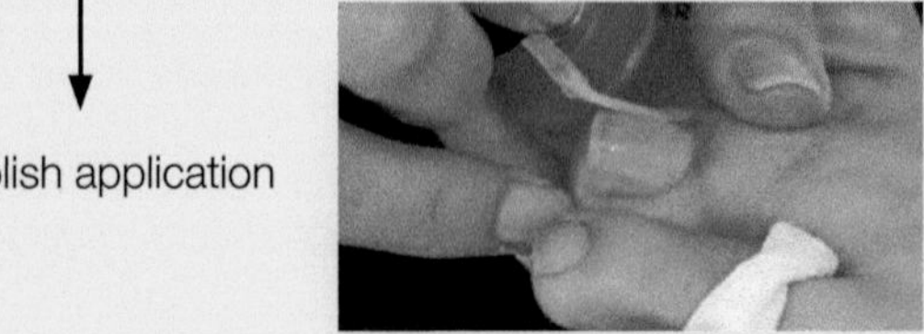

Equipment materials and products used in a basic nail service It is important that you understand the purpose of the different equipment, materials and products and any related health and safety practice related to their use. Read and follow manufacturers' instructions before using all nail service products. Have a Material Data Safety Sheet (MSDS) available for all products that you use in your service. Each beauty supplier is legally required to provide guidelines on how materials should be used and stored in compliance with the legislation: The Control of Substances Hazardous to Health (COSHH) Regulations 2002.

Item	*Use*	*Health and safety practice*
ELLISONS Sterilizing fluid	Sterilizing fluid that prevents the multiplication of microorganisms but does not kill all microorganisms Objects must be kept sanitary once sterilized	Could cause a slip hazard if spilt Might cause skin irritation and is toxic if swallowed Chemical sterilizing sprays are also used to sterilize the surface of nail tools. These should be used by following manufacturer's instructions and in a well-ventilated area, avoiding contact with flame and excessive heat
ELLISONS Manicure/pedicure bowl	Fill with warm water and add a pleasant smelling therapeutic nail soak to cleanse and soften the cuticles and skin	Clean after use with a detergent, disinfect, rinse and dry. Clean with a chemical disinfectant that will not damage the surface, i.e. if plastic When in use keep on a stable surface to avoid spillage
ELLISONS Nail file	A nail file used to shape the nails It usually has two sides; one side is coarser than the other	Use a new nail file or **emery board** for each client to avoid **cross-infection**. Throw away after use Use the coarser side to reduce the length of the nail Never use a sawing action when filing as you can cause the free edge to split Only file the nail straight across when filing toenails to avoid causing an ingrowing toenail
ELLISONS Orange sticks	Disposable wooden tools, usually with a hoof-shaped end for use around the cuticle and a pointed end for cleaning under the free edge They can also be used to remove the products from the containers	Never reuse the **orange sticks**: throw away after each service to avoid cross-infection Always tip with clean cotton wool if used to clean under the free edge to avoid injury to the finger Used incorrectly on the nail they could pierce the skin

Item	*Use*	*Health and safety practice*
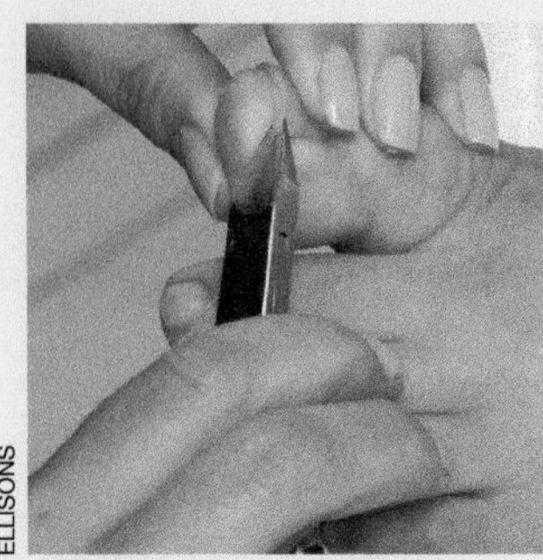 ELLISONS Nail clippers	Used to shorten long nails before filing Nail **scissors** are used on the fingernails and nail **clippers** on the toenails	Support the nails at the side of the nail plate with the other hand to avoid client discomfort and ensure that all pieces of nail can be collected and thrown away Sterilize nail scissors/clippers in an autoclave between each client to avoid cross-infection Store in the UV cabinet
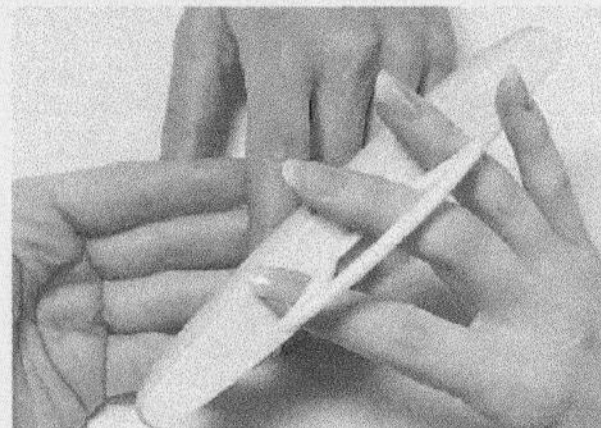 Buffers	Used in nail services to improve the surface appearance of the nail, stimulate blood circulation to the nail bed and impart shine to the nail plate. The **buffer** might have a plastic handle and a replaceable pad covered with soft leather. This buffer can be used with or without **buffing paste**. Also available are four-sided nail buffers, similar to a thick emery board with a choice of surfaces from slightly coarse to very smooth, these are used without buffing paste	Ensure that the soft leather cover is replaced for each client to avoid cross-infection. This means you will need more than one cover. Do not overuse the coarse buffer otherwise the nail plate will become thin and weakened Wipe buffing handle with disinfectant Wash buffing cloth in hot soapy water 60°C Place in UV cabinet when dry
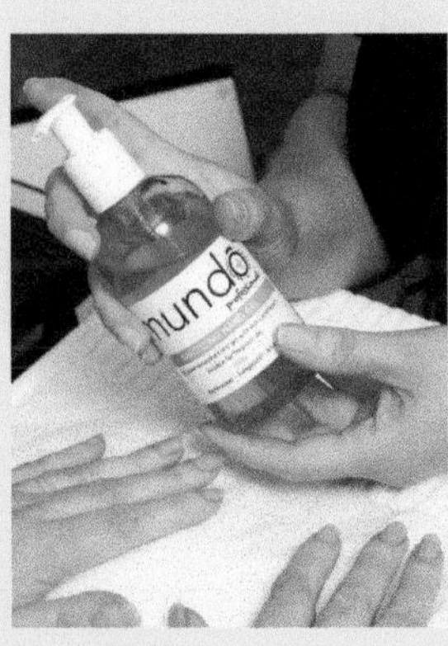 MUNDO Skin cleanser	A chemical that removes a number of harmful microorganisms from the client's skin that could cause infection. This cleansing process is called **disinfection** and an antiseptic product is often used. This is also termed **sanitization** cleansing or washing to an antiseptic level to prohibit bacterial growth	Antiseptics can be used safely on the skin but some clients might have an intolerance to them, leading to an allergic reaction Always check at consultation if the client has any known skin allergies
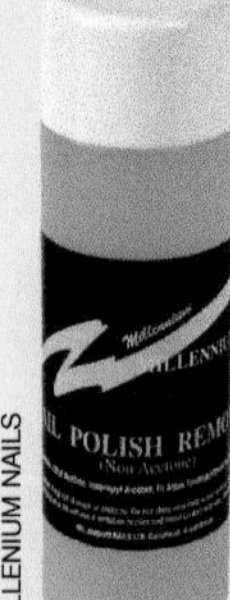 MILLENIUM NAILS Nail polish remover	A product that will dissolve and remove **nail polish** and grease and oils from the nail plate. The ingredient that causes this is called acetone	Nail polish remover can be drying to the nail as it also removes moisture and oils from the nail plate Store away from heat as it is highly flammable (may go on fire when heated)

Item	Use	Health and safety practice
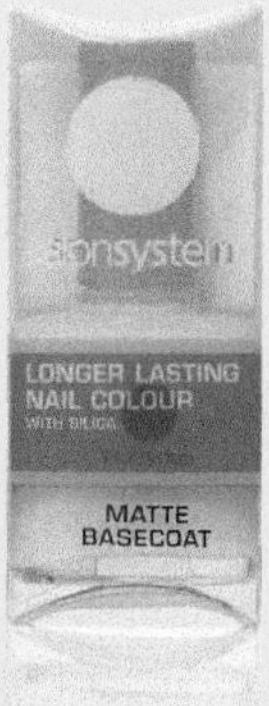 SALON SYSTEMS Nail polish: coloured, base coat, topcoat	Can be applied to improve the natural appearance of the nail, or add colour and protection	Always secure the lid tightly after use to avoid the product spoiling and accidental spillage Ensure that the client is not allergic; some clients have allergies to the ingredient *formaldehyde* in nail polish
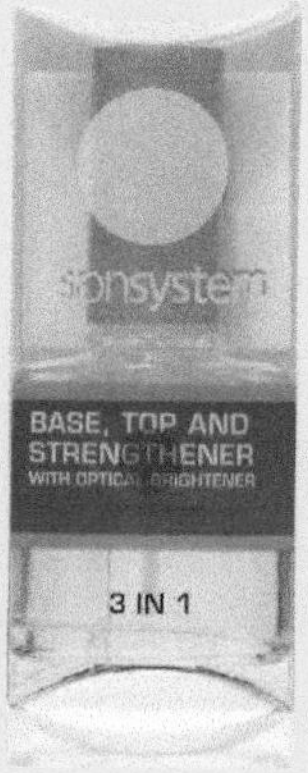 SALON SYSTEMS Nail strengthener	A nail polish product that strengthens a nail plate that has a tendency to split in layers, usually a dry, brittle nail	Check if the client has known allergies, some clients have allergies to the ingredient *formaldehyde*, which is sometimes found in **nail strengthener**
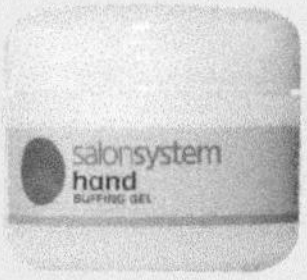 SALON SYSTEMS Buffing paste	A coarse cream containing ingredients such as pumice or talc to remove the surface cells of the nail plates, giving shine	Avoid overuse of the buffing paste to avoid thinning and weakening of the nail plate
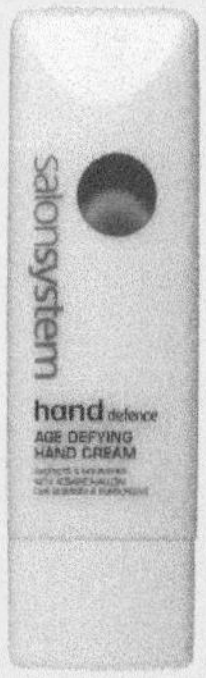 SALON SYSTEMS Hand/foot cream/oil/lotion	A mixture of waxes and oils with perfumes and preservatives to maintain its quality. Hand creams/oils soften the skin of the hands and cuticles and assist the application of **massage** movements	Some hand/foot massage products contain lanolin, a skin moisturising agent that can cause an allergic skin reaction Always check if the client has any known allergies before service, and know your product ingredients

Before service

Before service is carried out you will need to prepare the work area, yourself and the client for the service.

Equipment and materials Before carrying out the basic nail service, check that you have all the necessary equipment and materials to hand.

Refer to the equipment and materials checklist to make sure that you have all that is required to perform a basic nail service.

Tick in the box next to each item on the checklist to help you as you prepare the work area.

Equipment and materials checklist

		Hand	*Foot*
ELLISONS Manicure table	Nail service station or trolley on which to place everything	☐	☐
SORISA Towels	Medium-sized towels: three for manicure, five for pedicure	☐	☐
ELLISONS Small bowls	Small bowls lined with tissue (3) for clean cotton wool and putting products into	☐	☐
ELLISONS Cotton wool	Dry cotton wool to apply and remove products from the skin and nails i.e. to apply nail polish remover to remove nail polish from the nails	☐	☐
ELLISONS Manicure bowl	Manicure bowl for the client's fingers – to cleanse the skin and nails and soften the skin in warm water	☐	

		Hand	*Foot*
ELLISONS Pedicure spa	Pedicure bowl or spa for the client's feet – to cleanse the skin and nails and soften the skin in warm water. The bowl shown has a vibratory, stimulating effect when the feet are placed on the base of the bowl		☐
ELLISONS Emery boards	Emery board to file the nail free edge to shape	☐	☐
ELLISONS Orange sticks	Orange sticks, tipped at either end with cotton wool, to apply products to the nails and to clean the nail on and around the nail plate To gently loosen the cuticle To remove products hygienically from their containers	☐	☐
Nail scissors	Nail scissors used to reduce the length of the nails before filing	☐	
Toenail clippers	Toenail clippers to shorten the length of the toenails		☐
Buffer	Buffers to give the nails a sheen, improve the appearance of ridges when used with a buffing paste, and to increase blood circulation to the nail	☐	☐

		Hand	Foot
SALON SYSTEMS Buffing paste	Buffing paste, a course gritty nail product used to shine the nail plate when used with the buffer	☐	☐
ELLISONS Detergent	Detergent, to add to the warm water in the manicure bowl or pedicure spa to cleanse and refresh the skin	☐	☐
SALON SYSTEMS Hand cream	Hand cream, oil or lotion to soften and nourish the skin	☐	
SALON SYSTEMS Foot cream	Foot cream, oil or lotion to soften and nourish the skin		☐
MUNDO Skin cleanser	Skin cleanser to cleanse the skin before the service	☐	☐
MAVALA Base coat	**Base coat** polish to provide a base to apply coloured polish and to prevent nail staining	☐	☐

		Hand	Foot
ELLISONS Light coloured polishes	Light coloured polishes, a selection	☐	☐
MAVALA Topcoat	Topcoat to seal and protect nail polish colour providing durability	☐	☐
SALON SYSTEMS Nail strengthener	Specialist nail products such as nail strengthener	☐	☐
MAVALA Nail polish remover	Nail polish remover, to remove nail polish from the nail	☐	☐
CREATIVE NAILS Cuticle oil	Cuticle oil to soften and nourish the skin of the cuticle	☐	☐
Cuticle massage cream	Cuticle massage cream to soften and nourish the skin of the cuticle	☐	☐
ELLISONS Disinfectant solution	Small jar of disinfecting solution to hold small metal and plastic nail service tools	☐	☐

		Hand	*Foot*
ELLISONS Metal bin	Metal bin – lined with a disposable bin liner	☐	☐
ELLISONS Client's record card	Client's record card – to record the client's details before and after the service	☐	☐
Nailcare Aftercare ELLISONS Aftercare leaflets	Aftercare leaflets might be provided to the client on how to care for their nails	☐	☐

HEALTH & SAFETY

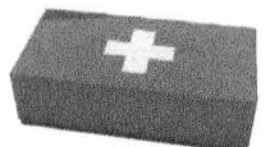

The autoclave

A sterilizing unit similar to a pressure cooker – creates steam as the water inside it boils. A temperature of 121–134°C is reached, which is sufficient to sterilize the items inside the autoclave. This process is only suitable for equipment that can withstand the heating process – always check first. When possible, use equipment that can be thrown away after use (disposable), e.g. emery boards and orange sticks.

Sterilization and disinfection It is important that good hygienic practice is considered before and throughout the client service. This will help prevent cross-infection – the transfer of harmful bacteria/microorganisms from one person to another. An **aseptic** condition should be aimed for in the workplace a situation where you are trying to destroy bacteria.

All equipment should be sterilized or disinfected using the most suitable method before use on each client.

Hygiene checks

- Ensure that all tools and equipment are clean and sterile before use.
- Disinfect work surfaces regularly.
- Use disposable items whenever possible. Discard immediately after use in a covered, lined waste container.
- Follow hygienic practices.
- Maintain a high standard of personal hygiene.

Preparation of the beauty therapist Make sure the service area is warm and comfortable, ventilation is adequate and that lighting is adequate to prevent eye strain and to enable the service to be performed competently. Check that the area is free from obstacles that could cause a fall.

Wash the hands to remove surface dirt, preventing cross-infection, this will also show the client you have good hygiene practice.

Follow the correct salon requirements for hygiene and personal presentation to ensure a professional image at all times.

TOP TIP

Work area

The work area should be left ready for the next client whenever a service is completed. Waste products should be disposed of correctly following local council waste disposal regulations. If you are free, help other colleagues to tidy the area after a service to maintain the work area ready for the next client.

HEALTH & SAFETY

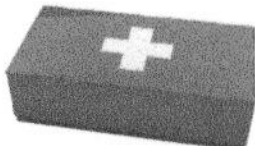

Nail Services: A Code of Practice

Habia has produced a Code of Practice in nail services that provides guidance on the correct hygiene procedures and working practices to prevent cross-infection and ensure a professional service and profile is achieved.

The code of practice is available to download from the Habia website: www.habia.org.

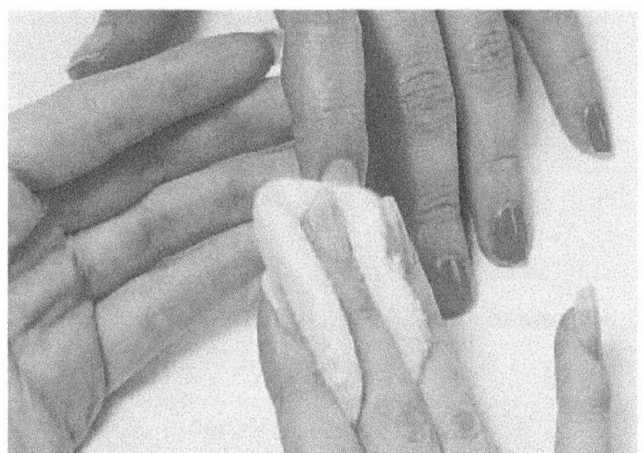

Removing nail polish to assess the client's nail condition

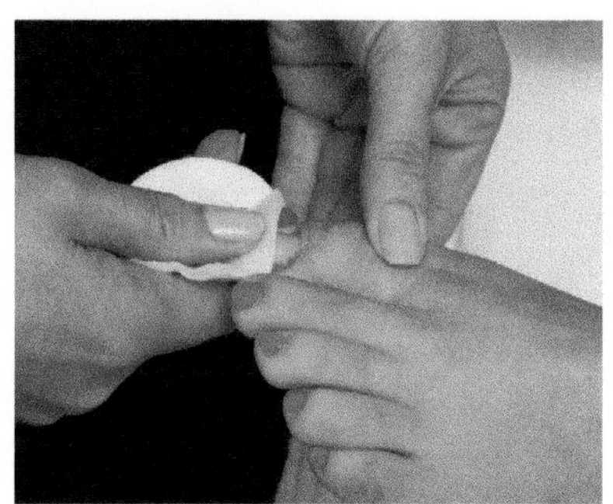

Removal of toenail polish

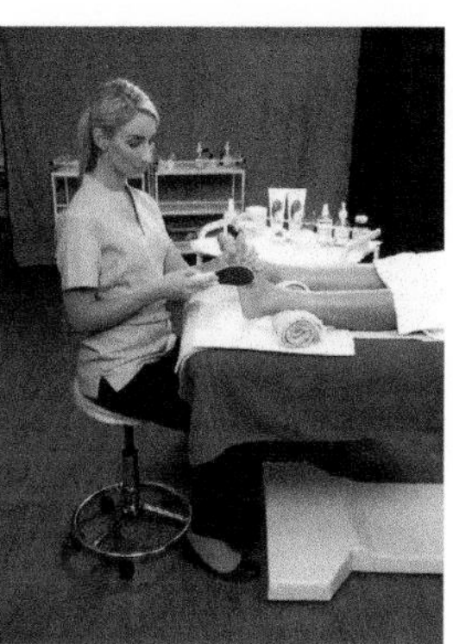

Work station setup for pedicure

Preparing the work area Check the work area to ensure that you have all the equipment, materials and products you require for the nail service. Use the checklist provided on pp. 204–208.

Hand nail service Place a clean towel over the work surface, then fold another towel into a pad and place it in the middle of the work surface. This will help support the client's forearm during service. Place a third towel over the pad.

The beauty therapist will need a small towel to dry the client's hands during the service.

A tissue or disposable manicure mat should then be placed on top of the towels, to collect nail filings. This is disposed of later to avoid skin irritation or cross-contamination from the filings.

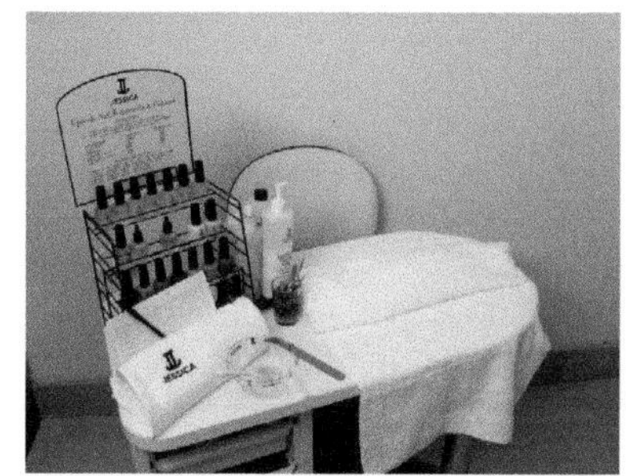

Work station for manicure

Foot nail service Ensure that the work station has everything to hand so that the client need not be disturbed during the service. The work area should remain in a condition for nail services during the working day. A towel should be placed on the floor between you and the client. The pedicure bowl or spa containing warm, soapy water should be placed on this towel. Towels should be available, one to cover your knee area for protection, another for drying the client's feet. Alternatively the nail service may be performed on a beauty couch or at a pedicure station. In this case towels are only required for drying and wrapping the feet.

Outcome 2: Consult, plan and prepare for nail services with clients

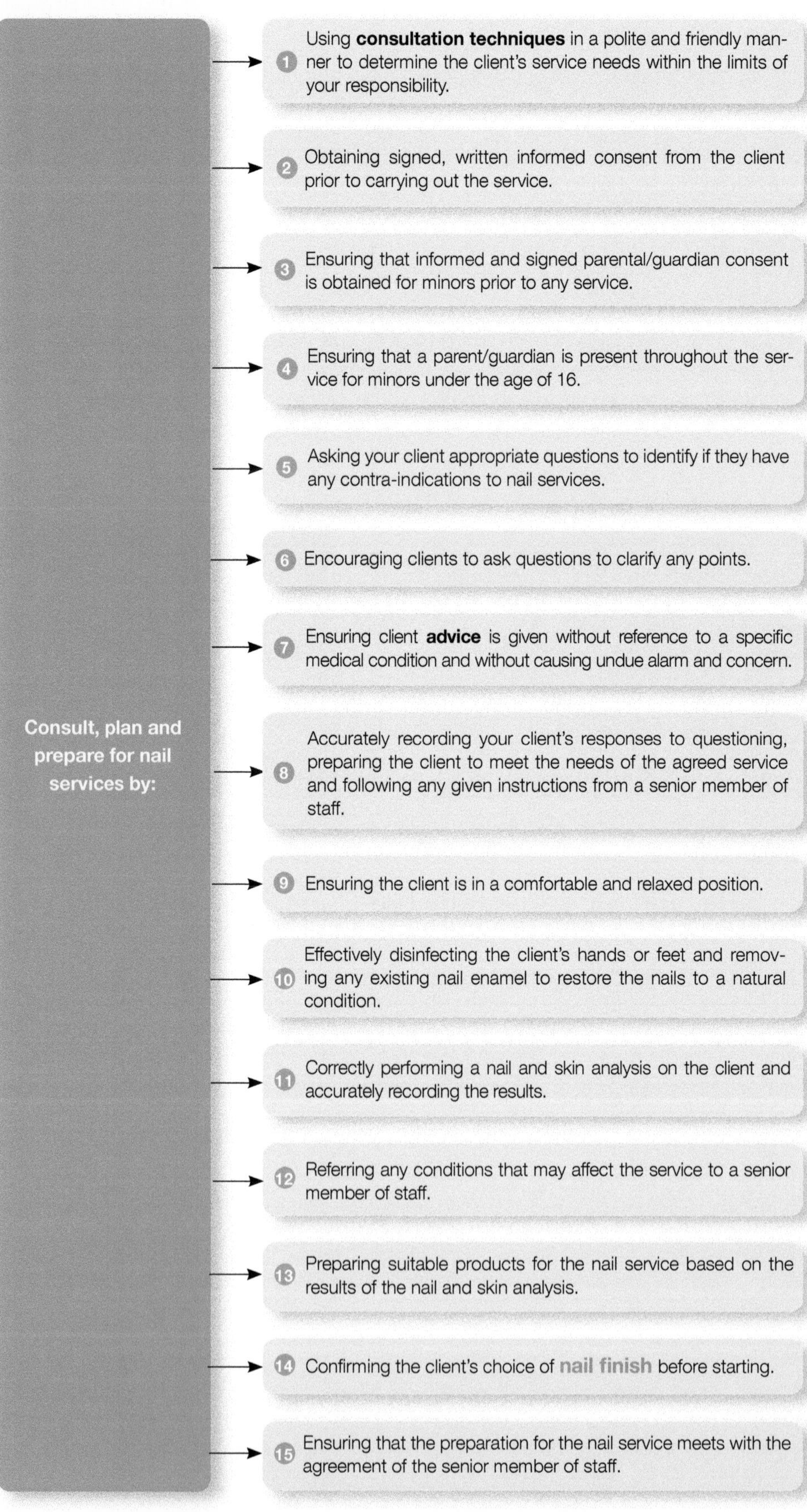

The consultation The consultation should be carried out in the privacy of the service work area. This takes place when the client first meets you at the start of the service and will take approximately 10 minutes. The **consultation** enables the beauty therapist to assess whether the client is suitable for the service or whether the service is contra-indicated in some way.

Ask the client specific questions about their current hand and foot home-care routine and about their general health. The client's answers will suggest to the beauty therapist what is required, and what is achievable from the nail service.

During the consultation the beauty therapist can also explain what is involved in the service and what aftercare and home care is required.

HEALTH & SAFETY

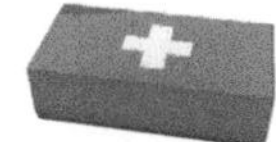

Contra-indications

Remember, you might be wrong when you think you have a client with a contra-indication. Always check with the senior beauty therapist – the client may be able to have the service after all.

Never diagnose, and try to avoid causing the client embarrassment. The senior beauty therapist may recommend that the client seeks medical advice before the nail service goes ahead.

Contra-indications to nail service

Certain nail, hand and foot skin conditions prevent or restrict you from performing the basic nail service. These are known as **contra-indications**. If, when looking at a client's hands and feet and nails before the service you think you recognize any of the following conditions, you must not perform the basic nail service. You will need to refer the client tactfully to the relevant person in the salon for confirmation that the service can go ahead (or not).

Contra-indications that prevent service

Many of the skin and nail conditions in the table below are contagious – they can be passed on to other clients and clients with these conditions should never be treated.

Name of contra-indication	*Cause*	*Appearance*
DR M H BECK Impetigo	A contagious **bacterial** infection caused by minute, single-celled organisms and which results in skin inflammation	The skin appears red and is itchy Small blisters appear, which burst and then form crusts
DR M H BECK Common warts **Common wart:** found on the hand **Plane wart:** found on the fingers or either surface of the hands	Contagious **viral** infection that results in abnormal skin growth A contagious **fungal** infection of the skin Fungal diseases of the skin feed off the waste products of the skin	Small skin growths, varying in size, shape, texture and colour Usually raised with a rough surface Found on the fingers, either surface of the hands

Name of contra-indication	*Cause*	*Appearance*
DR A L WRIGHT **Verrucae:** warts on the feet **Plantar wart:** found on the sole of the foot	Small skin growths Warts on the sole of the foot grow inwards, due to the pressure of body weight	Warts vary in size, shape, texture and colour Usually they have a rough surface and are raised
DR M H BECK Scabies or itch mites	Contagious condition caused by an **animal parasite** (something that lives off another living thing - which can cause it harm) that burrows beneath the skin and enters the hair follicles	Small lumps and wavy greyish lines appear on the skin. This is where dirt has entered, where the parasite burrows under the skin Found in warm, loose areas of skin such as in-between the fingers and the creases of the elbows
DR M H BECK Tinea corporis or body ringworm	A contagious **fungal** infection of the skin. Fungal diseases of the skin feed off the waste products of the skin	Small, scaly red patches spread outwards and then heal from the centre, leaving a ring May be found on the limbs
WELLCOME PHOTO LIBRARY Tinea unguium or nail ringworm	A contagious **fungal** infection of the nail plate	The nail plate is yellowish grey The nail plate becomes brittle and will finally start to separate from the nail bed
DR A L WRIGHT Tinea pedis (athletes foot)	A **fungal** infection of the foot occurring in the webs of the skin between the toes	Small blisters form, which later burst. The skin in the area can become dry, with a scaly appearance
MEDISCAN Diabetes	If a client has diabetes they are in danger of infection as they have slow skin healing Permission must be received from the client's GP before a service can be provided to a diabetic client to ensure they are safe to treat	Secondary infection can occur seen as pus, redness and swelling if the skin was accidentally broken during the service

Name of contra-indication	*Cause*	*Appearance*
WELLCOME PHOTO LIBRARY Broken bones	Injury – should be treated medically	The breakage might not be obvious. If the client is new, check that there have been no broken bones at the consultation. The broken bone must not be handled. Therefore, if one finger or toe is broken you must avoid this. Always check first with the relevant person in the workplace
WELLCOME PHOTO LIBRARY Severe nail separation–onycholysis	Lifting of the nail plate from the nail bed, may be caused by injury or infection to the nail or surrounding area	Where there is nail separation this appears as a greyish white area on the nail as the pink colour of the nail bed does not show
WELLCOME PHOTO LIBRARY Paronychia	Infectious bacterial infection can be caused by using non-sterile nail service tools where there is injury to the skin present	Swelling, redness and pus appears in the cuticle area of the skin around the nail
WELLCOME PHOTO LIBRARY Cuts or abrasions on the hands	Injury to the skin–treating the skin may lead to secondary infection seen as pus, redness and swelling in the area	Broken skin
WELLCOME PHOTO LIBRARY Severe psoriasis of the nail	An inflammatory condition where there is increased cell production and thickening of the nail	A pitting effect can occur on the surface of the nail plate like the surface of an orange Nail separation of the nail plate from the nail bed may also occur
WELLCOME PHOTO LIBRARY Severe eczema of the nail	Inflammation of the skin, which may cause differing changes to the nail	Ridges, pitting, nail separation and even nail loss may occur
WELLCOME PHOTO LIBRARY Severe ingrowing toenail	The sides of the nail penetrate the nail wall The client should be referred to a chiropodist for appropriate treatment	Redness, inflammation and pus may be present

TOP TIP

To prevent ingrowing toenails

The client should be advised to cut the toenails straight across and not too short. Clients who do lots of running are prone to both bruised and ingrowing toenails.

ALWAYS REMEMBER

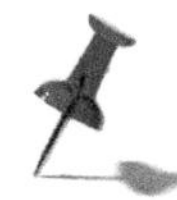

Broken skin

If a client has a minor, small scratch of the skin in the service area, service can usually go ahead by avoiding contact with the area, with permission of the senior beauty therapist. If the client has a cut, redness and swelling the service should not go ahead. If unsure, seek guidance from the senior beauty therapist first.

This could lead to paronychia.

Nail and skin conditions that might restrict service

The nail and skin conditions below are non-contagious and cannot be passed on to other clients. You can therefore treat a client with one of these conditions, although you might need to adapt your service application.

Name of contra-indication	*Cause*	*Appearance*	*Service*
DR A L WRIGHT Bruised nail	Damage to the nail (e.g. by trapping in a door)	Part or all of the nail plate appears blue or black	Avoid the nail that is bruised when carrying out the nail service
DR A L WRIGHT Onychophagy	Excessive nail biting	Commonly seen on the hands Very little nail plate The skin appears red and swollen due to biting of the skin around the nails	Regular weekly nail services to encourage nail growth and treat any dry skin and cuticle The client could try applying bitter tasting nail products at home to help stop nail biting
DR A L WRIGHT Pterygium	Neglect	Overgrown cuticles, tightly attached to the nail plate. When left untreated they often split and crack	Advise the client to have a nail service with a senior beauty therapist where the excess cuticle can be removed using specialized tools called *nippers* or ***clippers***. The client should be advised to apply a rich cuticle cream daily

Name of contra-indication	*Cause*	*Appearance*	*Service*
DR A L WRIGHT Ridges in the nail plate	Illness, damage or old age	Ridges in the nail plate running across or down the length of the nail plate, from the cuticle to the free edge. This can affect one or all nails	Buffing service to help to improve the appearance of the nail by smoothing out the ridges. A ridge-filling base coat can also be applied before nail polish application
DR A L WRIGHT Hangnail	Dry skin or cuticle that cracks Biting the skin around the nail	The skin around the nail plate cracks and a small piece of skin appears between the nail plate and the side of the nail (nail wall) Sometimes the area becomes red and swollen	Refer the condition to the senior beauty therapist for treatment. Specialized manicure service to soften the skin and cuticles Removal of the excess skin using cuticle nippers Advise the client to apply hand cream and cuticle cream to prevent dryness
DR A L WRIGHT Leuconychia	Damage to the nail plate due to pressure or hitting with a hard object	White spots appear on the nail plate, which grow out with the nail	Advise the client to take good care of the nails. Recommend the application of a coloured nail polish to disguise the white spots
DR A L WRIGHT Onychorrhexis	Poor diet Harsh chemical detergents. Incorrect choice/use of nail products	Split, flaking nails Commonly seen on the hands	Ensure a healthy, balanced diet Regular use of a hand cream. Protect the nails from chemical detergents, which dry the nails, always wear rubber gloves. Nail service base polishes can have specific effects to improve the nail. Incorrect use/choice can dry the nails causing the nails to split and flake
DR A L WRIGHT Non-severe skin eczema	Inflammation of the skin caused by contact with a skin irritant Often affects the inner creases of the elbows	The skin becomes red, swells and blisters can appear. The blisters burst, which then causes scabs to form on the skin	Ensure you find out what irritants make the eczema worse and avoid contact with such products, e.g. perfumed products The skin can benefit from massage lotion that contains soothing ingredients such as lavender Do not treat if the skin is broken

Name of contra-indication	*Cause*	*Appearance*	*Service*
DR A L WRIGHT **Non-severe skin psoriasis**	Cause unknown but becomes worse when the person is stressed often hereditary inherited from a parent	Itchy, red, flaky patches of skin, which can become infected if the skin becomes broken Found on the elbows	The skin can benefit from massage lotion that contains soothing ingredients such as lavender Do not treat if the skin is broken
WELLCOME PHOTO LIBRARY **Non-severe nail psoriasis**	Psoriasis of the nail can cause further nail disorders to occur. Cause unknown but becomes worse when the person is stressed. Often hereditary	Pitting and discoloration of the nail plate with possible increased nail curvature (where the nail curves over the end of the finger as it grows) and nail thickening	Take care when treating the nails It is advisable to keep the nails short
WELLCOME PHOTO LIBRARY **Non-severe nail eczema**	Inflammation of the skin, causing changes to the nail	Ridges and pitting of the nails	Take care when treating the nails It is advisable to keep the nails short

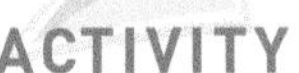

ACTIVITY

Skin conditions on the hand

What can cause the skin on the hands to become dry, chapped, irritated, rough or broken?

You need to ask the client questions to find out if there is a cause for the skin's appearance (look), and then you can give appropriate helpful recommendations.

Discuss with your colleagues common everyday causes that can lead to poor skin condition.

HEALTH & SAFETY

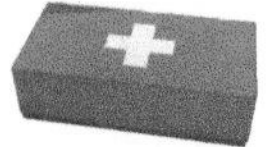

Recent skin disorders

Ask your client to consult their GP on the suitability of nail services.

Before treating any client, if at all unsure check with the relevant supervisor in the workplace.

Also during the consultation the client will:

- discover what services the salon can offer
- ask questions and receive honest professional advice concerning the most appropriate service
- confirm and agree the service aim.

All details should be recorded accurately on the client record card.

Preparing the client

1 Help the client into a comfortable and relaxed position for service. The chair should offer adequate back and knee support, be a suitable height for the work station and be comfortable. Unsuitable positioning of the client can cause the beauty therapist discomfort, and possibly even injury due to strain. For hand nail service your elbows should be able to rest on the work station without stretching. If the client is wearing long sleeves these must be turned up past the elbow to prevent soiling the clothes with the massage product during the service. A clean tissue may also be folded along the edge of the sleeve for further protection.

   For a foot service, if the client is wearing lower clothing that cannot easily be moved i.e. tight jeans these are best removed and a clean gown provided for modesty.

2 Carry out the client consultation, assess the client's needs using different techniques including questioning and natural observation. Complete the client record card, listing all details to ensure the client's suitability for the service.

If the client is a minor under the age of 16, it is necessary to have the parent/guardian permission for the nail service. The parent/guardian will also have to be present when the service is received. A client record card follows.

Sample client record card

Date | Beauty therapist name

Client name

Date of birth
(Identifying client age group.)

Home address

Postcode

Email address | Landline telephone number | Mobile telephone number

Name of doctor | Doctor's address and telephone number

Related medical history (Conditions that may restrict or prohibit service application.)

Are you taking any medication? (This may affect the sensitivity of the skin to the service.)

CONTRA-INDICATIONS REQUIRING MEDICAL REFERRAL
(Preventing **manicure service** application.)

- ☐ bacterial infections (e.g. paronychia/impetigo)
- ☐ viral infection (e.g. plane warts/plantar warts)
- ☐ fungal infection (e.g. tinea unguium/tinea pedis)
- ☐ severe nail separation
- ☐ severe eczema and psoriasis
- ☐ severe bruising
- ☐ broken bones

CONTRA-INDICATIONS WHICH RESTRICT SERVICE
(Service may require adaptation.)

- ☐ minor nail separation
- ☐ mild psoriasis/eczema
- ☐ recent scar tissue
- ☐ severely bitten nails
- ☐ severely damaged nails
- ☐ minor cuts or abrasions
- ☐ minor bruising or swelling

EQUIPMENT AND MATERIALS

- ☐ nail and skin service tools
- ☐ abrasives (e.g. buffing cream)
- ☐ nail and skin products
- ☐ nail conditioners (e.g. cuticle cream/oil)
- ☐ skin conditioners (e.g. hand cream/foot cream, oil or lotion)
- ☐ consumables (things thrown away after use e.g. cotton wool)

SERVICE AIM

- ☐ improvement of skin condition products used ____________
- ☐ improvement of nail condition products used ____________

NAIL FINISH

- ☐ buffing
- ☐ clear polish
- ☐ nail strengthener

NAIL, CUTICLE AND SKIN CONDITION

Nails	**Cuticle**	**Skin**
☐ normal	☐ dry	☐ dry
☐ brittle	☐ split	☐ hard
☐ dry	☐ overgrown	☐ rough
☐ weak		
☐ ridged		

MASSAGE MEDIUMS

- ☐ creams
- ☐ oils
- ☐ lotions

Beauty therapist signature (for reference)

Client signature (confirmation of details)

Sample client record card (continued)

SERVICE ADVICE
Basic hand/foot nail service – *allow 30 minutes*

SERVICE PLAN
Record relevant details of your service and advice given for future reference.
Ensure the client's records are up-to-date, accurate and fully completed following the service. Non-compliance may invalidate insurance.

DURING
Discuss:
- details that may affect the client's nail condition such as occupation
- products the client is currently using to care for the skin of the hands and nails and how often they are used
- the client's satisfaction with these products

Explain:
- relevant manicure procedures (e.g. how to file the nails correctly)

Note:
- any unwanted reaction (**contra-action**), if any occur

AFTER
Record:
- results of service
- what products have been used in the basic hand/foot/nail service
- the effectiveness of the service (were you, the client and senior beauty therapist happy with the result?)
- any samples provided (ask the client what they thought of them at the next appointment)

Advise on:
- product use in order to gain the best results from product use
- use of specialized products following manicure service for home-care use, such as nail strengthener
- general hand/nail care

Discuss:
- the recommended time between each service
- the importance of a course (more than one) of service to improve nail/skin conditions

RETAIL OPPORTUNITIES
Advise on:
- products that would be suitable for the client to use at home to care for the skin of the hands and nails
- other suitable services
- further products or services that you have recommended that the client may or may not have received before

Note:
- any purchase made by the client

EVALUATION
Record:
- comments on the client's satisfaction with the service
- if poor results are achieved, the reasons why

Note:
- if necessary, how you may change the service plan to achieve the best results in the future

HEALTH AND SAFETY
Advise on:
- the necessary action to be take in the event of an unwanted skin or nail reaction (contra-action)

Obtain the client's signature to confirm all details. This also enables continuity of the service and up-to-date tracking of services.

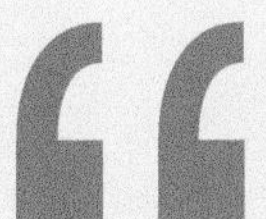

Treat nails as jewels whether it be a manicure or nail enhancements. They are fashion accessories.

Jacqui Jefford

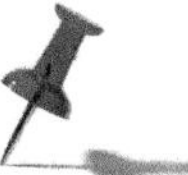

ALWAYS REMEMBER

Accurately record your client's answers to necessary questions to be asked at consultation on the record card.

1 If the client is wearing nail polish this must be removed to assess the client's nail condition. Use the following procedure:

   a Cleanse the hands/feet with an antiseptic applied with clean cotton wool or a spray to remove surface dirt and microorganisms.

   b Soak a clean piece of cotton wool in nail polish remover. Place over the nail plate and rest for 2–3 seconds to allow the nail polish to begin to dissolve. Apply firm strokes using the cotton wool over the nail plate surface to remove the polish. Any remaining nail polish left around the cuticle area should be removed using an orange stick tipped with cotton wool. Dip the cotton wool in nail polish remover and remove any remaining nail polish.

2 Assess the condition of the nails and skin:

   a cuticles – are they dry, tight or cracked, or are they soft and supple?

   b nails – are they strong, weak, brittle or flaking? Are they discoloured or stained? What shape are they – square, round, oval, long, short, bitten?

   c hands – is the skin dry, rough or chapped, or is it soft and smooth?

   d feet – is the skin dry, hard or rough, or is it soft and smooth?

3 Check with the senior beauty therapist that they agree with your nail service plan for the client.

4 Confirm and agree with the client the service aim and the client's choice of nail finish. Check that the preparation for the nail service meets with the senior beauty therapist's approval.

5 Ask the client to remove jewellery from the service area, to prevent it becoming soiled by the massage cream/oil or lotion. Place the jewellery in full view of the client, usually in a tissue-lined bowl or ask the client to look after it for safekeeping by passing the jewellery to them. Follow your salon policy.

TOP TIP

Dark nail polish

When removing dark nail polish from the nail it might be necessary to replace the cotton wool soaked with nail polish regularly. This is because dark nail polish tends to stain the nails and surrounding skin on removal.

TOP TIP

Service sales opportunities

If a nail is split, a nail wrap might be used to strengthen the nail. This should be performed by a senior beauty therapist.

ACTIVITY

Communication is important with your client

Communication includes talking with your client (verbal communication) and also what your body language is telling the client (non-verbal communication).

You might have given a client a great basic nail service but will you be asked to do it again if you are not bright, cheerful and helpful?

Think of three examples of communication used during a basic nail service to gain information about your client and find out if they are happy with the service being performed.

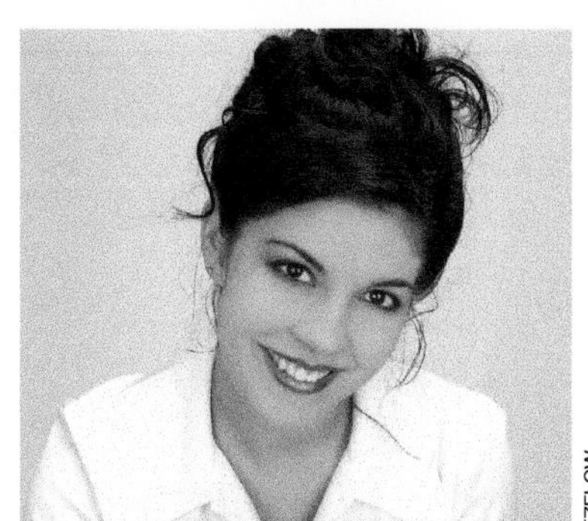

EZFLOW

Communication involves body language too. What does yours say?

Basic nail service procedure

Outcome 3: Carry out nail services

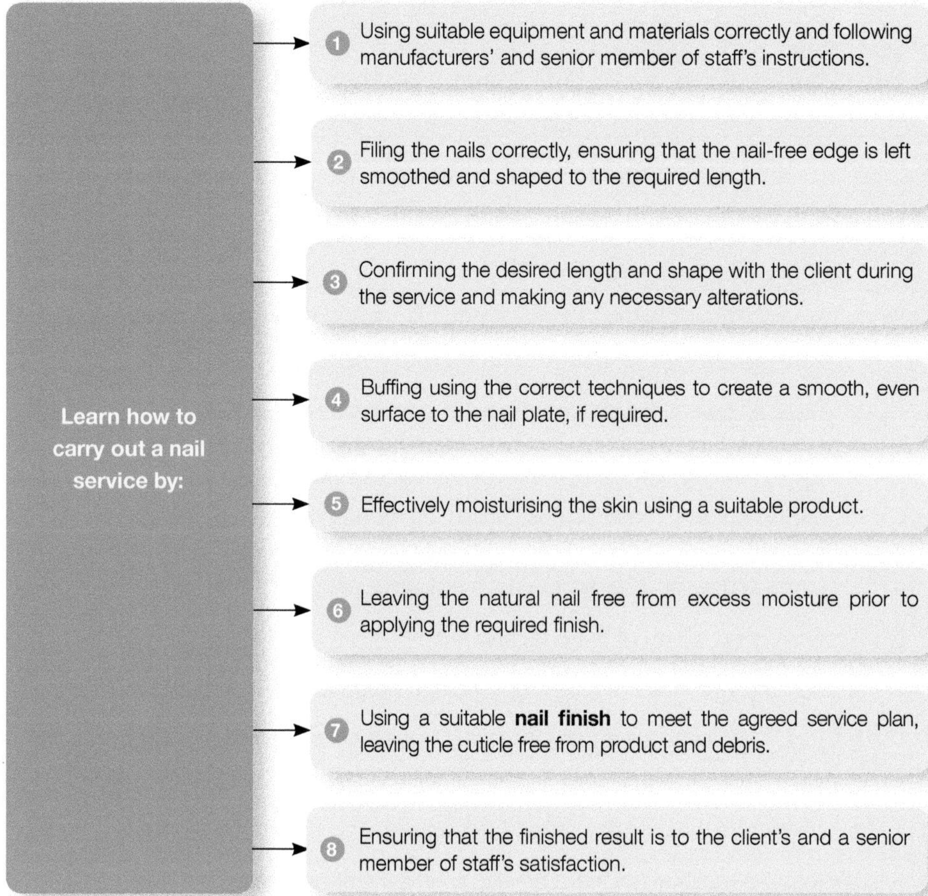

HEALTH & SAFETY

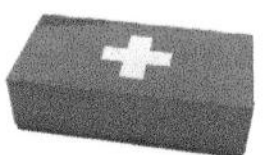

Follow manufacturers' guidelines

Use all products and materials in line with salon policy and manufacturers' guidelines.

Ensure health and safety best practice is considered throughout.

TOP TIP

Cutting the nails

It might be more practical to reduce nail length by cutting the nail at the free edge with nail scissors. These must be sterilized before use.

Support the nail at the sides with one hand of the free edge being cut. This minimizes client discomfort. Dispose of the trimmed nail plate hygienically.

Never cut the toenails too short at the free edge as this can lead to ingrowing toenails and cause pain and discomfort especially if the client takes part in active exercise, e.g. running.

Step-By-Step: Basic nail service procedure

TOP TIP

Filing the nails to suit the client's hands and nails

When filing the nails, ensure that the finished appearance suits the client's nail/hand.

If their fingers are long and thin, select a rounded/square shape and keep the nail length short.

If their fingers are short and fat, the nails should be filed into an oval shape and the nail length should be longer to make the fingers appear longer and slimmer.

ALWAYS REMEMBER

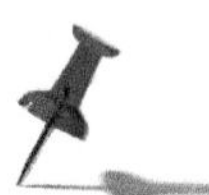

Filing the nails

Never file completely down the sides of the nails, as strength is required here to prevent breakage. Allow about 4 mm of nail growth to remain at the sides of the nail to provide strength.

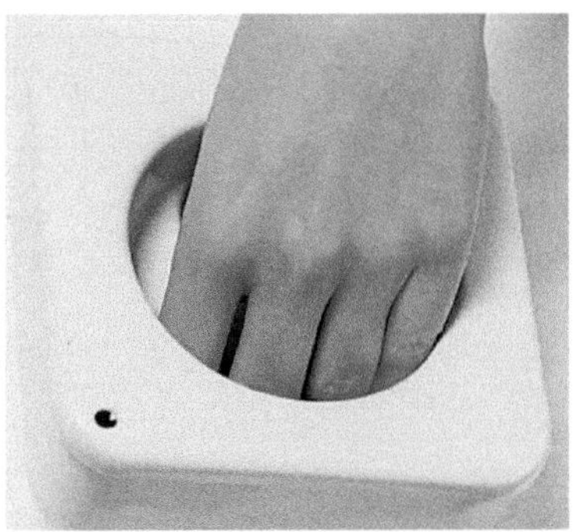

1 Cleanse the client's hands with an antiseptic applied with clean cotton wool or a spray to remove surface dirt and microorganisms. Use separate pieces of cotton wool for each hand to avoid cross-infection.

Cleanse both feet including between the toes with cotton wool soaked in skin disinfectant or a specialized hygiene spray for the feet. Use separate pieces of cotton wool for each foot to avoid cross-infection.

Soak both feet in warm water to which a mild liquid soap or similar suitable product has been added.

If the fingernails are dirty it might be necessary to soak them in warm water with a mild detergent before the service. An orange stick tipped in cotton wool can then be used to gently clean under the free edge of the nail; care should be taken when doing this.

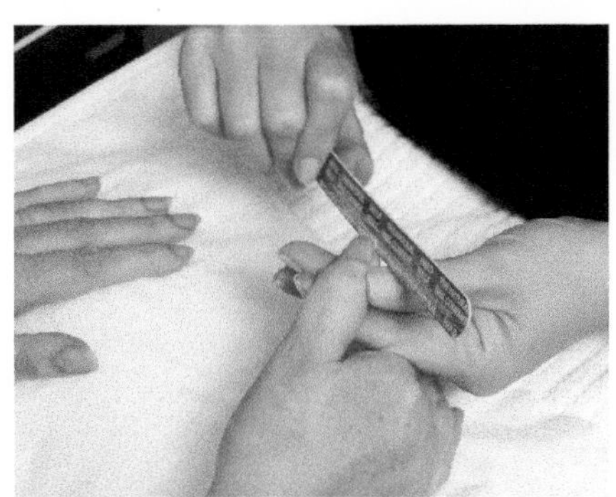

2 File the fingernails into the agreed shape and length; the part of the nail that is filed is the free edge. Use the lighter, fine textured side of the emery board when filing the nails into shape. The darker, coarser textured side of the emery board is used to remove length. File the nails from side to centre when creating an oval or round shape, with the emery board angled slightly under the free edge. To achieve a square shape, file straight across the top of the free edge in swift, strokes and gently curve the edges. File the nail length so that they are even in shape and length. Run your finger along the edge of the free edge to ensure they are smooth; any roughness should be removed using the fine side of the emery board in an upwards stroke. This is known as **bevelling**.

Cut the toenails straight across using toenail clippers or scissors.

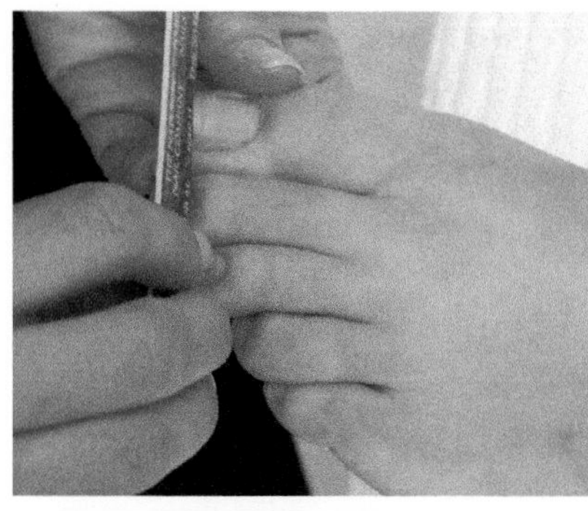

File the nails smooth with the coarse side of the emery board into a square shape, again do not shape the nails at the sides to avoid ingrowing nails.

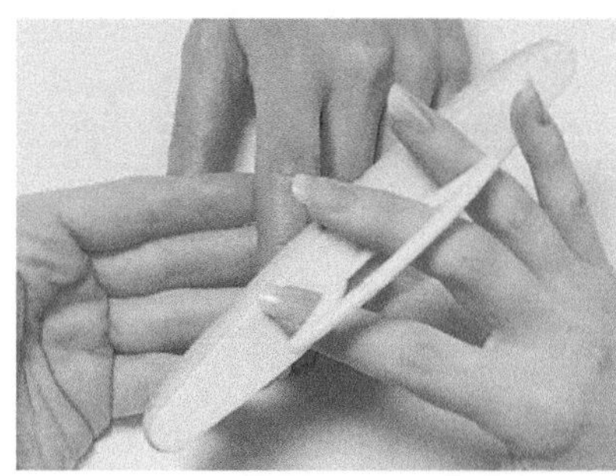

3 Buff the nails of the hands. Buffing is used to:

- give the nail plate a sheen
- stimulate blood supply to increase nourishment to the nail to improve the strength and health of the nail
- smooth surface irregularities on the nail plate, such as ridges.

Buffing is carried out after filing; it can also be used in preference to nail polish application, as in the case of a male nail service. If it is being used, buffing paste is applied: take a small amount from the container with a clean orange stick and apply this to each nail plate. With the fingertip, use downward strokes from the cuticle to the free edge to spread the paste over the nail plate, avoiding contact with the cuticle. Hold the buffer loosely in your hand, buff in one direction only from the cuticle towards the free edge. Approximately six strokes are applied to each nail plate.

It is not necessary to perform buffing on the toenails. A buffer can be used to smooth the surface of the nail plate and reduce the appearance of visible ridges.

4 Apply hand massage after buffing. Massage is applied to:

- moisturise the skin with hand cream
- improve blood circulation and nutrition to the skin, nails and muscles in the area
- improve lymph circulation, this helps the removal of waste products from the body
- relax the client
- help maintain joint mobility (how flexible our joints are)
- remove dead skin cells and improve the appearance of the skin.

Select and apply the chosen **hand cream/oil/lotion** for the client's skin type: dry skin or a male client with coarse body hair will benefit from an oil; normal skin will benefit from a lotion. Use the following procedure:

TOP TIP

Maintaining the quality of the nail polish

Clean the neck of the nail polish bottle after use to make sure that it is clean. This will ensure that the seal at the neck of the bottle is tight on closing, preventing the nail polish becoming thick.

Regularly clean the neck of the bottle with cotton wool and nail polish remover.

A product called solvent can be added to restore consistency to thick nail polish. Use according to manufacturer's instructions.

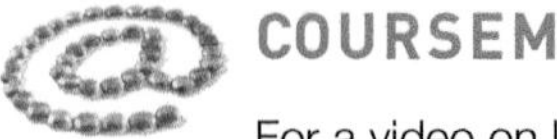

COURSEMATE

For a video on leg massage, please see this book's accompanying CourseMate.

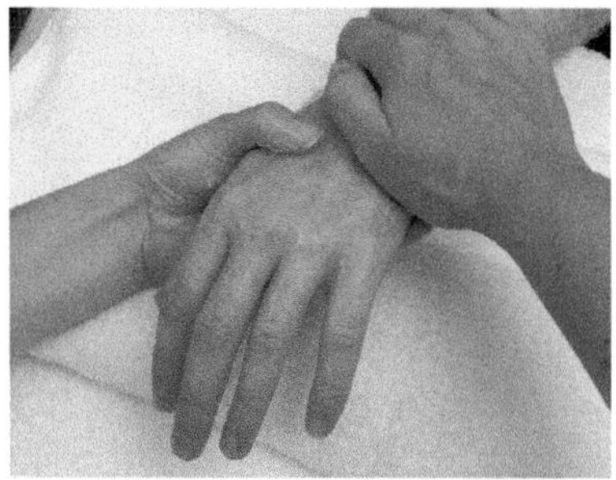

a Apply massage product using long sweeping strokes from the client's hand to the elbow, to both the inner and outer sides of the forearm.

Repeat five times.

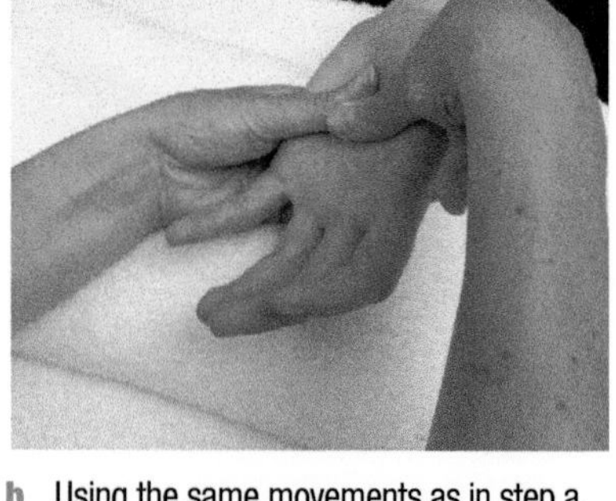

b Using the same movements as in step a, use the thumbs, one in front of the other move backwards and forwards over the palm and inner forearm.

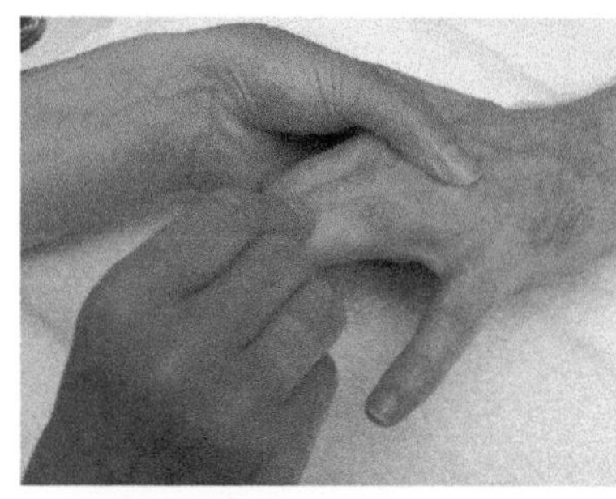

c Supporting the finger at the knuckle with one hand, hold the fingers individually and rotate the fingers clockwise and anti-clockwise.

Repeat twice.

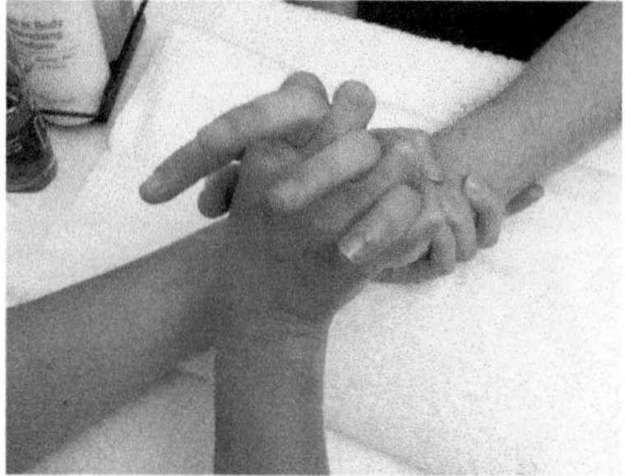

d Support the client's wrist with one hand and put your fingers between the client's fingers, grasping the hand. Circle the wrist clockwise and then anticlockwise. Repeat twice.

e Repeat step a five times.

5 As with hand massage, foot massage is carried out before nail polishing. The massage includes the foot and lower leg, and offers the benefits listed for hand massage.

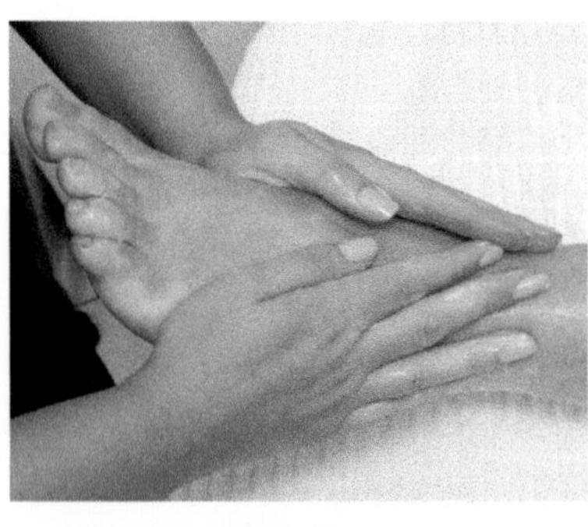

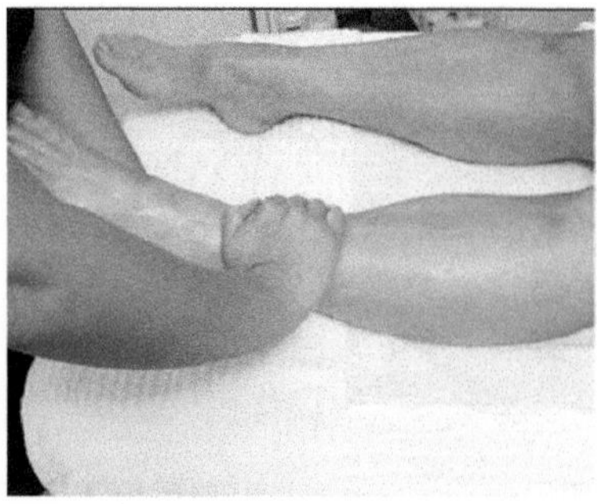

a Apply massage product using long sweeping strokes from the toes to the knee, moving on both the back and front of the leg.

Repeat five times

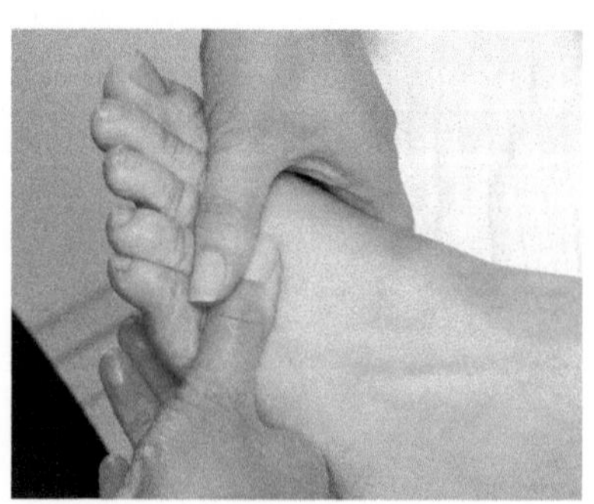

b Using the thumbs, one in front of the other, move backwards and forwards in a gentle sawing action. Move from the toes to the ankle, then slide back down to the toes.

Repeat twice.

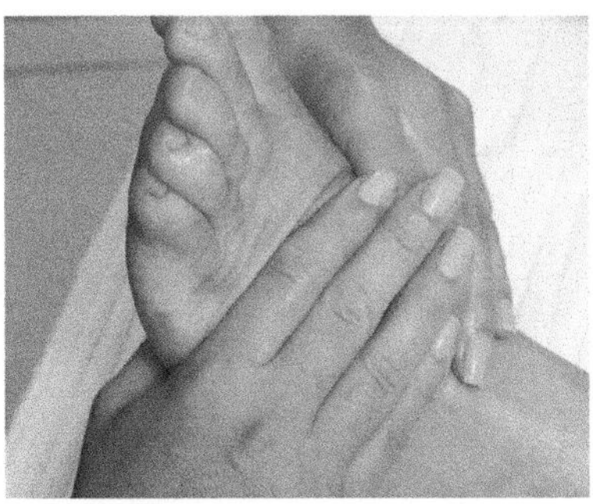

c Use the same movement as in step 2, but on the sole of the foot.

Repeat twice.

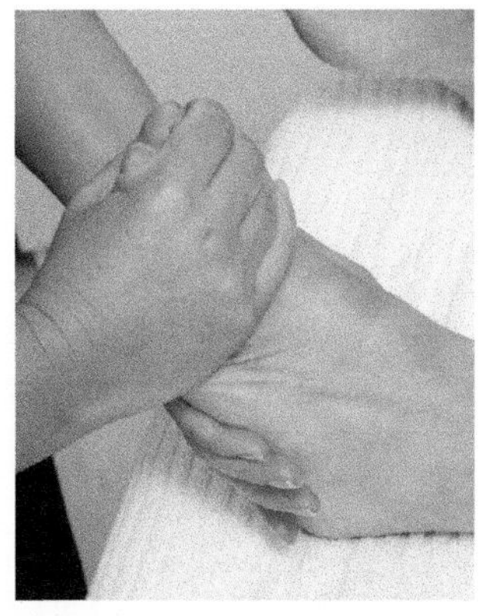

d Place the hand either side of the toes; gently press together and rotate all the toes three times clockwise and three times anti-clockwise.

e Repeat step 1 to finish the massage to the lower leg and foot.

TOP TIP

Too much polish

Avoid having too much polish on the brush during nail polish application.

A thick application of polish will increase the time the nail polish takes to dry and could cause it to run onto the surrounding skin. Two thin coats are better than one thick coat.

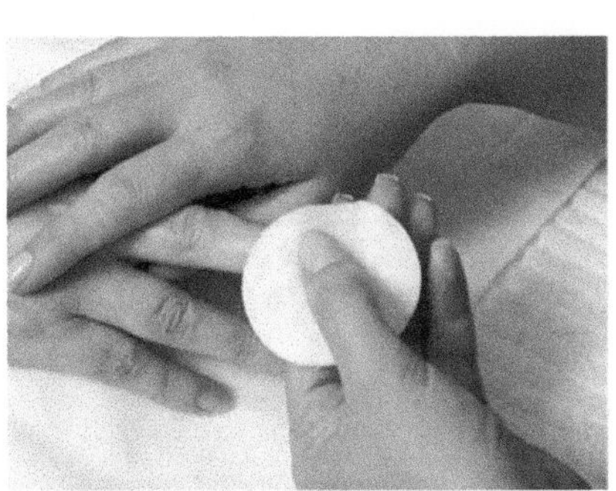

6 Remove excess oil/cream lotion from the hand or foot. The client might find it convenient to put her jewellery back on and pay for her service at this stage of the hand nail service to avoid damage to the nail polish after application.

Remind the client that adequate time must be allowed to allow the nail polish to dry for both the hands and feet dependent upon which nail service has been received.

If treating a male client or if the client does not wish to wear polish a final buff may be given to the nails to provide a shine. This may also be applied to the toenails to provide this natural nail finish.

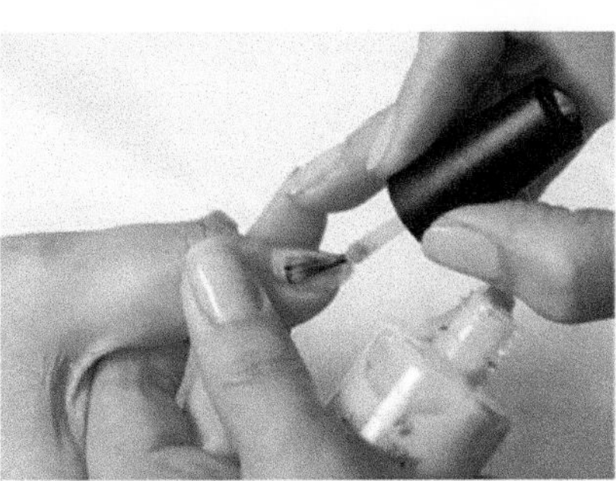

7 Nail polish application: nail polish is applied to coat the nail plate for the following reasons:

- for cosmetic improvement to the nail's appearance
- to disguise stained nails
- to add strength to weak nails
- as a specialist nail service, e.g. nail strengthener and ridge filler polish.

Use the following procedure:

a Remove excess grease remaining on the nail plate following the massage by applying nail polish remover to the nail plate surface with clean cotton wool. This will help the nail polish stick to the nail plate.

b Check that the edge of the nail is still smooth and even, re-file as necessary.

c Choose and apply nail polish following the manufacturer's instructions. The correct nail polish application technique is shown below.

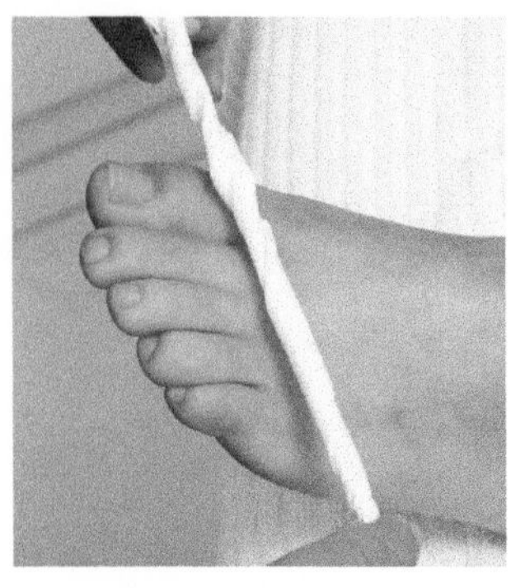

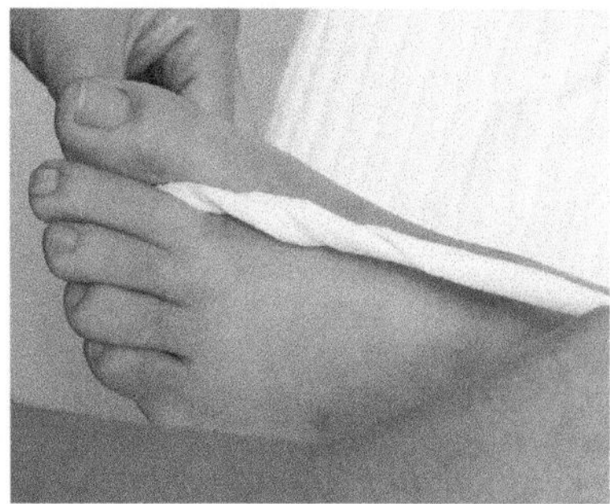

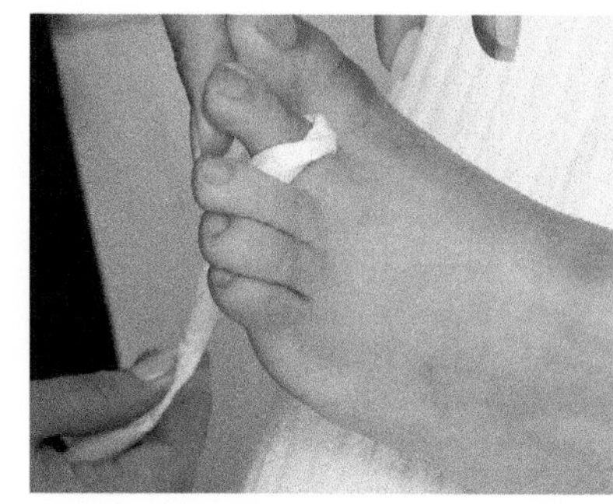

For the feet separate the toes using a hygienic method, i.e. disposable toe separators or other hygiene equivalent to separate them and facilitate polish application.

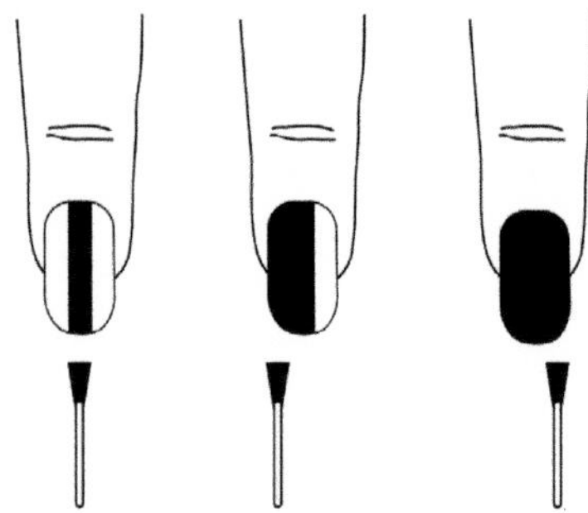

Correct polish application

TOP TIP

Fast drying spray

A fast drying spray product can be applied to reduce the drying time of the polish.

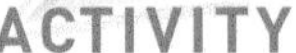

ACTIVITY

Client dissatisfaction with the service

Examples of reasons why clients may not be happy with the service they have received include:

- the service start time was delayed
- the service was rushed
- poor beauty therapist communication skills: good communication skills helps the client to relax and enjoy their service and feel confident to ask you questions about their service
- poor hygiene practice.

Can you add further reasons to the list why a client may not be happy with their service?

Remember, an unhappy client may not return to the salon!

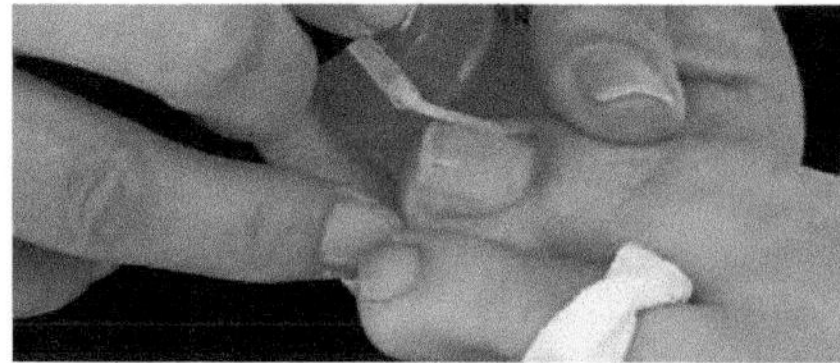

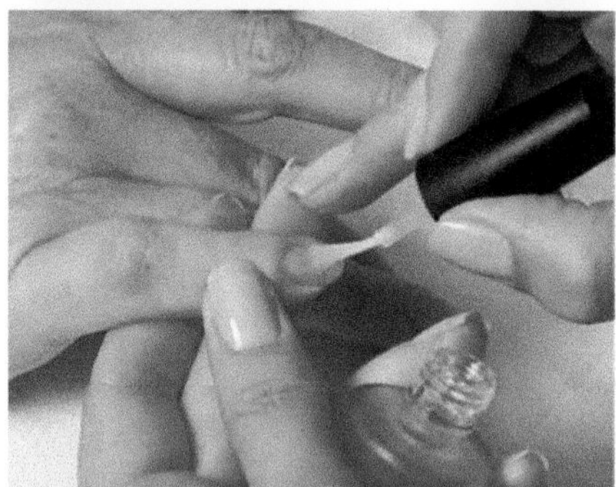

d Select a base coat or nail strengthener polish to suit the nail condition.

e Unscrew the bottle top to which the brush is attached. Wipe the brush on one side against the neck of the bottle, turn the brush around and apply the side of the brush with polish to the nail.

f Start with the thumb or large toe, apply three brush strokes down the length of the nail towards the cuticle, but avoid contact with the cuticle. The first stroke is down the centre of the nail and then down each side.

g Apply one coat.

h If polish comes into contact with the skin, remove with an orange stick tipped in clean cotton wool and dampened with nail polish remover.

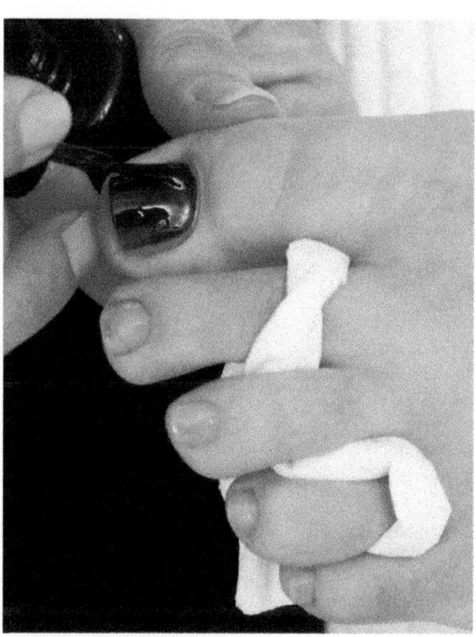

If agreed, apply coloured polish in the same way:

a Apply two coats of a cream polish and three coats if pearlized (frosted).

b A light, neutral colour is suited to short nails. Stronger, darker colours are suited to healthy longer nails and if a dramatic effect is required.

HEALTH & SAFETY

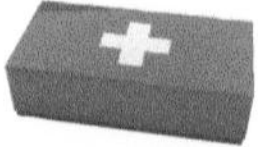

Ensure the area is well ventilated to avoid inhalation of excessive fumes from nail polish product.

Lighting should be good to avoid eyestrain.

Additional light, i.e. from a table lamp is a good idea when painting the nails.

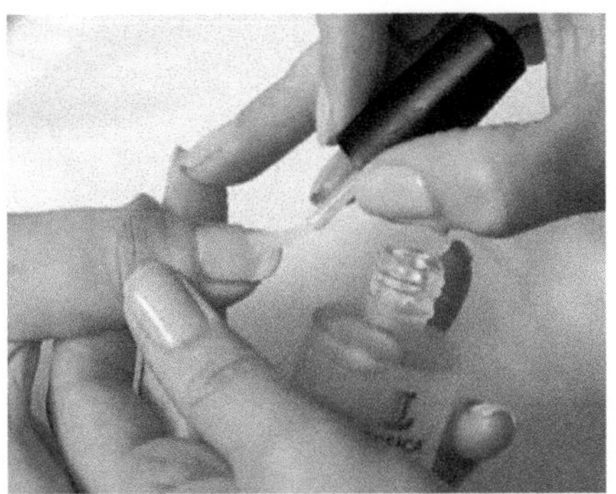

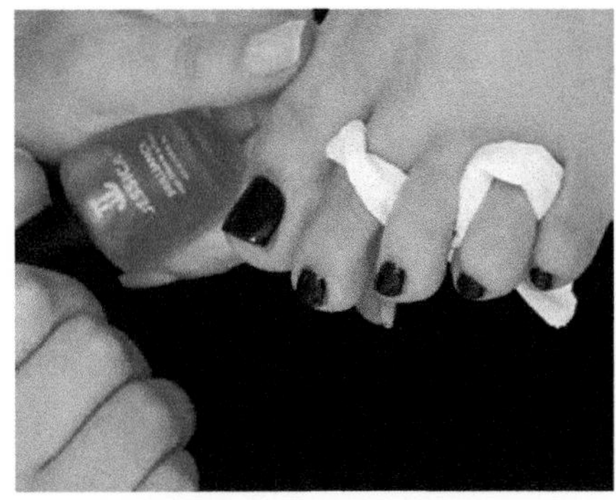

c Apply a topcoat. If using a pearlized polish, a topcoat is not applied.

d Check the result meets with client and senior beauty therapist's satisfaction.

Practise your nail service until you can complete it in the allocated time. This is important to ensure the service is cost-effective and clients are not delayed.

TOP TIP

Maintaining the appearance and hygiene of the work area

It is important that you work in a hygienic, organized manner and that you leave the work station neat and tidy, with all waste materials removed both during and at the end of the service. This will provide a professional, efficient service.

> Always know the main benefits of all products and services used in the salon.
>
> **Jacqui Jefford**

Completing nail services

Outcome 4: Provide aftercare advice

Learn how to provide aftercare advice which supports and meets the needs of your clients' service by:

1. Giving **advice** and recommendations accurately and constructively.
2. Giving your clients suitable **advice** on basic nail care.

At the end of the service, make sure the client records are up-to-date. This is important because you will need to look at these in the future. The record card should then be stored securely.

The client should be given home-care advice on how to care for the nails and surrounding skin at home. This will differ for each client, depending on individual needs.

Basic home-care advice

- Hands – wear protective rubber gloves when washing up.
- Hands – wear protective gloves when gardening or doing housework.
- Dry the hands/feet thoroughly after washing.
- Feet – foot sprays containing peppermint or citrus oil to cleanse and refresh are useful to apply to the feet during the day.
- Apply hand/foot cream regularly to moisturise the skin and nails.
- Hands – avoid harsh, drying soaps.

ACTIVITY

Design an aftercare leaflet

Design an aftercare leaflet for your client that they can read to learn how they should look after and care for their nails/hands/feet at home.

ALWAYS REMEMBER

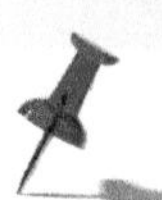

Offering advice to your clients will make them aware of the retail products you have to maintain the professional result achieved.

This beauty therapist is recommending an exfoliant service for the client's next nail service to improve her dry foot condition and has a retail product the client may use at home too!

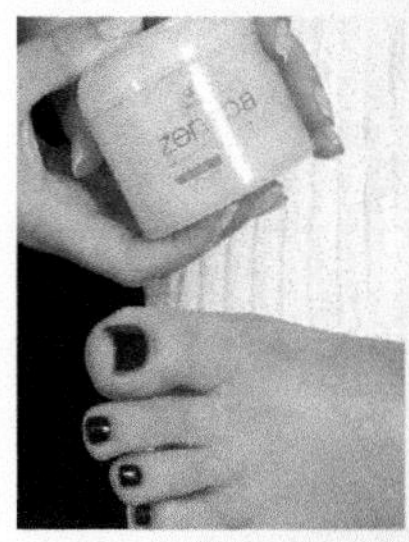

HEALTH & SAFETY

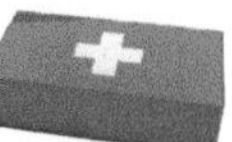

Skin disorders

Allergy symptoms do not necessarily appear on the feet. In the case of nail polish allergy the symptoms show up on the face.

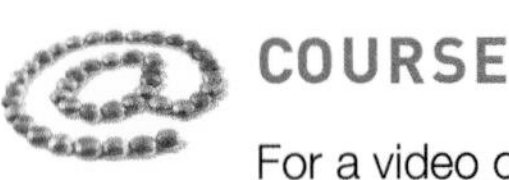

COURSEMATE For a video on dark polish application, see this book's accompanying CourseMate.

Hands – do not use the fingernails as tools, this causes the nails to weaken and split and break.

Advise the client how to file their nails on the hands/feet to keep them healthy and strong.

- Advise the client what action to take if a contra-action occurs such as an allergic reaction to products used.

Advise the client that the interval between nail services is usually 7–10 days.

Advise the client on a service plan to improve the nail/skin condition as necessary, and what other professional services you could recommend within the **limits of your authority**.

> You can only sell if you believe in what you are selling.
>
> **Jacqui Jefford**

Promoting products Providing advice also gives you the opportunity to recommend retail products, such as nail strengthener and hand cream. This enhances the salon's retail sales and profit.

Contra-actions Ask clients to contact the salon immediately and speak with the senior beauty therapist if any unwanted reaction to the service occurs. Such contra-actions (e.g. an allergy, recognized by redness, swelling and inflammation) should be noted on the client's record for future reference.

Ensure the client's service card is completed accurately with all details of the service recorded. Store the record card securely in compliance with the **Data Protection Act 1998**.

TOP TIP

Gloves provide great protection

Gloves provide a barrier to protect the hands and nails from chemical detergents that could cause the skin and nails to become dry and chapped. They also prevent the nails from becoming dry, causing peeling and breaking.

GLOSSARY OF KEY WORDS

Aftercare advice recommended advice given to the client following the service to continue the benefits of the service.

Aseptic a situation described as trying to destroy bacteria, and one that you should strive to achieve in the workplace.

Base coat a nail polish product applied to protect the natural nail and prevent staining from coloured nail polish.

Bevelling a nail filing technique used at the free edge of the nail to ensure that it is smooth.

Buffer a nail tool used to improve the appearance of the nail plate and stimulate blood to the nail bed area.

Buffing paste a coarse cream with a gritty texture; it removes surface cells from the nail plate.

Clippers nail tools used to shorten the length of the toenail before filing.

Consultation assessment of a client's needs using different assessment techniques, including questioning and natural observation.

Contra-action an unwanted reaction to the service occurring during or after the service.

Contra-indication a reason or condition that prevents or restricts you from performing a service.

Cross-infection the transfer or passing of contagious microorganisms.

Cuticle the part of the skin found around the base of the nail.

Data Protection Act 1998 legislation designed to protect client privacy and confidentiality.

Dermis the inner part of the skin, situated underneath the epidermis.

Disinfection the removal of micro-organisms by chemical or physical means which inhibits or slows the growth of disease.

Emery board a nail file used to shape the free edge of the nail.

Epidermis the outer layer of the skin.

Free edge the part of the nail that grows beyond the end of the finger.

Hand cream/oil/lotion a cosmetic mixture of waxes, water and oils applied to soften the skin of the hands and cuticles.

Hygiene the recommended standard of cleanliness necessary in the workplace to prevent cross-infection and secondary infection. The minimum standard laid down in law.

Industry Code of Practice written procedures specified by the workplace.

Limits of your authority the extent of your responsibility as specified in your job description and workplace policies.

Massage movements applied to the skin using the hands to improve its condition and functioning.

Matrix the growing area of the nail, found at the bottom of the nail.

Nail protective, hard shield found at the end of the fingers.

Nail bed the part of the skin covered by the nail plate.

Nail finish the product finally applied to the natural nail to enhance its appearance, i.e. choice of nail polish type/colour.

Nail plate the nail plate is a tough hard covering on top of the nail bed, the part of the skin upon which the nail plate rests.

Nail polish a clear or coloured nail product that adds colour/protection to the nail.

Nail strengthener a nail polish product that strengthens the nail plate, which has a tendency to split.

Orange stick a disposable wooden tool for use around the cuticle and free edge of the nail.

Organizational requirements beauty therapy procedures issued by the workplace management.

Sanitization cleansing or washing to an antiseptic level to prohibit bacterial growth.

Scissors nail tools used to shorten the length of the nail before filing.

Topcoat a nail polish product applied over another nail polish to provide additional strength and durability to the finish.

ASSESSMENT OF KNOWLEDGE AND UNDERSTANDING

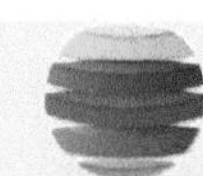

FUNCTIONAL SKILLS

Having covered the learning objectives for **assist with nail services** – test what you need to know and understand by answering the following short questions below.

The information covers:

- organizational and legal requirements
- how to work safely and effectively when assisting with nail services
- contra-indications and contra-actions
- client consultation and service planning
- anatomy and physiology
- nail services
- aftercare advice for clients.

Organizational and legal requirements

1 What is the Habia Industry Code of Practice for nail services?

2 Why must minors not be given services without informed and signed parental/guardian consent?

3 What is the recommended service time for completing a basic nail service?

4 Why must accurate up-to-date records of the client's service be kept?

5 Why is it important to follow the senior beauty therapist's instructions for service application?

6 Why is it important to complete the nail service in the given time?

7 Where should a client's record card be stored on completion of service?

How to work safely and effectively when assisting with nail services

1 Give examples of methods which can be used to sterilize and disinfect tools and equipment for nail services.

2 What is the difference between sterilizing and disinfecting tools and equipment?

3 What is the importance of having the necessary environmental conditions for nail services, i.e. lighting, heating, ventilation and general comfort?

4 Why it is important to maintain standards of good personal hygiene?

5 What condition should your work area be left in following each service and why is this important?

6 Why is it important that existing nail polish is removed before the service starts?

7 Why is it important that you wash your hands thoroughly before the service starts? Give two reasons why.

8 How should you position yourself when performing basic nail service? Why is your working position important?

Contra-indications and contra-actions

1 What is the importance of, and reasons for, not naming specific contra-indications when encouraging clients to seek medical advice?

2 Name a fungal, viral, bacterial and parasitic infection to the skin and nails. How do you recognize them?

3 What types of nail/skin conditions and disorders may restrict the nail service?

4 State a contra-action that could occur after nail services and what advice are you able to provide.

5 Name three contra-indications to basic nail service.

Client consultation and service planning

1 Why is good communication essential to ensure your client's nail service needs are met?

2 What type of questions would you need to ask in order to find out information from your client? Open or closed?

3 Why it is important to allow time following the consultation for your client to ask questions?

4 Why it is important to record client responses to questions asked?

5 What is the purpose of the client consultation?

6 Why is it important to talk to your client during the service?

Anatomy and physiology

1 Draw a cross-section of the nail to show the parts:
   - a matrix
   - b cuticle
   - c free edge
   - d nail plate
   - e nail bed.

2 Briefly describe the function of each part of the nail listed above.

3 Briefly describe the epidermis and its structure. Name **four** structures found in the dermis. Research and explain the functions of each.

Nail services

1 Name 10 items required when setting up the work area for a basic nail service and explain the purpose of each.

2 Name the **four** different nail shapes shown:

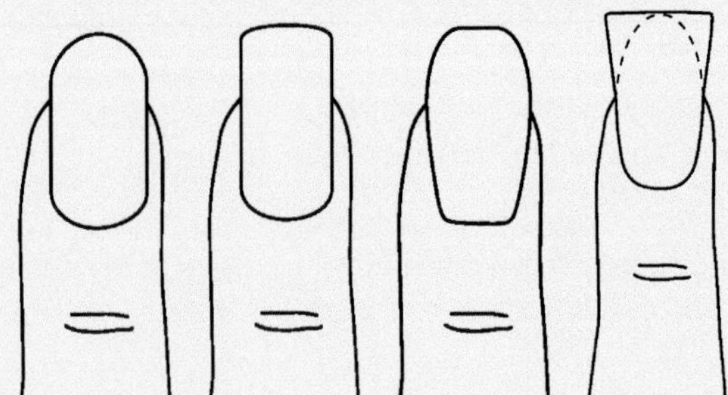

3 How does buffing improve the appearance of the nails?

4 Which side of the emery board is used to reduce the length of the nails?

5 How is a square nail shape achieved when filing?

6 State **three** effects of massage used in a nail service on the hands/feet.

7 What is the purpose of:
   - a base coat?
   - b top coat?

8 State two effects that could be caused by incorrect technique when filing.

9 When would you select to use a nail strengthener?

Aftercare advice for clients

1 State **three** pieces of home-care advice that could be given to a client for both hands and feet.

2 What retail product could you recommend to a client for the hands and feet?

3 What advice would you give a client about contra-actions to service?

4 Why is it important to explain how to correctly use nail tools and products at home?

5 What is the recommended time interval for nail services? Why is it of benefit to the client to receive regular nail services?

Index